D1128646

FLORIDA STATE
UNIVERSITY LIBRARIES

MAY 19 1995

TALLAHASSEE, FLORIDA

DIALOGUES ON PERCEPTION

BELA JULESZ

DIALOGUES
ON PERCEPTION

A Bradford Book
The MIT Press
Cambridge, Massachusetts
London, England

BF
311
J85
1995

© 1995 Massachusetts Institute of Technology

All rights reserved. No part of this book may be reproduced in any form by any electronic or mechanical means
(including photocopying, recording, or information
storage and retrieval) without permission in writing from
the publisher.

Set in Galliard.
Printed and bound in the United States of America.

Library of Congress Cataloging-in-Publication Data

Julesz, Bela.
  Dialogues on perception / Bela Julesz.
    p.   cm.
  "A Bradford book."
  Includes bibliographical references and index.
  ISBN 0-262-10052-5
  1. Perception. 2. Psychobiology. I. Title.
BF311.J85 1994
152.14—dc20   94-8883
                                    CIP

Dedicated to the memory of the scientific heroes of my youth, to my co-workers, and to Margit.

CONTENTS

PREFACE

A farmer, his wife, and their young son Johnny are visiting the zoo for the first time.

Johnny: Dad, why does the elephant have such a big trunk?
Father: I haven't the foggiest idea, son.
Johnny: And why does the giraffe have such a long neck?
Father: Only God knows, son.
Johnny: Dad, why does the lion roar so loud?
Father: I don't know, son.
Mother: Why do you pester your tired father with so many silly questions?
Father: That's all right, my dear, let the child ask—that's the way he learns!

The ancient maxim that there is no royal road to mathematics (or to science) is attested daily by our frustrated attempts to understand scientific articles outside of our fields of expertise. As we live in the Tower of Babel built by overspecialization, it is one of the great pleasures that a few intellectual pursuits still remain that we can grasp without undue effort.

Indeed, we can enjoy a haunting melody without a background in musical harmony, relate to a painting without studying the history of art, or laugh at a joke spontaneously. Strangely enough, it is just these "bootstrapping" features, such as a good metaphor, an artistic comment, or a humorous quotation, that scientific journals remove from articles in the name of compactness. This insistence on terseness and forced scientific jargon alienates the experts from a wider readership, whereas a redundancy of 20 or 30 percent might have greatly increased the accessibility of any paper. This thriftiness is particularly paradoxical in view of the fact that it is now possible to store an entire encyclopedia on a single ROM disk.

Until we see the emergence of more verbose (but still strictly edited) scientific journals that capitalize on the digital media, the scientific monograph will remain the best medium for making one's knowledge palatable to a wider readership.

Because in visual perception—besides the usual intellectual channel—there is a direct channel between the author and the reader, I tried to share the many visual demonsrations that illustrate, demonstrate, and occasionally enchant. To this end, a stereoscope is provided with the book to help the reader who cannot freely fuse to view the stereo pairs. After all, a stereo image is worth two thousand words!

This book was written in the form of a series of dialogues to make reading more interesting and retention easier. Because each dialogue is an independent essay some crucial material is repeated (usually in different contexts). A reader who is annoyed by repetitions should skip those parts. However, one who reads the dialogues in sequence will see the book's internal logic, and will be rewarded with many unexpected associations.

Dialogues is a scientific monograph for colleagues interested in psychobiology, written by a worker in visual (and occasionally in acoustical) perception. It is aimed at the scientist educated in psychology, neurophysiology, neurology, machine vision, and artificial intelligence. (Psychobiology, once called "physiological optics," is nowadays known as physiological psychology or brain research. While these various names might evoke slightly different connotations in some readers, I use them interchangeably.) It can be read by mathematicians, physicists, philosophers, and engineers who are interested in problems of brain research. Although care was taken to make it self-supporting, familiarity with certain psychobiological and mathematical concepts is taken for granted. (A glossary of technical terms is included, however.)

Part I contains essays on general topics, such as the creative process, the roles of mathematics and theories in psychobiology, the irrelevance of metascientific questions, and the importance of maturational windows and cortical plasticity. Part II, which addresses more specific topics related to current work and its relation to my past findings and ideas, contains an essay on some important strategic questions that can be solved with existing tools. This essay (dialogue 8) is particularly recommended to my colleagues in perception and to Ph.D. students in search of thesis topics.

As to the value of reading books in psychobiology, a rather premature scientific field, the joke in the introduction tells it all.

ACKNOWLEDGMENTS

Here I list and thank the friends and colleagues who helped me with this monograph. I pay detailed tribute to the benefactors of my life in appendix A.

First, I thank my friend and longtime associate Dr. Thomas Papathomas, who conceived the International Conference (entitled Linking Psychophysics, Neurophysiology, and Computational Vision) that was held in my honor at Rutgers University in the spring of 1993. (This conference was attended by more than 200 colleagues from all over the world. Its proceedings, entitled *Early Vision and Beyond,* will be published by The MIT Press.) Having stipulated that my 65th birthday be seen merely an excuse for a symposium, and that no explicit tributes dilute the quality of the gathering, I decided to enjoy the conference without actively participating in it and instead to write a monograph as a gift to my colleagues. (However, I wrote a last chapter in the proceedings.)

Working with the organization committee, and particularly with our secretary, Carol Esso, Thomas spent many months bringing the conference into being. The conference was a great success. and I enjoyed the talks immensely. They reflected my many interests in psychobiology, and I was particularly pleased that so many of the distinguished speakers were my former postdocs.

I am also most obliged to the editors of *Spatial Vision*—particularly Adam Reeves and the guest editor, Jeremy Wolfe—for devoting two special issues (1993, no. 2; 1994, no. 2) to the celebration of my birthday. I am very honored by the contributions to the conference proceedings and the special issues of *Spatial Vision*.

I finished two invited papers—for three different readerships—just prior to writing *Dialogues*. The first, which appeared in *Reviews of Modern Physics* under the title "Early vision and focal attention" in 1991, was the backbone of *Dialogues*. The second, "Some strategic questions in visual perception" (in *Representations of Vision: Trends and Tacit Assumptions in Vision Research,* ed. A. Gorea (Cambridge University Press, 1991)), was intended for psychobiologists and epistemologists. In the second article I used some material from another invited article of mine: "Consciousness and focal attention: Answer to John Searle," which appeared in *Behavioral and Brain Sciences* in 1993 after a long delay. The many favorable comments I received from the readers of these precursor articles encouraged me to write the present book. I thank Dr. Gérard Toulouse for inviting me to write in *Rev. Mod. Phys.*, and Dr. Francis Crick for his encouragement after reading the manuscript. I also thank Dr. Andrei Gorea for inviting me to the Paris conference.

Dialogues was read in several earlier versions by many colleagues. I thank them for their useful advice on matters ranging from strategy to English style. I am particularly grateful to Dr. George Hung, who advised me to divide the essays into two parts—that indeed made the reading much smoother. I also thank Drs. Bart Anderson, Jochen Braun, Jih Jie Chang, Itzhak Hadani, and Ilona Kovacs. I received many useful comments from my colleagues at Caltech, and I thank Professors John Allman, Christoph Koch, and Terry Sejnowski for their encouragements. My special thanks go to Dr. John T. Bruer, president of the James S. McDonnell Foundation, for reading the manuscript and recommending to me Mr. Harry Stanton, executive editor of Bradford Books.

As I glance through the references and see how many colleagues—whom I admire and from whom I learned so much—I have not quoted, I feel I owe them my deepest apologies. The only excuse I have for these omissions is that for years I have been working on a textbook, *The Enjoyment of Vision by Eye and Intellect,* in which I refer to hundreds of important articles not cited here. *Dialogues* is a highly individual monograph related mainly to my own research interests and to some work that caught my fancy.

Twice in my life—in 1969–1971, when I wrote *Foundations of Cyclopean Perception,* and now—I have had the interesting experience of having my thoughts just pop out (then on a remote typewriter, now on the screen of a monitor). In contrast, for several months in 1987, when I was recovering from a car accident, each time I put pen to paper all that materialized was an inkblot. Once I read an interview with Jean-Paul Sartre, who at age 70 was almost blind and had stopped writing. When asked why he did not dictate his thoughts to a stenographer, he said that without the feedback between his fingers and his mind ideas would not flow. The ability to write a book should not be taken for granted, and I regard it a special grace of fate.

EDITOR'S NOTE

This is indeed, as the author says, a highly individual book. For that reason the dialogues are presented with minimal editing.

Unbracketed text is to be understood as the speech of one of the dialogue partners, **A** and **B**; bracketed information is supplementary.

HOW TO VIEW
STEREO IMAGE PAIRS

Because a stereogram is worth two thousand words, and the thrill of watching the emergence of the monocularly hidden surfaces is worth sharing with the reader, a stereoscope is provided with the book. Ninety-eight percent of the readers have functional stereopsis and should be able to enjoy the fusion of the stereo pairs. As a matter of fact, many readers will be able to fuse the stereo pairs by just crossing (or diverting) their eyes.

Whether one fuses the stereo pairs without or with the stereo viewer, one should always wear one's reading glasses. Astigmatism is automatically corrected by cylindrical lenses added to spherical lenses, and astigmatism greatly diminishes stereopsis (stereoscopic depth perception). This is the more serious when the difference between the angles of distortion in the left and right eyes is more than 45°. Many readers who have good vision and do not wear glasses (and are not stereo blind as a result of "lazy eye" or some other visual handicap) could improve their stereopsis by wearing glasses

with the proper cylindrical corrections. (An inexpensive solution is to buy two neutral contact lenses without any diopters, since these perfectly spherical lenses worn over the corneas are filled with tear fluid, and astigmatism is caused by deviation of the corneas from spherical shape.) Restoration of stereopsis by correcting astigmatism might benefit millions of viewers. Furthermore, the fusion of random-dot stereograms (RDSs) often takes some time, but after success, it is commented, years later one can fuse them in a jiffy. Viewers have also commented that their perception of plasticity has been heightened after the fusion of RDSs. The fusion of RDSs is an unfakeable test for stereopsis in human and monkey infants and adults. Cross-eyed infants sometimes can be helped to restore their stereopsis when diagnosed early; adults can decide to stay away from professions for which stereopsis is a must.

Figure A shows a typical RDS that portrays a triangle hovering over the background after bi-

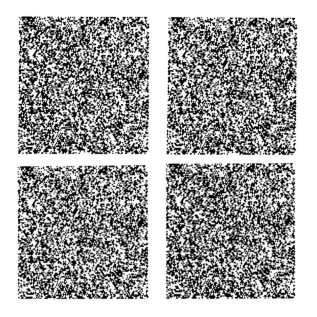

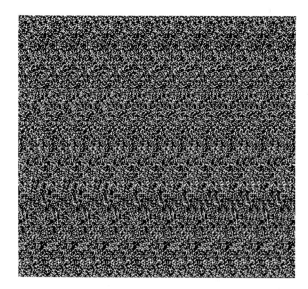

nocular fusion when viewed by the stereoscope. Figure B is similar to figure A except the two images are interchanged, so nasalward disparity becomes temporalward. Thus, when figure B is fused with the stereoscope the diamond recedes. Free fusers who divert their eyes temporalward will perceive the triangle in figure A in front; those who cross their eyes in the nasal direction will see it recessed.

The use of the stereoscope is straightforward. The flat stereoscope has to be folded twice to become T-shaped. The septum, between the two lenses, has to be placed perpendicularly between the gap that separates the left and right images. After placing your nose in the cutout, check that each eye sees its image in full. After a brief time the hidden image will emerge in depth.

Figures C and D are "autostereograms" generated by Jih Jie Chang. These can be fused without aid. If you can fuse figures C and D, you should also be able to fuse freely figures A and B.

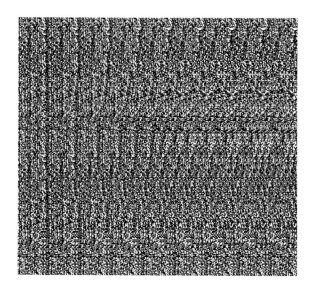

INTRODUCTION

Graduate student: Professor, could you advise me about the length of my thesis?

Professor: Certainly. If you were Dr. Dirac, one page would suffice; in your particular case, it should be 480 pages!

Unfortunately, psychology is not as mature a discipline as physics, nor am I a Dirac. I also think that I am smarter than the student in the story, so this monograph is slightly less than 480 pages. Psychobiology—including my field, visual perception—is most likely in the primitive state where, say, molecular biology was prior to the discovery of the double helical structure of DNA by Watson and Crick. Indeed, workers in visual psychophysics, neurophysiology, and neuroanatomy cannot agree on fundamental problems; what is more, some would even deny that we have adequate knowledge at present to formulate a fundamental question. Just take the problem of "sensations" (also called "qualia"). Wherever neurophysiologists probe the brain with their microelectrodes, they seem to re-cord similar histograms of neural spike activity, regardless of whether the corresponding sensations are brightness, color, pitch, itch, temperature, pain, pleasure, anxiety, hunger, or contentment. Most likely there must be subtle differences in the spatio-temporal spike or chemical activities in neural pools for these various perceptual modalities, which are still shrouded in mystery. This is just one illustration of the extent to which we do not know the "code of the brain," if there is such a thing at all. (The problem of sensations will be discussed in dialogue 6 together with other metascientific questions.)

Of course, not all research in molecular biology was worthless before the discovery of the DNA helix and the genetic code. On the contrary. Darwin's theory of evolution is probably the greatest scientific insight so far, and Mendel's experiments paved the way to the concept of the gene. In a similar vein, as I approach the respectable age of 65 (an almost miraculous event by itself, in that I had a low probability of survival on several counts), I had the good fortune to be a witness to the great discoveries in visual neurophysiology and psychobiology, from the concept of the columnar organization of the cortex and the finding of specific neural analyzers to the split-brain paradigm. I feel particularly privileged to have been able to contribute to these developments by introducing into psychobiology the techniques (involving computer-generated random-dot stereograms, cinematograms, and textures) that eventually led to the subfield of human psychology called now "early vision" and made it possible to link psychophysical data to the neurophysiology of early cortical stages observed in the monkey.

In 1987, on the very day a party was planned to celebrate my election into the National Academy of Sciences, I suffered an almost fatal car accident. A severe depression ensued. In my tormented mind, a detractor materialized, who started to mock me and to question everything I cherished. Whatever I thought to be self-evident, or believed to be one of my few original ideas, was scrutinized and turned upside-down by my opponent. This reminded me of Galileo's famous *Dialogo* involving Simplicio (who believes in Aristotle), Salviati (who represents Galileo's views), and Sagredo (an intelligent and neutral arbiter), and it was my humble person playing the role of Simplicio. I had almost finished my second monograph; however, at the insistence of my internal opponent I decided to rewrite it totally. I hoped that I would be able to remember the arguments and to rewrite the manuscript as a series of dialogues between me and my internal critic. I also suspected that this would be an enormously difficult enterprise, like trying to play chess against oneself. Luckily, after a few months, I suddenly flipped out of my depression

and back to my usually optimistic former self, and an interesting cognitive conversion took place. Much as the inverting goggles of G. M. Stratton and Ivo Kohler eventually resulted in perceptual correction, the upside-down arguments of my opponent suddenly flipped right-side-up and became similar to my own; they were converted into doubts of the sort that a scientist should have.

B: So far I have not cared for how you have wasted your time. Obviously I would have enjoyed it more if we had gone on a year-long trip around the world instead of writing this book. But calling me your "detractor," a sort of "devil's advocate," and your "tormentor" goes too far. I really have to protest! We both thought after the accident that we would die, and I always felt uncomfortable about the way you carried around your scientific achievements as if they were decorations for everyone to see. I wanted you to face your last days in dignity without the unnecessary trimmings of human vanity, so I seriously raised the doubt in your head that your scientific achievements were not very substantial. After all, you must agree with me—even now that you are your former self—that your best-known scientific feat, the computer-generated random-dot stereogram, is just a variant of the camouflage invented by Nature millennia ago. That, say, Helmholtz did not make such a stereo pair from sandpaper with a pair of scissors is just a lucky break for you, and, as you mentioned in your first monograph, Aschenbrenner (1954) did something similar. Your second "paradigm," with your conjecture that "iso-second-order texture pairs cannot be discriminated without scrutiny," was so abstract that nobody bothered to disprove it, so you had another lucky break. Fate permitted you to disprove it yourself, and you covered up this defeat by presenting it as a triumphant discovery of the textons. As a matter of fact, I let you go ahead with this monograph to amuse myself. I wanted to see how you could convert such meager accomplishments into a respectable story. That is the reason why I will control myself in the next chapters. If you are not bragging much I will remain silent, but I will not tolerate exaggerated claims or bombastic statements from you. Perhaps the reader should interpret **B** as Bela—your better self, somewhat more hedonistic but certainly more honest than the Author, who will be referred as **A**. I still would have preferred if you had taken me for an exotic trip along the Silk Route than on this ego trip of yours!

A: I am glad that you are willing to collaborate with me, and I will regard you for the time as my partner and not my opponent. I also notice that you are rather stable, and that in my up-and-down moods I judge you sometimes my opponent but more often my partner. In spite of that, I am sure that after your outburst most of my readers will appreciate that their alter egos are more accommodating. As a matter of fact, during my depression, some of my colleagues noticed that I was not sure of myself and my scientific theories, and tried to distance themselves from me. For instance, during this period I received two papers to review from

the editors of *Nature* that criticized my texton theory and recommended in its place some linear filters in a Laplacian pyramid, followed by some nonlinear operation. (By the way, such a model was proposed years earlier in Julesz and Bergen 1983.) I regarded these papers as excellent, but I pulled a joke on their authors. I submitted to "News and Views" (the section of *Nature* in which the two papers were to be published) a manuscript written with Ben Kröse, a postdoc of mine at Caltech (Julesz and Kröse 1988). Kröse and I used the same Laplacian pyramid the other authors had used, but in the very hierarchical stage their models deemed the most relevant we placed a uniformly gray stimulus and then performed the inverse operations (figure I.1). As we expected, the resulting texture pair was as easily discriminable as the original one in spite of the missing stimulus at the stage of spatial resolution the other authors considered the most crucial. (This trick, called the "missing fun-

Figure I.1

(a) The original texture pair. (b) Its decomposition by the Laplacian pyramid, followed by squaring the output of the Laplacian filters. Because of the limitation of the photographic reproduction, only levels 0–5 are portrayed. The largest blob-contrast difference occurs at level 3. (c) Reconstructed image, with the Laplacian pyramid in reverse but with levels 2–4 changed to uniform gray. As can be seen, the resulting image is a highly discriminable texture pair even though it lacks the levels (frequency bands) that contain the large energy differences in b. From Julesz and Kröse 1988.

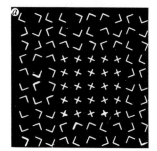 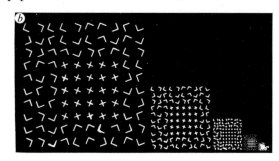 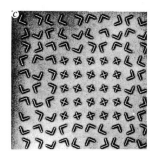

damental" in acoustics, is often used to show how the nonlinearity of the auditory system restores the missing pitch from combination products of higher harmonics.) For the initiated this was a sure sign that I had finally recovered, and my friends felt reassured that I had regained my confidence. I mention this episode merely to illustrate two important things. In psychobiology many of the accepted research topics are merely fashions, depending more on the persuasion of some charismatic individuals than on some deep scientific truth, and therefore the scientific community expects these individuals to believe in their own work. If they start to have doubts, why should the rest believe them? After all, they should know better!

B: In this case I agree with you—the more so since I know for sure that you genuinely esteem your scientific critics. Because I am the fun-loving one, what could be more fun than reversing a critical comment in a scientifically correct way that is also humorous! It was a particularly sweet joke, since, after all, a critical paper about a not-too-important detail of the work of an old friend could have been published in some specialty journal instead of in the highly visible *Nature*. I made these comments merely to clarify my role in these dialogues. My problems with the author are not related to his vanity, pride, and other human weaknesses I share with him as his alter ego. While he is writing this book, I will interfere with **A** only when I regard some of his statements as half-baked or as too pompous for my taste.

A: That's a deal! However, you raised an important point about scientific critics. Let me quote from the preface of the beautiful book *Experiments*

in Hearing, by one of my scientific heroes, Georg von Békésy (1960): "One of the most important features of scientific research is the detection and rectification of errors. . . . A way of dealing with errors is to have friends who are willing to spend the time necessary to carry out a critical examination of the experimental design beforehand and the results after the experiments have been completed. An even better way is to have an enemy. An enemy is willing to devote a vast amount of time and brain power to ferreting errors both large and small, and this without compensation. The trouble is that really capable enemies are scarce; most of them are only ordinary. Another trouble with enemies is that they sometimes develop into friends and lose a great deal of zeal. It was this way that the writer lost his three best enemies."

I also want to add that whenever I am not the first or the sole author of a paper I try to avoid concepts of my personal metatheories. For instance, I was careful not to drag into the texton theory those postdocs of mine who were somewhat skeptical of it, and in our joint papers we used in place of, say, "texton gradients" the less committal term "texture gradient." I hope this interlude might clarify the role of the two participants in these dialogues.

You also mentioned that, prior to the introduction of computer-generated random-dot stereograms into psychology (Julesz 1960), a handmade RDS was published by Aschenbrenner (1954), which he seemed to have created during World War II. Computer-generated RDSs permitted *ideal* camouflage (without imperfections, which could yield monocular cues), and computers made the generation of RDSs a practical enterprise. Both Aschenbrenner and I were aware of the technique of "breaking camouflage by stereopsis," generally known to experts in aerial reconnaissance. However, Aschenbrenner, who published his findings in a specialty journal (unknown to me and to other psychologists), was unaware that this truth was not known to workers in psychobiology. Therefore, I regard as my main contribution the historic fact that I was the first to bring the message that *no camouflage is possible in three dimensions* to the awareness of psychologists.

My recovery coincided with my department's move, in January 1989, from Bell Labs to the newly created Laboratory of Vision Research at Rutgers University. After this move, my co-workers and I cleared a number of scientific hurdles that had stood in our way for years. The recent insights are so important to me that I have devoted all of dialogue 12 to them.

There is, in addition to the story recounted above, another story behind the writing of this book. As I worked on *The Enjoyment of Vision by Eye and Intellect*—a textbook for advanced undergraduate and graduate students—I was struggling with advanced topics that I was not quite sure about but nonetheless found important. Textbooks are usually written in a declarative style, with the author speaking as an authority and presenting facts without raising doubts. It occurred to me to take out these sophisticated sections and convert them into a dialogue format.

The dialogues address a series of unconnected topics. The reader is assumed to take part in the discussion, by agreeing with **A**, or with **B**, or with neither. (Unfortunately, in psychobiology there is no Sagredo who could serve as a detached and wise debate leader.) Indeed, I hope that the reader will have a third opinion, orthogonal to the ones expressed, and will come up with an entirely novel idea. After all, the only justification for a scientific monograph is to be a catalyst and to help others to clarify their own ideas and bring into their consciousness some unexpected new insights! I tried to select topics that are of interest not only to me but to my friends and colleagues as well. If in return, some of my unsolved questions will be answered by them, I will be rewarded beyond my expectations.

I
DIALOGUES ON GENERAL TOPICS

DIALOGUE 1
THE ENTERPRISE OF
VISION RESEARCH

Author: So tell me, Georg, what do you think happiness is?

Georg von Békésy: That is easy, Bela. Happiness is a good experiment.

Honolulu, January 1968

A: This first dialogue could have been conducted on scientific research in general; however, as a practitioner of vision research, I will restrict myself to my specialty. I will speculate on the enterprise of scientific research in its entirety, beyond its main goal of furthering human knowledge.

I start with the distinction between the "museum pieces of science" and the "daily conduct of science," even though the two are intimately interwoven. In the first category are the many valid facts, theories, and tools (still accepted, while others have already been proven false) that are found in textbooks and archival journals: the existence of the blind spot, the waterfall illusion, the stereoscope, Fechner's law, the theory of trichromacy, and so on. As with museum pieces of art, certain pieces are exhibited and others go into storage as certain styles become fashionable or lose popularity. For instance, the pseudo-problem of how the retinal upside-down image be inverted by the brain was clarified by George Stratton (1896), who showed that wearing inverting prisms for a few days did revert the image if the observer could freely move around. For decades, each generation wanted to retest this finding, at ever-increasing speeds. The most recent example was Ivo Kohler (1941, 1951), who drove his motorbike through the streets of Innsbruck wearing inverted goggles. I have no doubt that someone will try this experiment at Mach speeds!

B: I think Kohler used prisms that mirrored images, so left-right became right-left. After he had worn them a few days, he commented that the directional flow of the moving world became correct but the license plates of the cars still remained their mirror images. Also, Kohler found real perceptual plasticity, beyond mere proprioceptive rearrangement. He observed that prisms caused chromatic fringes (due to their bad chromatic aberrations), but after wearing them for a few days these color fringes disappeared. They reappeared for a while after the prisms were removed.

Also, Stewart Anstis attached in front of his eyes a device that inverted the luminance distribution of the outside world. Blacks became whites, whites became blacks, dark grays became light grays, and so on. Such negatives are rather confusing; one can hardly recognize a familiar face or object. Anstis wanted to know whether one could adapt to negatives the same way as to inverted images. That is, could one learn to become familiar with negative images the same way as with positive images?

A: Thank you for that scholarly comment. [Adaptation experiments of this kind can be performed in a few minutes by all of us under less dramatic conditions. For instance, Harris (1980) used a wedge prism over an eye (with the other closed) and asked his observers to hit an object with their outstretched arms. Observers would make lateral mistakes for a few minutes, but eventually learned to compensate for the lateral error caused by the prism. After Harris removed the prism, observers made the opposite lateral error for a few minutes until the proprioceptive adaptation wore off. Such proprioceptive adaptation requires active participation by the organism, as was shown in the classic study by Held and Hein (1963). They had two kittens explore the world after birth. One kitten could actively explore the world; the other sat passively in a gondola yoked to a harness worn by the active kitten. The active kitten learned to move swiftly in its environment; the passive kitten, after its release from the gondola, had to learn from scratch to move. With respect to efforts to adapt to negative images, so far such attempts have been negative. If you had not mentioned them, I certainly would not have broken my stream of thoughts by referring to unsuccessful experiments.]

An important difference between artistic and scientific museum pieces is that the former are more tightly coupled to their creators. When a beautiful painting is discovered to be the creation of a lesser-known student, it loses much of its value in most people's minds. On the other hand, the discoverer of a scientific fact or the creator of a scientific theory is often contested or ignored. His theory may be disguised by his contemporaries, only to be rediscovered decades later by others. Indeed, trichromacy—one of the most important scientific theories of visual perception [attributed to Thomas Young (1802), later refined by Hermann von Helmholtz, and now known as the Young-Helmholtz theory]—was originally postulated by George Palmer. Palmer stated the theory in 1777; his publications are reprinted in MacAdam 1970 and are reviewed in Barlow and Mollon 1982. Similarly, whether the stereoscope was first discovered by Wheatstone in 1838 or had already been used in the form of binocular microscopes generations earlier [e.g., by a French Capuchin friar, le Père Cherubin of Orleans (see Jabez Hogg 1854)] is not significant for scientists. *Perhaps the greatest tribute to a scientific discovery is when people suddenly regard it as a fact of their own culture, so that it becomes a "scientific folk song," regardless of who invented or discovered it.*

Of course, science is quite different from art, even though the human mind underlies both creations. In the arts, the viewer, listener, or reader is usually less concerned with the problem-solving side of the artist than with his opus. Very seldom are we concerned with the problem of who introduced, say, three-dimensional perspective in painting, or who introduced the sonata form in chamber music; instead, we pay tribute to a Vermeer painting or Bach's Brandenburg concerti as the final manifestation of a given style that could not have been detached from the creator. On the other hand, in science the solving of problems is the creative act, and the nature of its execution is less interesting. [In modern art there is a tendency to emphasize the problem-solving aspect at the expense of the actual production of exhibition pieces, which leads to the alienation of the public.]

From the foregoing it must follow that doing science cannot have its rewards in seeking fame, but mainly that *doing science is fun*. Obviously doing science also helps us to earn our living, although for the effort most of the other occupations are usually more lucrative. However, for a person who is tormented by easily becoming bored and is endowed with a creative and disciplined mind, the solving of scientific problems is perhaps the highest form of being original. In turn, such a person is rewarded by understanding something for the first time in history. Whether mankind celebrates the scientist for this first encounter or disputes its importance or originality should be of minor concern to the scientist. Indeed, while human vanity can explain why such scientific giants as Newton and Leibniz could have had such bitter disputes about the priority of the discovery of calculus, there is a real difference in their notations, and we are most indebted to both.

What really matters is that, relative to many other professions, perhaps a scientist still has a "future" at an older age. At 65, I still go to my laboratory with the same excitement as decades ago, and mingle and enjoy working with colleagues who could easily be my grandchildren. Indeed, while one's old friends in retirement or in routine jobs are reminiscing or engaging in hobbies, scientific interests permit us to have our work also be our hobby. This is a unique reward, and when young people ask my advice on career choice I always ask them two questions: Are you artistically gifted? If not, are you good at mathematics, or do you enjoy scientific problems? If the young person is artistically exceptional, I always encourage him or her to pursue an artistic career, since I regard science as a substitute for the arts. If the person is not artistic but is endowed with a scientifically inquisitive mind, I always encourage him or her to enter a scientific field, even though other professions might yield more monetary rewards or a more secure existence.

B: I have listened to your personal opinions with patience. But do you have to drag your private life into these dialogues, even if they are related to your 65th birthday? I might listen to your scientific problems, and if these appeared to be interesting I would argue with you. But could you spare me the incidental details of your life? After all, I might be willing to read another monograph from you, but an autobiography in disguise is really going too far!

A: It is impossible to spare you from some anecdotal stories from my own life. It is my firm belief that a scientist's published works in archival journals are just the visible part of the iceberg. Motivations, beliefs, suggestions, half-baked ideas, metaphors, humor, encounters with important persons, historic coincidences, and all the other aspects of a scientist's life are censored out by reviewers and editors according to prevailing custom. It is the monograph format that could bring a colleague alive. Indeed, when one is reading Hermann von Helmholtz's monumental monograph, written a century ago, he appears almost alive, and even though much more is now known about human perception his monograph is still fresh, exciting, and inspiring. On the other hand, I doubt that many colleagues would read scientific articles by Helmholtz that appeared in archival journals which are now defunct. [Since Helmholtz, thousands of new findings and concepts have been reported. A recent handbook edited by Boff, Kaufman, and Thomas (1986) is highly recommended. Yet this handbook, containing an enormous volume of new material, was written by many individuals and lacks the uniformity and intimacy of Helmholtz's.] Of course, there are only a few geniuses like Helmholtz. Even so, when some esteemed colleague whom I have not met in person retires or dies, I feel somewhat less of a personal loss if he has left behind a few monographs. It is not the inconvenience of searching for scattered papers in the literature; it is the individual's personality that is lost forever. Often the best one can hope for is a few inaccurate recollections by intimate students and co-workers. Let me note that I do not confuse monographs with autobiographies. While autobiographies by famous scientists and mathematicians (e.g., Erwin Chargaff, Stanislaw Ulman, and Mark Kac) have given me great pleasure, by its very nature this genre is primarily aimed at a broad readership, sacrificing scientific content. Furthermore, while an autobiography is interesting only if written by a charismatic individual of exceptional scientific achievements, I regard many monographs by outstanding but less famous colleagues as still fascinating.

B: You still have not convinced me that writing a monograph as you have described is not just an ego trip by someone suffering from a delusion of grandeur. Please continue, anyway.

A: After three decades of doing basic research in psychobiology and interacting with dozens of colleagues, postdoctoral fellows, students, and readers of my articles, book chapters, and monographs, there is one problem that I regard as fundamental. The problem is the eternal "student-master relationship." Obviously, a master tries to recruit students by giving them his best ideas and sharing with them his dreams, insights, scientific tastes, sophisticated equipment, etc., with the hope that the students will carry on the master's quest, even becoming active members of the master's paradigm circle. With postdoc there is no problem, since it is to their advantage to publish joint papers with their better-known masters. I always strove to arrive at some scientific problem that neither of us had pursued before joining forces, so that my postdocs would be regarded as independent thinkers aided by an experienced helper. The problem starts later, when a former student finds an academic position and wants to break away from his master—especially since tenure committees and funding agencies

like to reward original work. Should one compete with one's former student; or should one be satisfied that his thoughts are being further developed by a creative younger brain, even if the former student or colleague might not give deserved credit? In this hard choice I have chosen the second alternative, greatly aided by the formative years I spent as a member and then for 25 years as a department head at Bell Laboratories. Since the purpose of an industrial laboratory is to solve problems and gain novel patents, regardless of supervisors' sensitivities, the slogan at Bell Labs was "Either do things yourself or give credit where credit is due!" I regard it as more important to see a novel idea put forth during my lifetime than to be concerned with priority issues that arise because of human vanity.

Of course, some vanity is part of the normal human condition. During the weeks I spent in intensive care after my automobile accident, I did not feel any pride in my election to the National Academy of Sciences a few days earlier. What is more, I did not feel any indignation when I received the first edition of the influential book *Parallel Distributed Processing* (Rumelhart et al. 1986), the first chapter of which reproduced a basic computer-generated random-dot stereogram from my monograph and attributed it to David Marr (who had used the same figure of mine in his book *Vision*, even though he had given credit to me). Here I was dying, and my best-known contribution was attributed to another colleague, already dead. For months I had no interest in establishing priority for the AI community. I assumed that my friends and colleagues knew the genuine facts, and about the rest I did not care. But after my slow recovery, vanity prevailed; I protested to the editors—the more so since the RDS from Marr's book was identical, dot by dot, with the one in my 1971 book. In a few weeks a second edition of *PDP* was issued, with proper credit finally given to me. I bring up this story because I think that it is normal, healthy, and ethical that a scientist (and his students and friends) should be concerned about priority, and mistakes of this kind should be avoided.

B: That episode was to my liking. Who cares about the origins of applying camouflage to psychology? Of course, if someone improperly attributes the invention of the computer-generated RDS to the wrong person, then indeed he casts a shadow on the scholarliness of other materials in a poorly edited book. While you can be sensitive about the editors of a book, you must forgive your many colleagues who do not call your stimuli "Julesz' RDSs" or "Julesz patterns" but simply RDSs. You have achieved the ultimate a scientist can strive for: during your lifetime your creation has become an accepted way of doing science. Indeed, you have created a scientific folk song. I know that you have always liked the idea of the mathematical school of Bourbaki (with its many talented but anonymous members), so you should be proud that you were a catalyst. But chemical compounds are not named after the catalysts that helped in their creation! At this point I would turn to a related problem that is of concern to you when you select postdocs: the problem of having selected the wrong person.

A: I was very lucky, but I was also prudent. Usually I selected as my postdocs young colleagues who had written their theses under the supervision of some of my highly esteemed senior colleagues and friends and whose thesis work not only was excel-

lent but also differed from the usual interests of my friends, so that I was assured of the creativity of the candidate. So, I am happy to state that I had only a few failures in my choice. Almost all of my postdocs stayed in my field or went into related fields and became well-known scientists. In a few cases a former postdoc had some doubts about his creativity or became disgusted with the competitiveness of struggling for grants and went into medicine or finance. In these instances I was somewhat sad for having lost a valuable person for science, but I realized that for mankind an excellent physician or financial expert might be of more value than a disenchanted researcher. Furthermore, the research we did together was of excellent quality and enriched my life. However, twice it occurred to me that a candidate who had worked with me on an exciting and promising project left me without our having written a joint paper. I regarded such behavior as most disappointing. It happens that both of these individuals went into secure jobs in machine vision and did not need papers in visual perception to further their careers. Nevertheless, I could have easily found more honest postdocs. Now that time is my most valuable asset, such a breach of trust is a severe blow.

The first case of the former postdocs mentioned above still owes me an important paper; however, before leaving, he rewarded me with one of my most important joint papers. In the second case, however, we had already published some material, such as an abstract in some proceedings, but none of this research was ever written up in an archival journal, so I regard almost two years of joint work as a total loss. [Although most colleagues ignore abstracts that are not followed by a published article in a refereed journal, I make an effort in appendix B, where I comment on my own abstracts, to point out which of them were followed by detailed articles.] If you assume that after these experiences I refrained from trusting postdocs with engineering backgrounds, you are mistaken. I come from an engineering background, and many of the best scientists in perception started as engineers.

Of course, I often supported some mature scientists by giving them postdoc positions when I could not do better, and I encouraged them to work on their own projects under their own names. But it was a tacit understanding that we were to publish one or two good papers together, and so we did.

B: While I understand your frustration when two of your postdocs broke their promises and no published papers resulted in spite of investing your time and resources, I cannot blame anyone but you. I bet that the selected projects in both cases were not in your strongest areas of expertise. Otherwise you would have finished these papers yourself. If we are discussing some darker side of research, what is your opinion of scientific fraud in your field?

A: Since I never had more than three postdocs at a given time, I was able to follow their research intimately. It is also my custom to publish results only if I was an informal observer myself. Nevertheless, since I stopped programming computers myself and since the systems became immensely complicated, I have always been ill at ease as to whether some inadvertent mistake was committed—whether the afterglow of the phosphor was correctly stated on the monitor, or the luminance value of the stimulus was correctly measured, or the

clock time of the computer was well adjusted, or some programming bug was lurking. I always relaxed when, years later, some colleagues repeated my experiments and confirmed the findings.

Besides inadvertent mistakes, there are sometimes deliberate efforts to tamper with truth. In my youth in Hungary, during the end of the dark years of Stalin's rule, I watched how a librarian was instructed to paste a section called "Bering Sea" over the section called "Beria" in a volume of the *Soviet Encyclopedia*, making this feared leader of the secret police instantly a nonperson. The reader might assume that such "warping" of history can occur only in dictatorships, but unfortunately it can occur in science too. A case in point is the third edition of Helmholtz's monumental *Treatise on Physiological Optics* (1896).

It is hard to reconstruct historical facts of over 100 years ago, but somehow I knew that Helmholtz, in his *Handbook of Physiological Optics,* already had shown that humans can move their focal attention without eye movements, and I was surprised that in English-speaking countries this finding was attributed to rather recent work (see, for instance, Posner 1980). In vain I consulted the last (third) edition of *HPO* (translated into English by J. P. C. Southall, published by the Optical Society of America in 1924, and reprinted by Dover Publications in 1962), and I was unable to find any hint of this work. After many years, the mystery was solved when Nakayama and Mackeben (1989) referred to this classical experiment in the second (1886) German edition of *HPO,* which was never translated into English. The first German edition was published in 1866, and Helmholtz wrote his foreword in Heidelberg. However, he wrote the foreword to the second edition in 1885 in Berlin. In

1896, two years after Helmholtz's death, a revised second edition was published with a foreword by Arthur König. Both the second edition and the revised second edition contain several passages that did not appear in the first edition. These passages probably could be attributed to König's influence, since there are several references to him. Indeed, in the foreword to the second edition Helmholtz acknowledged König's additions and explained the need for a second edition. Helmholtz regarded this second edition as superior to the first, since it contained a large amount of new material that improved and clarified many statements he had made in the first edition. In order to help the reader find the places that were new or that deviated from the first edition, Helmholtz put "n" in the margin. Nevertheless, the third and final edition was based on the first edition, as if the committee responsible for the final edition did not want to have anything to do with König's version (or with the earlier second edition, which Helmholtz regarded as superior to the first). Indeed, W. A. Nagel (in the preface to the third German edition (1909), and in its English translation) makes the following apology for selecting the first edition as the ultimate (third) edition, instead of choosing the second: ". . . the next question was whether to use the text of the first or second edition. Undoubtedly, the natural thing was to select the later version for this purpose. How could an editor choose to disregard any alterations or additions which had been made by the author himself? . . . Curiously enough the changes and additions which were introduced in the second edition seem to be called in question and discarded to a far greater extent than the contents of the first edition. . . . Thus at present time it is not only easier but wiser to undertake the revision on the safe basis of the first edition instead of attempting to reconcile the tentative investigations in the second edition." I am not implying that this was an intentional tempering with scientific history; nevertheless, the epoch-making study of focal attention was suppressed for scientists who did not understand German for almost a century! This unusual reversal of history is most unfortunate, and I hope that an English translation of the 1866 edition will inform the English-speaking public of the full scope of Helmholtz's monumental heritage.

B: You made much ado about the Helmholtz story, at least as the omission of focal attention goes. But you probably neglected an article by one of your favorite colleagues, the Dutch researcher Engel (1971), who certainly could read German and English and who found in the translated English text of *HPO* (thus, in the first edition) some hint on searching with focal attention in stereoscopically fused images during a brief flash. Helmholtz repeated the classic experiment by Dove (1841), who used a tachistoscopic flash produced by an electric spark to illuminate stereoscopic images and whose finding was reported on page 455 of the Dover reprinted edition of *HPO* as follows: ". . . in case of complicated stereoscopic photographs with numerous details, the spectator does not get a clear impression of the whole scene at once, and it may take several sparks to reveal it all. It is a curious fact, by the way, that the observer may be gazing steadily at the two pinholes and holding them in exact coincidence, and yet at the same time he can concentrate his attention on any part of the dark field he likes, so when the spark comes, he will get an impression about objects in that particular region only. . . . Thus it is possible, simply by conscious and voluntary effort, to focus the attention on some definite spot in an absolutely dark and featureless field. In the development of a theory of attention, this is one of the most striking experiments that can be made." It was Engel (1971), over a century later, who embarked to study the size of the "conspicuity area" that one can inspect in a brief flash, and how attention can increase it, and how this area depends on the conspicuity of the stimulus (embedded in texture). You would call now Engel's "conspicuity" concept "texton gradient strength." It is the more curious that you seem to have forgotten about Engel since with a Dutch postdoc of yours, Ben Kröse, you spent considerable effort to continue his work (Kröse and Julesz 1989). I did not want to embarrass you with your forgetfulness, but merely to illustrate how futile it is to write a book. Had you recalled Engel from the beginning, your monograph might be quite different from the present version. Continue, however, with your thoughts on scientific priorities.

A: I did not forget the Helmholtz quotation in Engel's paper; only my attention has fluctuated. The omitted passage in the second edition of *HPO* is more general and detailed than the one in the third edition. [I brought up this omission merely to find a possible explanation why the English-speaking circle of psychologists did not know about Helmholtz's work on attention, but after your remark I have no excuse.] By the way, Dov Sagi and I showed that when an observer had to identify a target (say, a T or an L) away from fixation—a difficult task—this perceptual act sensitized the target's neighborhood, permitting the detection of a

tiny dot that otherwise would be invisible (Sagi and Julesz 1986). We called this enhanced area the "aperture of focal attention," and we measured its shape as a function of eccentricity (i.e., the distance from the fixation point).

Recently one of the lost diaries of Leonardo da Vinci was found, and we learned that he even invented the ball bearing. This fact seemed merely a historic curiosity, since inventors whose work had a direct impact on human affairs "count." I mention this fact because many things about vision have been discovered and rediscovered by several generations, at intervals of 30 to 60 years. Over such time spans, a generation of scientists vanishes from the scene. Many of the younger generation—who refrain from reading the old literature—then rediscover some obscure phenomena that fit into some recent theory and are unaware that, for similar reasons, one or two generations ago someone else reported the same phenomenon. In my first monograph (Julesz 1971) the reader will find half a dozen hyphenated pairs of names. The first is the name of the researcher who rediscovered the phenomenon and who is assumed to be the discoverer; the second is the real discoverer (usually decades or generations earlier). Of course, there might be even earlier discoverers of some curious phenomena not yet identified by historians. Nevertheless, my inclusion of the rediscoverer's name is the acknowledgment that, if someone could get away without anyone's mentioning the real discoverer for many years, then a genuine contribution was made to science, bringing into awareness a forgotten fact.

In essence, when it comes to science in the making, the motives of workers in this enterprise cannot be separated from the motives that drive humans in any other pursuit. From curiosity and playfulness to vanity and greed, all possible forces come into play. Scientists are similar to most other human beings in this regard, but they channel all of their emotions and drives into a unique quest: acquiring new knowledge. The idea of organizing seemingly *ad hoc* findings into some coherent structure by some principle, called a theory, checking and rechecking the theory as new data become available, and replacing the theory with a better one is the most important aspect of science—a unique human activity. Although we humans are mortal, our science is immortal, at least as long as mankind is not wiped out by some disaster and is able to continue its scientific activity without interference by some foreign force (like religious intolerance, or dictatorial zeal by some group, party, or government).

B: I am glad that you finally stopped metatheorizing about science and started to talk about the essence of science: the role theories play in research. Indeed, I found your analogies between art and science quite *ad hoc*. Science and art are two very different and important aspects of humanity. At one point you esteem artistic creations above scientific ones. Then you regard the interaction between scientific theories and data as one of the most important of human activities. You probably wanted to draw attention to the artistic aspects of science, particularly to the "museum pieces" of science. Shall I assume that you want your reader to study the history of psychology, much as certain artists are preoccupied with the history of art?

A: You may be right that I was vague about my thoughts on scientific museum pieces. When it comes to the arts, the most important criterion is originality. The most beautiful artistic creation seems worthless if it is executed in an obsolete tradition. Who would like to listen to chamber music by a contemporary composer who wrote it, say, in a Baroque style? [Fritz Kreisler, however, forged such music and attributed it to some unknown Baroque musicians he had discovered. He got away with his "creations," since they became part of the popular repertory before the public learned that they were forgeries!] Such a quest for originality is less important in the mature sciences, since one has to wait for the jigsaw puzzle to become adequately dense in order to find a creative solution. In less mature sciences, including psychobiology, much of the research is based on some fashionable ideas that are posed by a few "original" individuals and the rest jump on the bandwagon. Therefore, it is important to be scholarly and remember the old museum pieces of psychobiology. If certain facts and theories did not work generations ago, then it is unlikely that they will be of importance today; of course, there are always surprises.

Now I turn to psychological theories. Many colleagues believe that psychobiology has more facts than necessary and that it is time to have a few good theories that would organize these facts in some tractable structure. While I partly agree, I think that some of the really fundamental facts are not yet discovered. On the other hand, without a good theory there is no way to tell fundamental facts from irrelevant ones. Also, good theories seldom are overthrown—particularly if they are adequately general and simple, thus appealing to memorization. Even in physics, where accuracy of predictions is measured by many decimal points, Newton's theory is still taught even though Einstein's relativity theory has "falsified" it. In daily affairs one seldom encounters the bending of light by gravitation or the perihelion changes of Mercury. In psychology (in contrast with physics) one can seldom perform experiments that could decide between conflicting theories, since the accuracy of such experiments is crude. Usually the simpler or more elegant hypothesis carries the day. I will spend considerable time on the few theories in psychology which I regard as "scientific," particularly on the theory of focal attention. I will address this problem in detail in dialogue 3, starting with an epigram by Karl Popper, whose other motto that "genuine scientific theories must be falsifiable" had a great influence on my generation. [See my comments on Popper's maxim in Julesz 1981.]

B: I have listened to you carefully, and I am unable to get your take-home message. Could you help?

A: Perhaps what I wanted to say implicitly was that, in addition to the real business of doing science, there are some important background issues that are not explicitly mentioned. I was venting some of my thoughts about these officially ignored topics that are an important part of the research enterprise. I imagine that most young researchers acquire this knowledge only after they have selected science as their profession. I think that bringing some of these issues into the open might help my young colleagues. Most important, I want to remind all my colleagues that in psychobiology many of the trends are just fashions. Our activities are in the spirit of Hermann Hesse's "Glass Bead Game," so we should enjoy the "game" and should not take ourselves too seriously!

DIALOGUE 2
THE CREATIVE
PROCESS: CONJUGACY
VERSUS SCIENTIFIC
BILINGUALISM

Even mature scientists know little more than the names of most branches of science. . . . The amplitude of our cultural heritage exceeds ten thousand times the carrying capacity of any human brain, and hence we must have ten thousand specialists to transmit it. To do away with the specialization of knowledge would be to produce a race of quiz winners and destroy our culture in favor of a universal dilettantism. . . . But how can anybody compare the scientific value of discoveries in, say, astronomy with those in medicine? Nobody can, but nobody needs to. All that is required is that we compare these values in closely neighboring fields of science. Judgments extending over neighborhoods will overlap and form a chain spanning the entire range of sciences.

Michael Polanyi (1969)

A: We all agree that the study of the human cortex is so complicated that a range of disciplines—including sensory, perceptual and cognitive psychology, neurophysiology, neurology, neuroanatomy, embryology, neuropharmacology, mathematics, engineering, information theory, neural network theory, and physics—are necessary to study its workings. The question arises as to how any individual can cope with such a variety of different fields. A likely answer is given by Michael Polanyi (1969), as quoted in the epigraph above.

This "manifold view" of spreading knowledge between overlapping scientific disciplines occurs unconsciously, similarly to the cooperation between members of a beehive. The only requirement is that specialists working on the brain do not have too narrow specializations, so they can indeed communicate with other specialists in overlapping areas of shared knowledge. Novel applications of technical breakthroughs are special cases of progress by such cooperation. For instance, in the 1940s electrical engineers started to develop special low-noise amplifiers that enabled neurophysiologists to record spike potentials in individual neurons. Another example is the development of surgical techniques to reduce epileptic seizures by splitting cortical hemispheres, which enabled Sperry (1982) and his collaborators to study the mental competences of the separate hemispheres.

Are there ways to make this slowly accumulating knowledge more conscious, thus accelerating progress? This question is intimately related to the essence of scientific creativity. While there must be many ways to create a new paradigm or get a novel insight, here I will briefly discuss "conjugacy" and particularly "scientific bilingualism" as two approaches that can be used to advance science in general and brain research in particular.

Conjugacy is the "trick" of establishing an equivalence relation between a difficult (or unexplored) task (operation) and a familiar one whose solution is already known. This is depicted in figure 2.1, where the difficult task O is to transport an object from point A to B through an impenetrable obstacle (wall). A possible way to complete this task is to drill a hole with shaft S at point A, drill a tunnel T under the wall (assuming that drilling is a routine operation), and finally drill an inverse shaft S^{-1} to point B. One case in point is facilitating the operation O of multiplication (division) by introducing the logarithmic transformation S and its inverse, which reduces the task to the much simpler operation T of addition (subtraction). Similarly, convolution (or cross-correlation) O of two functions can be reduced to the simple multiplication of the Fourier transforms S of the two functions, followed by taking the inverse Fourier transform. As a matter of fact, when the neurophysiologists discovered Mexican-hat-shaped (Laplacian of a Gaussian) receptive field profiles of a concentric circular kind in cat retinal ganglion cells (Kuffler 1953) and an oriented elongated kind in cat and monkey visual cortex of (Hubel and Wiesel 1960, 1968), it was apparent that these spatial filter responses had to be convolved with the visual image (brightness distribution cast on the retina). However, neurophysiologists were not at home in the convolution domain, so it took the psychologists Blakemore and Campbell (1969) to show that sinusoidal luminance gratings would selectively fatigue the detection of such gratings when the test grating had spatial frequencies similar to those of the adapting grating. In figure 2.2 it is apparent that the visibility (response) function to a sinusoidal grating, called the modulation transfer function (MTF), is a decomposition of perceptually weighted Dirac functions in the Fourier domain, which in turn is the Fourier transform of the neuro-

---

Figure 2.1

The equivalence relation "conjugacy" (O = STS^{-1}), or how to solve a difficult task by transforming it to an already-familiar task. From Julesz 1991.

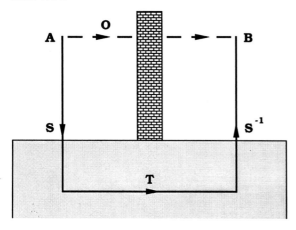

physiologically measured receptive field profiles. Had researchers been more familiar with Fourier analysis or with convolution techniques, they could have discovered the luminance grating adaptation paradigm years earlier, when the first neurophysiological findings were obtained. I do not want to dwell on the use of conjugacy further, since anyone can make a long list of instances in which a novel unexplored task was transformed by some ingenious application of conjugacy into an already familiar task. [See Melzak 1976.] However, an equally effective way to gain novel insight, based on scientific bilingualism, is less well appreciated, even though it appears analogous to linguistic bilingualism.

Now imagine that a cat is waiting in vain in front of a mousehole. Another cat passes by and suddenly starts to bark. The mouse thinks that a dog chased away the cat, and comes out of the hole. The newly arrived cat zaps the mouse and turns to the other: "Isn't it handy to speak a second language!"

A person who speaks foreign languages in the same language family as his native tongue—say, Russian and French besides English—cannot appreciate the intellectual thrill of learning a language in a different language family. For a Hungarian child it was customary to learn an Indo-European language at early age. (Hungarian belongs to the Finno-Ugric language family.) When I learned German, I was quite surprised by the existence of the passive voice. In Hungarian one has to memorize the name of, say, a lecturer. Announcing that "someone will give a lecture on stochastic processes at noon" sounds comical even in Hungarian, while in any Indo-European language one can easily announce that "a lecture on stochastic processes will be given at noon." The noncommittal passive voice, a great invention, is taken for granted by speakers of Indo-European languages, while Hungarians, Finns, and Estonians have to struggle with knowing concretely who did what.

In 1959, after I arrived at Bell Laboratories as a young communication and radar engineer, I started to learn psychology. I had joined a group dedicated to reducing visual information in pictures without perceptual deterioration, and I thought that some familiarity with human vision would be beneficial. Obviously, pictures have a lot of redundancy in them, and the human visual system does not require half-tone images in their full detail. (For instance, it can recognize objects merely from their outlines—a fact exploited by cartoonists.) But what is an outline (contour)? Could one design a machine (algorithm) that could emulate a skilled cartoonist by extracting meaningful contours from patches of various grays?

The idea of using the second spatial derivative (the Laplacian) for extracting contours, proposed and discussed by Ernst Mach (1886), was revived by David Marr (1982) and his followers, who averaged the image luminance with a Gaussian filter followed by the Laplacian. Convolving the image

Figure 2.2

An illustration of conjugacy in brain research. The neurophysiologically determined double-Gaussian-shaped receptive field profiles and the psychophysically determined modulation transfer functions (obtained by measuring the visibility thresholds to spatial luminance gratings with changing spatial frequencies) are related by the Fourier transform. From LeDoux and Hirst 1986.

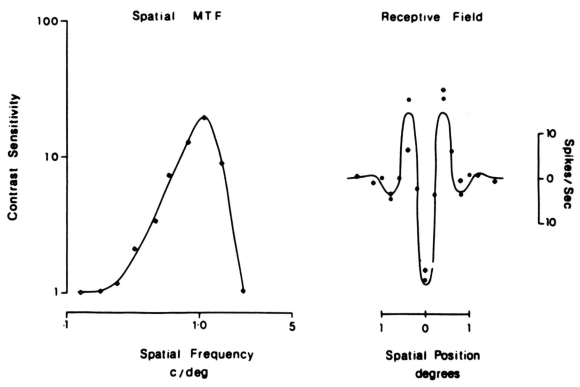

with the Laplacian of a Gaussian is almost identical to the double Gaussian (or Mexican hat function) receptive field profiles found by the neurophysiologists in concentric form in retinal ganglion cells and in elongated form in the striate cortex of cat (V1) (figure 2.2, right). [These receptive field profiles are also quite similar to the cosine and sine functions weighted with a Gaussian envelope—now called Gabor functions, in honor of Dennis Gabor (1946), who derived these functions as the optimal solution to carry information simultaneously in both the spatial and temporal domains.]

Such simple linear operators applied to an image are surely inadequate to find contours and segment overlapping objects. A rabbit sitting in front of a fence has ears that could belong either to the fence or to the rabbit, and a great amount of familiarity with rabbits and fences is needed to separate the face from the background. Furthermore, the existence of the "subjective contour" phenomena, discovered by Schumann (1904) and elaborated by Kanizsa (1976) (figure 2.3), shows clearly that subjective contours exist in uniform areas

where no luminance gradients occur, based on the linear continuation of quasi-collinear line segments. In the cognitive psychology literature, this phenomenon was regarded as a complex task of completing line segments by some higher-order reasoning. Luckily, as neurophysiologists have recently shown (von der Heydt et al. 1988), the completion of subjective contours occurs in V2 (an early cortical stage in the monkey cortex).

In essence, as I got acquainted with the psychological literature in 1959, it became apparent to me that the extraction of contours was intimately linked with the segmentation of objects, which in turn was based on the enigmatic cues of semantic memory. So when I suggested that stereoscopic depth perception (stereopsis), based on horizontal disparity, be used to segment objects, it was pointed out that in order to find in a crowd the corresponding faces in the left and right retinal projections one would first have to recognize the faces—a complex feat whose execution is shrouded in mystery. Already with four targets, not knowing which retinal projections correspond to each other (figure 2.4), one can make 16 localizations, of which only four are correct; the rest are false (phantom) targets. With N targets, the number of phantom targets increases as $(N^2 - N)$. Thus, monocular form cues and contours were believed to be essential for stereopsis—a belief shared even by the the period's leading expert on binocular depth perception, Kenneth Ogle (1964). As a former radar engineer, I knew that this view of the psychologists could not be valid. After all, in order to break camouflage in aerial reconnaissance, one would view aerial images (taken from two different positions, called *parallax*) through a stereoscope, and the camouflaged target would jump out in vivid depth. Of course,

Figure 2.3

Subjective (illusory) contours as first described by Schumann (1904) and elaborated by Kanizsa (1976). One sees a triangle with a sharp boundary even though no luminance contours exist at most places. After Kanizsa 1976.

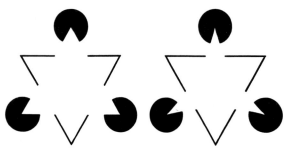

in real life there is no ideal camouflage, and after stereoscopic viewing one can detect with a single eye a few faint cues that might discriminate a target from its surroundings. So I used one of the first big computers, an IBM 704 that had just arrived at Bell Labs, to create ideally camouflaged stereoscopic images as shown in figure 2.5a. Here the binocular disparity is an integer multiple of the randomly selected (but correlated) black and white dots (pixels) that make up the left and right arrays. Therefore, these images, when viewed monocularly, are only aggregates of random dots with, no break or gap between areas of different disparities. However,

when binocularly fused, the correlated areas segregate in vivid depth according to these monocularly invisible disparities (Julesz 1960, 1971). [For more detail, see Bernstein 1984; Hunt 1993; Julesz 1986a, 1990a,b.]

Figure 2.5b is similar to figure 2.5a, except the density of the RDS is reduced to a few percent. It is as easy to fuse as the dense RDS, and it is interesting to observe that the visual system interpolates a surface in depth where there are no dots present (as if it were a "convex hull"). [This "filling in" phenomenon inspired many model builders of early vision; see Grossberg and Mingolla 1985.]

Figure 2.4

Binocular matching, or the problem of false-target elimination. The four identical targets (dots) yield 16 possible localizations, of which only four are correct. Without monocular labeling (primitive tokens), only global constraints (such as cross-correlation) can eliminate the false matches. From Julesz 1971.

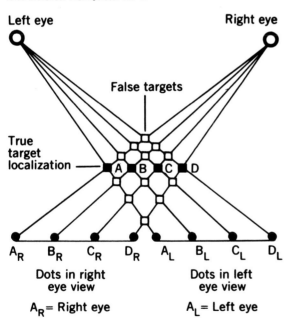

Figure 2.5

Random-dot stereograms: (a) with 50% density, (b) with 5% density. When viewed monocularly the arrays appear to be random aggregates of dots, but when they are binocularly fused a triangle (a) or a square (b) jumps out in vivid depth. After Julesz 1960, 1971.

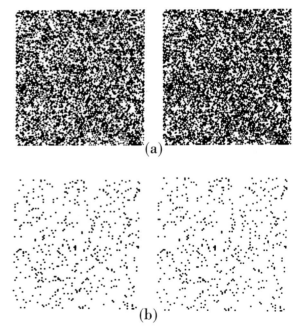

I have dwelt on this historical account merely to stress the point that the introduction of the RDS to psychology was due to a lucky realization by a radar engineer that the common knowledge in aerial reconnaissance that camouflage cannot exist in three dimensions was unknown to psychologists. It was this scientific bilingualism that led to the discovery of the RDS, although there must have been dozens of stereo photographs taken from balloons or airplanes of densely textured scenes that emulated random-dot stereograms quite well. [Babington-Smith 1977 reprints a British aerial reconnaissance photograph of Cologne, taken from two different vantage points, in which one can see the floating ice on the River Rhine. When binocularly fused, the pieces of ice portray interesting surfaces in depth—particularly in the vicinity of the piers of a bridge, where the ice flow is altered.] Of course, the arrival of computers permitted ideal camouflage with absolute stimulus control. Nowadays one can generate a dynamic RDS at 30 frames per second or faster, portraying moving surfaces in depth, whereas in a monocular view only dynamic noise ("snow") is perceived.

The essence of these somewhat personal comments is that, although science usually progresses unconsciously through overlapping fields of disciplines, more conscious contributions can be made if a scientist is willing to learn two remote disciplines and apply his scientific bilingualism to the study of brain research. For instance, physics and psychology together provide an excellent background for psychobiology, as do physics and neurophysiology.

B: I have no doubt that conjugacy and scientific bilingualism are excellent vehicles for creative ideas, but I doubt that the creative process can be put in the straitjacket of two methods. What is so exciting about creativity is the startling way it jumps out of one's head. When Kekule dreamed about the benzol ring, was it conjugacy or bilingualism? It was, rather, some rich, unconscious, perhaps parallel process that came to the surface, beyond logical thought. Creativity seems to me the most unfathomable act of the human mind—even more enigmatic than consciousness, whose very essence is shrouded in mystery.

DIALOGUE 3
THE ROLE OF
THEORIES IN
PSYCHOBIOLOGY

It is not the accumulation of observations which I have in mind when I speak of the growth of scientific knowledge, but the repeated overthrow of scientific theories and their replacement by better and more satisfactory ones.

Karl Popper (1963)

A: I am an experimentalist by choice, and I prefer a good experiment to most theorizing. Of course, if one is to know what a good, revealing experiment is, there must be an underlying theory, except if the experiment is so fundamental that it gives birth to a brand- new theory. My underestimation of theories is only for psychobiology, since I think that field has only a few real scientific theories—trichromacy being one of them. I admire some of the grand theories of physics, such as the electromagnetic theory of Maxwell (described by his equations), quantum theory (described by the Schrödinger equations), and Einstein's theory of general relativity (described by the Einstein-Riemann equations). However, physicists have a knack for ignoring "dirty" problems, such as computing the shape of a puddle of spilt milk on a kitchen floor (Sperling 1978). When they are forced to compute the shape of a plasma in a magnetic bottle, they are confronted with the same difficulties as their colleagues in psychobiology. Indeed, a "thought" might correspond to the shape of a puddle of cooperating neural pools of a certain activity.

By the way, these famous theories of physics are described by partial differential equations whose solutions—for simple, usually linear cases—are now routine. The difficulty starts with nonlinear cases. Let me ponder for a while on linear versus nonlinear problems. My first maxim is that linear problems in psychobiology cannot be fundamental,

since a linear transformation always has an inverse operation that can undo it and hence no decision is made. A system that does not perform a decision is merely a window glass. Perhaps a bundle of optical fibers is a better analogy, since one can scramble a function until an inverse fiber bundle unscrambles it. I can see the usefulness of such a spatio-temporal scrambling operation in many cases; for example, one can build a secure lock by cutting a scrambled fiber bundle (with hundreds of optical fibers) and then use the broken piece as a key. Spatio-temporal linear filters can perform such a useful scrambling prior to some nonlinear operation. However, unless a nonlinear operation follows the linear ones, such a system has no biological significance, since no decision occurred and thus no information was lost. I am always puzzled when a colleague of mine is proud of having been able to find a linear perceptual phenomenon. This, in my eyes, only shows that something insignificant has been observed!

B: Your statement about linear systems' limited significance is an exaggeration. After all, Hook's Law [stating that the displacement of stretching rods is a linear function of the rod's length] is one of the foundations of mechanics, as Weber's Law is the foundation of psychophysics. Let me add that Newton's second law, $F = ma$, is the foundation of physics and describes a rich variety of phenomena, from the movement of cars to that of comets.

A: You forget that Hooke's law is governed by a linear equation, while Newton's law is a linear differential equation in which a is the second temporal derivative of a space vector. For such differential equations that appear linear, there is a theorem, stated in the classical paper by Zadeh and Ragazzini (1950): If any of the parameters (e.g., *m* in Newton's law) of a seemingly linear differential equation describing a system's behavior are varying in time, then the behavior of the system is nonlinear. Newton's law is interesting only when applied to real-life situations, such as nonlinear friction, or when the "psychology" of a fly is added as a force term. [Werner Reichardt glued a fly to a torsion meter and rotated a cylinder with a grating around the fly, measured the torque as the fly homed on the moving grating, and regarded the deviation from Newton's law as the behavior of the fly.]

I am glad that you brought up Weber's Law. Obviously we like it if a transducer between two phenomena is a linear function such that the incremental change in intensity that can be sensed (called the *just-noticeable difference,* or j.n.d., and also denoted as ΔI) increases linearly with the Δ amount of the background intensity (I). So, $\Delta I = kI$, where k is a constant. Such a "linear" transducer relationship yields *logarithmic* dependence between the two phenomena to be coupled, as stated by Fechner's law. Fechner made the ingenious suggestion to regard $\Delta I/I$ as equal to ΔS, where S would be the psychological dimension of "sensation." After integration of ΔS, $\int \Delta S = S$ yields $S = c\log I$, where c is some constant. For more than 100 years it has been generally accepted that our sensations of loudness, brightness, pressure, heat, and electric shock are logarithmic function of the physical forces of sound pressure, luminance, mechanical pressure, temperature, and voltage, respectively. Nevertheless, there are problems with Fechner's Law, which is the integral of Weber's Law.

First, Weber's Law j.n.d. is linear only in a limited range. At large stimulus force, transducers start to become nonlinear (i.e., become overloaded). Even iron rods start to "flow" and disobey Hook's Law. For very small stimuli the central nervous system approximates an "ideal observer," so the mean/standard deviation ratio counts; thus, Weber's Law does not hold, since the incremental sensation (j.n.d.) becomes the *square root* of the stimulus. The second problem with Weber's Law and Fechner's Law is more recent; it originates with Stevens' Power Law. Stevens observed that sensations (S) were related to the physical stimulus (P) as $S = P^N$, where N often would be less than 1, but in several cases would be greater than 1, so the departure from Fechner's logarithmic law would be total.

I do not want to dwell on the technical details of how one should proceed in obtaining Weber-Fechner-type psychometric functions or Stevens-type power functions. Textbooks of the past decades were preoccupied with such measurements. To my knowledge, it was my friend Donald MacKay who first made a daring proposal, illustrated by figure 3.1, for reconciling these two theories. He assumed that the the simplest sensation requires both bottom-up and top-down processes, connected by two transducers (obeying Fechner's logarithmic system function) and a comparator. The physical intensity through the first (top-down) transducer is connected to the comparator, while the (top-down) transducer gets its input from a "sensation generator (S)," a mysterious box in which qualia are generated. According to MacKay, one can vary the strength of this internal S qualia, which is also connected to the comparator until the two inputs of the comparator are matched.

Because I am championing early vision and ignoring top-down processes, MacKay's idea that the simplest sensations require a top-down stage that contains a qualia generator is not very appealing, yet I regard it an interesting possibility.

𝔹: It seems to me that you are among the few who took this idea of MacKay's seriously. Perhaps colleagues who do not want to separate top-down from bottom-up processes have a better conscience than you have and do not wish to refer to a model that appears to postulate a mind-brain duality. However, MacKay's point, that one cannot separate the human brain into bottom-up and top-down processing stages but these have to work in unison even for the simplest perceptual tasks, is a good proviso.

𝔸: From a philosophical point of view I could not care less whether one believes in a dualistic or a monistic mind-body concept, since these beliefs are irrelevant in pursuing brain research.

So, I turn now to the role theories play in psychology. [In dialogue 5 I will discuss some detailed theories of stereopsis.] With some added assumptions one can explain fundamentally very different phenomena of stereopsis, and the only criterion is the psychobiological plausibility of these assumptions. As one goes from perceptual phenomena to more cognitive ones, the testability of psychological theories becomes even less feasible—as I will illustrate with focal attention.

𝔹: Before you go into focal attention, could you explain what this term means and why you want to discuss it so early?

𝔸: I think focal attention is one of the most interesting phenomena of psychology. It fits into an early discussion of psychological theories because it illustrates how careful one has to be to clarify the many meanings of a concept and, in turn, to show to what extent each concept depends on some subtle experimental outcome. It is also sobering that some of these experiments could only be performed by the most recent technological innovations. Decade-long arguments could only be resolved recently, and others wait for illuminations

Figure 3.1

MacKay's derivation of Stevens' Power Law from Fechner's Law.

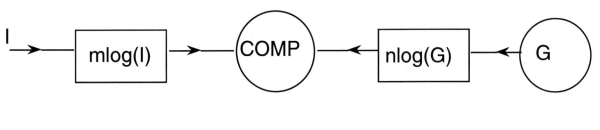

$$mlog(I) = nlog(G)$$

$$G = I^{m/n} = I^{k}$$

after the non-invasive techniques for brain scanning are further improved.

Focal attention conjures up several meanings. For Helmholtz (1866) it meant a "searchlight" enabling him to move his "mind's eye" over any portion of a retinally stabilized image (achieved by burning an afterimage on the retina with a brief flash). For James (1890) focal attention meant "divided attention" that enabled limited mental resources to be concentrated on one or more places or modalities. For some others focal attention means the miraculous ability to switch our stream of thoughts to different items and at will return to the original thought. Furthermore, throughout our lives we are bombarded by trillions of visual scenes, events, and thoughts whose storage might fill our heads with trivial information. So, attention is a bottleneck or filter. All the unattended information will be regarded as "ground" (or "nothing"), and the few attended information is treated as "figure" (or a "thing") that can be also stored in long-term memory. This string of attended and stored memories is the very essence of our personal history and tells our life apart from others. So far the many ideas about focal attention from searchlight to distributed type are not models but merely metaphors.

While all these aspects of focal attention are important, throughout these dialogues I will concentrate on another unique property of focal attention, which I will call "release from crowding." When a text of alphanumeric characters becomes dense, the characters cease to "pop out" spontaneously, and to detect a character requires element-by-element scrutiny. As a matter of fact, the point at which this crowding effect (due to lateral inhibition of adjacent elements) starts to operate is the

point I call "texture formation." In this case the crowded array of letters forms an alphabet texture. If the letters are in "texton equilibrium" (i.e. there are no local conspicuous features that would pop out), letter-by-letter scrutiny (called also rapid scanning or "reading") is needed to isolate the individual characters from neighborhood inhibition. I will use the term *focal attention* to denote this fundamental process that liberates elements from crowding in dense text and textures. Whether this scrutiny is letter by letter or whether some larger aperture of attention permits several adjacent letters to be released from crowding is also an interesting question. [This will be discussed in the last dialogue.]

We also know (from Sagi and Julesz 1986, among other studies) that attention drawn to a certain place can sensitize the area around it so that faint stimuli around it can be better seen.

If the elements in a display are far from each other and are individually resolvable, then the way one can read out these letters either sequentially or in parallel is not my main concern. [See, however, Saarinen and Julesz 1991 and Hung et al. (in preparation).]

There is another important function of focal attention: the selection of different scales. One can inspect a visual scene in three different zooming ranges without having to change his distance from the target (Julesz 1980). One can look at a face at medium range, as one face among several other faces. Then one can zoom on the face and inspect all the fine details, such as unshaven whiskers. Finally, one can regard the face as a small object in a large room, and lose all the details of the face. As I pointed out, these three zooming ranges correspond to the three spatial-frequency channels that when two octaves apart are not interfering with each other (see also Stromeyer and Julesz 1972), and only three such independent channels fit into the 0.5–30 cycles/degree range in which a human can see spatial gratings. This mental switching to these three scales is perhaps the most important aspect of focal attention, and we have studied this in some detail (Papathomas and Julesz 1984).

B: Your comments on focal attention were too detailed for my taste, although you showed the difficulty of understanding and falsifying psychological theories insofar as this term can mean so many different phenomena. While I understand that the focal attention metaphor is incompatible with the divided attention metaphor, your concepts of "release from crowding" and "zooming on different scale" appear to me the same. After all, when one is attending a coarse scale, dense arrays appear crowded, and as one attends to the high-spatial-frequency channel the dense array can be resolved in its detail. However, you drifted very far from the role theories play in the sciences. If you have anything to say about this topic, you have your chance here; otherwise you should turn to another topic.

A: OK. I used to think of Nature as a complex game, and on a greatly simplified scale I would think of, say, a physicist as kibitzing a game of chess or *go* and trying to understand the rules that were completely unknown to him before. It is not at all certain that the physicist would be able to reconstruct all the rules of the game by just watching thousands of games played by experts, but let us assume that eventually he accomplished such a prodigious feat. He might even learn some of the strategies that yield good moves and interesting

games. However, he could never predict an actual game. After all, this depends on the random preferences of the players. All he could do is to tell whether an actual game played to its very end was a genuine game according to the rules of the game. Thus, the *history* of a game is very different from the rules of the game. Before quantum mechanics, physicists believed that they could solve the outcome of a game from some given boundary conditions; we know now that this is impossible, even in physics, because of the probabilistic nature of quantum events. In the life sciences (and, of course, in psychobiology) this split between the rules of Nature and some actual outcome of an evolutionary game was always a fundamental distinction. As a matter of fact, *the most interesting questions of the life sciences and psychobiology go beyond the rules of the game and into the history of the game, including its enigmatic boundary conditions.* For instance, we know more or less the rules of life on Earth, but we do not have the faintest idea how the proper boundary conditions came into existence (the "egg" or the "chicken") from which the cycle of conception, embryogenesis, and maturation of a given individual of a given species would unfold. Moore (1961) has an important theorem (not well known) that every self-reproducing automaton must have a "Garden of Eden" configuration that cannot be derived from the rules of the automaton. Whether the alphabet of DNA is an *ad hoc* historical accident or whether it belongs to the rules of Nature is a metascientific question. It seems to me similar to another metascientific question: whether *Homo sapiens* evolved from mammals only because dinosaurs were wiped out by some catastrophe.

It seem to me quite obvious that our visual system evolved through many evolutionary dead ends. Who knows what visual stimulus that was crucial for the survival of an amoeba or a fish is still preserved in our nervous system in ways completely unknown to us! Physics might also develop similarly to the life sciences by asking what other kinds of universes could have evolved after the Big Bang, with what kinds of rules or histories. Obviously, this is not my concern. However, the fact that in psychobiology the very structure of an actual game (the human central nervous system) is the basic question, while the rules of the game (assumed to be physico-chemical in nature) are of less concern, sets our quest apart from that of the physicists in a fundamental way.

B: Knowing of your interest in epistemological questions, I will be surprised if this dialogue is not very lengthy. For instance, I recall that you often voiced the opinion that psychological theories are difficult if not impossible to overthrow.

A: The dialogue will be short, because it is difficult to discuss the role of theories in my field in a general way. [The next dialogue, in which I discuss the role of mathematics in psychobiology, is much longer.] After all, mathematics usually enters a field when it has some theories that can be made concrete. The few theories that exist in psychology are so vague that it is difficult to falsify them. Psychologists like crisp statements, and the more modifications are introduced the less they like them. For instance, there is the cognitive theory that is referred to as "the magic number of seven plus, or minus two," after a seminal paper by George Miller (1956), and its precursors (Pollack 1952, 1953). It is assumed that this "theory" refers to the maximum number of items one can handle at once. For instance, we can quickly count ("subitize") four stones presented in a flash without a mistake, but when five or more stones are flashed we start to err. While this wide limit of 5–9 items is not as accurate as some constants of physics that are precise to many decimal places; nevertheless, it makes a general statement about some performance limits of the human mind. The problem with this limit is that there are ways it can be overcome. For instance, four pebbles can be perceived as a higher perceptual *chunk,* called a *4-gon* (e.g. a square), and then one can perceive four such squares. Thus, it is possible to perceive 16 pebbles. It is well known that chess masters can reconstruct an entire chessboard from memory, but only if it represents a genuine chess game. If it is a random configuration they do as poorly as a beginner, who can remember only about four pieces. The grandmaster constructs complex chunks, such as "a king is being castled and the left knight is pinned down by a bishop," and usually four such complex chunks are enough to reconstruct an entire board. Without an explicit statement of a person's ability to generate and later recognize such a high cognitive chunk, the "magic number of seven" is not a very useful insight. A chess master, or a master of the English language, might have constructed a special vocabulary of 10,000–100,000 words (chunks), while most of us know only a few thousand.

Here, then, is a typical example of a simple, compact statement about the limitation of our mind. Yet it is not clear how one could falsify such a statement. What is a simple item for one individual is an entire page of complex relationships for another. That theories—what Kuhn (1972) calls paradigms—die hard is true even in physics. However, in psychology some of them probably will never be overthrown.

B: I recall your habit of telling your friends "science fiction" stories about the brain at various intervals during your career in order to sum up your understanding of psychobiology in the light of progress that was made in other fields, particularly in physics. What would be your "science fiction" story this time?

A: Mankind usually tries to understand brains by the most complex devices that became available for making some analogies—clockworks, Fourier-transform holograms, computers, neural networks, nonlinear fluids and optics, etc. When the first Fourier-transform holograms became feasible, years after Gabor invented holography and Leith and Upatnieks (1962) used the first coherent light sources (lasers) to generate them, Keith Pennington and I were among the first, if not the first, to point out the similarity between distributed memories in brains and in holograms (Julesz and Pennington 1965). After our observation many researchers either quoted us or rediscovered this analogy at a time when we regarded this observation as almost trivial except for the fact that this analogy was the first time when several seemingly *ad hoc* properties of memory systems in brains were brought together in holograms too. Whether these similar structural properties were just a coincidence or were based on a deeper structural similarity that followed from some common design principle is still unknown. Therefore, the story of "similarity between brain storage and holograms" can be regarded either as a fairy tale or as a cognitive theory,

depending whether one regards it a metascientific statement or believes that some neurophysiological or psychophysical experiments can be invented and performed to compare the two processes in detail. As a matter of fact, this example clearly shows the limits of some theories in psychobiology. [I will discuss another "fairy tale" of mine in a later dialogue, where I regard the eye and the cortex as two lenses that constitute a virtual optical telescope, which in turn presents all objects at physical infinity. Such a system can explain why objects are perceived in constant position while our eyes move, if we assume that the mind's eye looks through this telescope. If we regard this rather unlikely explanation as an isomorphic model to any complex explanation for perceptual constancy, then there is not even a need for an experiment. The telescope model can be regarded a comical fairy tale or a thought experiment, and some elaborate other explanation—based on a visual system that could compute absolute depth—might be accepted merely because this could be finally tested in detail and falsified]

My science fiction story serves several purposes. First, it shows how can one "snow" colleagues by one's mathematical or theoretical physics knowledge, particularly if the one is a charismatic individual with a well-established record of serious contributions to science. Second, the story has to be novel, unexpected, nevertheless about something credible, and part of the zeitgeist. Third, it should show the narrow line between a creative idea that might be corroborated and some charlatanism that has no foundation whatsoever. It reminds me of an amusing statement by Sigmund Freud: that if one were to claim that the inside of the moon contained seltzer water he might be left alone (after all, we know of geysers next to volcanos), but if one were to insist that the moon contained marmalade he would probably placed in an asylum. My science fiction story has some precursors. Indeed, in recent years, several colleagues with excellent scientific reputations believe that the way the brain's operation is based on stable neuronal oscillations in the 30–70 Hz range, and these oscillation can be phased locked over remote distances. I quote Christof Koch (1993) verbatim: "These high-frequency oscillations and, in particular, the presence of stimulus-dependent synchronization among groups of neurons have given rise to a subculture of modelers and theoreticians arguing that these fast dynamic phenomena are the Rosetta stone of the brain and play a crucial role in figure-ground segmentation, perception, and consciousness." Now, in nonlinear hydraulic and optical systems there is a new excitement about the exploitation of *solitons* (stable solitary waves) for practical purposes. As a matter of fact, AT&T Bell Labs, a pioneer in soliton research, is now exploiting solitons to send packets of waves thousands of miles without dispersion, over transoceanic fiber cables. Solitons were first described early in the nineteenth century by Scott Russel as he rode his horse along a canal and observed a wave of very long duration. For an excellent introduction see Zabusky 1984. As I learned from Norman Zabusky, the nonlinear Fermi-Pasta-Ulam lattice (composed of tiny nonlinear oscillators of masses and springs) can be described in asymptotic limit by the Korteweg-de Vries (KDV) equation (here in one dimension):

$$\partial_t u(x,t) + u^p(x,t)\partial_x u(x,t) + \partial_{xxx}u(x,t) = 0.$$

The second is the nonlinear term, and p can be on the second and third power for solitons to exist.

The most important is the third spatial derivative in the third term to have a soliton solution. The x can also be a two- or three-dimensional vector. This is the reason why curvature, based on the third spatial derivative, plays such a prominent role in visual perception. Whether a neural net with its active neurons and refractory periods can be still modeled by a nonlinear hydrodynamical or optical (glass) medium, and, if not, whether in neural nets solitons do evolve, and whether such solitons could be regarded as stable solutions of certain mental states that last for weeks or years, are questions about which I am not worried, since I am telling a fairy tale here. Let me note that solitons became practical only after sliding filters were found (Desurvire 1994) that absorbed the many small waves but let solitons through. There are several periodic structures in the brain whose functions are mysterious. For instance, the cerebellum has only inhibition as its output. Could it be that its main function might be to act as a sliding filter to be transparent for solitons by filtering out noise?

B: I liked your quotation from Freud about the guy who believed that the inside of the moon was made of marmalade. I think your fairy tale about solitons belongs to the same category. I just hope that your colleagues will regard it as a warning to be more critical about half-baked ideas, instead of believing that deep down you might harbor such nonsense!

DIALOGUE 4
MATHEMATICS AND
HUMAN PSYCHOLOGY

As to your question why I myself am not a mathematician, I shall give you the reasons. I did not conceal my high opinion of mathematics. . . . As a matter of fact, I am also sort of a mathematician, only of a different kind. An inner voice, you may call an oracle, to which I always listen carefully, asked me many years ago: "What is the source of the great advances which the mathematicians have made in their noble science?" I answered: I think the source of the successes of the mathematicians lies in their method: the high standard of their logic, their striving without the least compromise to the full truth; their habit of starting always from first principles, defining every notion used exactly, and avoiding self-contradictions." My inner voice answered: "Very well, but why do you think, Socrates, that this method of thinking and arguing can be used only for numbers and geometric forms? Why do you not try to convince your fellow citizens to apply the same high logical standards in every other field? . . . From that time, this is what I have always tried. . . .

Alfred Rényi (1964)

A: I have always liked both mathematics and Socrates (at least in the interpretation of Plato, whose *Apologia of Socrates* was the only book I carried with me when I escaped from Hungary in 1956). I am also a great admirer of Alfred (Buba) Rényi, one of the best mathematicians I ever met and a man whose untimely death we all lament. It was my early encounter with Hungarian mathematicians — in particular my dear friend and mentor Rózsa (Rose) Péter [of recursive function fame and the leading mathematical pedagogue of her generation]—that exposed me to the intellectual vista of mathematics at the age of 16. At the same time, she gave me insight into my intellectual limitations, saving me from becoming a frustrated mathemati-

cian. Although I thought of myself as "globally clever," with some creative ideas, I knew that I lacked the additional "local cleverness" of the gifted mathematician, who is able to balance a dozen facts and lemmas and fit them together into a unified proof. Without such a local fitting of the parts into a valid structure, all my grandiose ideas seemed to be only daydreams. After much searching through several disciplines, I finally found my proper profession and became a physiological psychologist in human auditory and visual perception. Here I could try some of my global ideas without being defeated by the local scrutiny of mathematical rigor.

The introduction of random-dot stereograms and cinematograms, in 1960, was based on my familiarity with the stereoscopic techniques used in aerial reconnaissance to break camouflage. Surprisingly, these techniques were unknown to psychobiologists. My interest in them was related to the correlation of stochastic signals, my former thesis topic. Thus, my most important scientific contribution did not require much mathematical insight. Nevertheless, my work in perception helped me to acquire some standing among my mathematically gifted colleagues at Bell Laboratories, who were kind enough to take some of my mathematical questions and conjectures seriously, pursuing them in a mathematically rigorous way. One of my questions in 1961–62 concerned the possibility of generating stochastic texture pairs with identical Nth-order statistics but different $(N + 1)$th-order statistics. This was the question that led to my ideas about textons [as I will explain in dialogue 7]. While the importance of textons in psychobiology is now questionable, the hectic activity of the mathematicians who strove to provide answers to my question resulted in a new paradigm in random geometry that is still pursued. Ed Gilbert, Jonathan Victor, and I generated iso-third-order texture pairs using two-dimensional cellular automata (Julesz et al. 1978). [Cellular automata were originally proposed by John von Neumann.] The abundance of novel methods led to a large class of texture pairs with identical second- and even third-order statistics. This, in turn, led to my now-defunct conjecture that the preattentive texture-discrimination system cannot discriminate between textures having identical second-order statistics (hence identical autocorrelations, and thus identical power spectra).

So, here are the two most important scientific paradigms of my life: the random-dot correlogram and the paradigm by which iso-Nth-order texture discrimination without scrutiny can be studied. The first, without the need of mathematical sophistication, became a rather important tool and yielded valuable insights; the second, which required some of the most sophisticated tools of integral geometry, had much less impact. I use these examples to illustrate that it is not the mathematical sophistication that determines the importance of a psychological innovation!

B: Listening to you, I might assume that you do not believe that the maturity of psychobiology and the deciphering of the brain's code, with its highly nonlinear processes, are crucially dependent on very sophisticated mathematical methods. If problems of physics, which are many orders of magnitude simpler than those of brain research, require linear and nonlinear partial differential equations (of the Maxwell and Schrödinger kinds), how can you believe that a mature psychobiology could be treated with simpler mathematical tools?

A: Problems of brain research might require very sophisticated mathematical machinery that has yet to be discovered. However, some rather fundamental problems of psychobiology might be solved without the aid of mathematics. Instead, it is probably more important to discover the *canonical level of complexity* that describes the phenomena to be attacked. When a canonical problem is raised in brain research, mathematical problems often become simplified or vanish. Fundamental insights will probably be gained by the discovery of a novel way to look at some emerging property at the "proper" level of complexity that allows us to understand something that was previously not understood! Indeed, much of the action in modern molecular biology can be understood at the phenomenological level of folding and unfolding of proteins, without computing the many-body problems of van der Waals forces. Thus, working *below* or *above* the proper level of proteins, amino acids, and nucleotides would have prevented us from understanding what life is, and no mathematical sophistication could have provided the deep insight that was given by the epoch-making discovery of the double-helical structure of DNA by Watson and Crick. Even the genetic code turned out to be a redundant three-letter-long code, instead of the complex error-correcting code envisaged by information theorists. This does not mean that some insights from theoretical physicists, particularly from experts in complex adaptive systems, might not be crucial for psychobiology. Of course, I cannot even guess whether a similar breakthrough (such as finding the functional language of the brain) will ever come, or whether a universal organizational principle exists at all.

B: You seem to be too pessimistic. Several workers in psychobiology claim that the brain code exists and that we already know it! Indeed, some believe that a "population vector" can be derived from the responses of a large number of active neurons that relate to the input stimulus (Georgopoulos et al. 1988; Zohary 1992). Földiák (1992) claims that the large number of cells necessary to derive reliable estimates using population vectors is due to the inadequate nature of the "population vector" method, and not to the highly distributed nature of the neural representation. Instead, he suggests a method of *Bayesian statistical inference* that allows us to "read the neural code." His method is based on repeated recordings of neural responses to known stimuli that can estimate the conditional probability distribution of the responses given the stimulus, P(response/stimulus). Using Bayes' Rule, the conditional probability distribution of the stimuli given an observed response from a neuron or a group of neurons, P(stimulus/response), can be derived. Földiák claims that this distribution contains all the information present in the response about the stimulus.

A: I do not wish to dwell on the mathematical problems of the Bayesian method. The difficulties of the Bayesian method, known as the problem of the "*a priori* probability," is discussed in my favorite little book by Woodward (1960). Since the Bayesian method is one of an inverse (ill-posed) problem, and the *a priori* probability distribution of the stimuli is unknown, the solution in general cannot be obtained. Nevertheless, by restricting the incoming signals to a narrow subclass of targets (airplanes) one can derive some "ideal" radar systems. Whether the primate visual system can be also restricted to a useful subset of targets spanning its behavioral repertoire remains to be seen. So, this method is based on the shaky assumption of "Bayes' axiom" that every state occurs with equal probability. It is almost comical that the only stimuli for which the Bayesean method seems proper are my random-dot stereograms, cinematograms, and textures!

B: In essence, then, you do not regard mathematics as a panacea for brain research. What about fractals, catastrophes, chaos, neural nets (with backpropagation), and similar complex theories, such as information theory? You need an excellent mathematical background to understand them, and are you skeptical about their relevance to psychobiology?

A: You have touched a sensitive chord here. I believe that one of the important outcomes of mathematical literacy is not to be snowed by complex but inappropriate mathematical ideas. While I am not competent to judge the mathematical or scientific values of some of the fashionable mathematical theories you asked about, I will tell you my opinion about their applicability in psychobiology. Years ago, when catastrophe theory entered the scene, I was fascinated by René Thom's proof in differential topology that in four dimensions (three spatial and one temporal) only seven types of discontinuities can exist (cusp, swallow-tail, etc.), which he called "catastrophes." I found this result perhaps even more fascinating than the proof that only five regular polyhedra can exist in 3-D. I pondered its implications for embryology, where the same developmental algorithm could construct, say, different cactus varieties depending on which of the seven discontinuities we selected at various arborizations. Yet, on second thought, it occurred to me that for computers (and perhaps for brains), for which memory is based on a *single kind* of discontinuity (a jump from state 0 to state 1 and vice versa, called a "cusp catastrophe"), which kind of the seven catastrophes the hardware designer could have incorporated is irrelevant. After all, the selected catastrophe occurs millions of times a second, as the algorithm that is executed by the computer unfolds. So, the algorithm is the only significant event. So much for the application of catastrophe theory to psychobiology.

I was even less excited by the advent of chaos theory. I found Feigenbaum's insights into finding some general principle behind many different deterministic systems' chaotic behavior unexpected, but not as unfamiliar as it might have been for a physicist accustomed to well-behaved pendulum and planetary movements. Indeed, over decades I used to get access to the largest (unclassified) pseudo-random number generators with the longest cycles of repetition. I used the same pseudo-random generator to create both the left and the right image of a dynamic RDS, and even after millions of such stereograms (composed of 1000×1000 pixels) one could stereoscopically fuse them provided the computer did not make some error. This should drive home my point that computers are deterministic systems that can exhibit complex behavior that resembles chaos but in fact cannot generate randomness! [Of course, some genuinely random generator, governed by quantum theory, could be inserted in the computer, but this goes beyond the scope of these dialogues.]

These remarks were made mainly to stress the fact that chaos is not more than deterministic quasi-randomness, while brains work more as analog systems and are most likely to be genuinely random. So, chaos theory may not be applicable to brain research. However, as a metaphor it could appeal to some. Indeed, I am impressed by the chaotic behavior, exhibited as fractals, at the boundaries between stable domains in the phase space of complex adaptive systems. It is suggested by Stewart Kauffman, among others, that learning (e.g. evolution of life) does take place at "the edge of chaos." Might some of the emerging higher states of human thoughts occur at such chaotic boundaries? [Certainly my own seem to originate from a chaotic cloud.]

B: I think your ideas about catastrophe theory miss some of the value of this idea. Indeed, while catastrophe theory may have not been a good mathematical tool to deal with neurons, Koenderink and van Doorn (1991) have used it very effectively to understand how geometric singularities come into and go out of existence as we change vantage points. So I think you prematurely dismiss the value of this theory.

With regard to chaotic systems no one suggested that computers were not deterministic (except for some microcircuits that operate at quantum levels). The really important question is whether there are psychological phenomena that exhibit apparently random behaviors that are actually deterministic.

A: I am quite sure that some of my smartest colleagues would not waste their time on trivial theories; however, I am too old to experiment with ideas I am not comfortable with. Now I turn to neural nets, one of the most fashionable paradigms in psychobiology.

Since the brain is a network of neurons, and neurons can be emulated by artificial devices (as we know, starting from the pioneering work of McCulloch and Pitts), it is an obvious statement that brains can be studied by means of computer-simulated neural nets. The real problem is to understand an organizing principle of how these neurons are connected, and what individual and ensemble properties emulate the states that resemble our mental states. This problem is still shrouded in mystery. We all know about the quick rise and fall of Frank Rosenblatt's perceptron idea (1958), whose linear version was brought down by the lack of an adequately powerful learning rule (such as backpropagation) and the primitive state of the available computers. The severe critique of Minsky and Papert (1969) was only the last nail in the coffin. Of course, linear perceptrons are rather simple devices. They should be imagined as classifying objects and events by cutting the N-dimensional space by an $(N-1)$-dimensional hyperplane for each yes-no question and asking which side contains them. Of course, even an earthworm is superior to such a decision device that can segment only polyhedra-bounded regions. Although Rosenblatt proposed nonlinear perceptrons too, he had no mathematical theorem that could handle convergence of learning for such sophisticated devices. Two decades passed before the unexpected analogies between human memory and the spin glass drawn by Hopfield (1984) brought nonlinear perceptrons back into fashion and inspired psychobiologists to search for some hidden structures or organizational principles in the brain. However, the AI researchers' models based on nonlinear perceptrons are metaphors rather than deep analogies to brains. Thus, the physicist should be warned that

the perceptual system, particularly its modules (transducers) of early vision, is not similar to a spin glass or a parallel computer, as devotees of parallel distributed processing might like us to believe! However, it is intellectually exciting that the higher association areas (outside the scope of this discussion) might be modeled by neural computation that exhibits flow to attractors of the network dynamics. Of course, my magnetic spring-coupled dipole model of stereopsis (Julesz 1971) exhibited such properties years before such models were called neural nets!

Because connectionism—particularly its representation by neural networks of the PDP kind (Rumelhart et al. 1986)— is popular among physicists who are not familiar with facts of brain research but who understand "Hamiltonians," "strange attractors," "thermal annealing," and so on, one should be particularly alert. While the invention of "hidden layers" and convergence theorems of learning through "backpropagation" extended the processing power of "perceptrons" considerably, it should be noted that the simplest network with a hidden layer implements the "exclusive or" (with three gates) and that to learn this logical function from scratch requires more than 500 trials. Now, let us assume that the number of trials for learning a task increases monotonically (linearly, polynomially, or exponentially) with the number of gates. A special way of genetic learning (evolution) is to change the connectivity of neurons in a brain of a given species at each mutation. So, to develop the human brain, with its 10^{15} gates (synapses), might require eons. Even at a high mutation rate, the time of life on Earth would be too short to accomplish this feat by PDP techniques. This criticism of mine hinges on the monotonic increase of learning time with the number of synapses in a neural net; it would evaporate if one could prove that learning time stays invariant with the size of the network (an unlikely event). Stephen Judd (1987) gives a proof that, in general, supervised training in connectionist networks is NP-complete, so that learning time goes up exponentially with the number of synapses (gates, or nodes) in a network. He shows that, even for very restricted networks, teaching (loading) time to set the connectivity of the gates requires polynomial time. So, my criticism against connectionist neural networks—based on the learning (loading) time being a polynomial or exponential function of 10^{15} gates, thus orders of magnitude larger than the age of our universe, where the unit of each learning step is "one tick of the clock of mutation" for a given species—seems to be correct. Because humans are particularly bad at logical tasks of the exclusive-or kind, one could argue that my criticism of PDP is irrelevant, since neither people nor machines are good at this task. Of course, I could have selected hundreds of form recognition tasks in which people excel and PDP algorithms fail miserably. [For a deeper critique, see Pylyshyn 1984 and Fodor and Pylyshyn 1988; and for discussions of the "top-down versus bottom-up paradigm" in neurophysiology, cognition, and PDP, see Churchland 1986 and Churchland and Sejnowski 1992. For an interesting discussion of evolution, brain research, and AI models, see Edelman 1989.]

B: Are you equating mathematical thoughts in psychobiology with AI research?

A: The role of mathematics in psychobiology obviously goes much deeper, and it predates by a

century the relatively young discipline of artificial intelligence. Most of us, since Helmholtz, used mathematical models in psychology decades before the term "artificial intelligence" was coined. As a matter of fact, I regard myself as an experimental psychologist, and to my surprise I was awarded the MacArthur Prize in 1983 for my work in perception *and* AI. This indicates that mathematical model building in psychobiology is believed by some to be similar to AI. In my view, good work in psychology always tried to find good models, and poor work in AI proposed models that were psychobiologically implausible. Of course, a dollar bill changer does not have to recognize the face of George Washington. If it did, a photocopy of a bill might fool it. It is a much better idea to analyze the chemical compositions of pigments at preselected sites on the bill, as most bill changers do. For such a nice AI solution, however, we pay a price. Such a machine will be never able to extend its pattern-recognition capabilities in ways we humans can.

By the way, AI researchers became separated from psychobiological modelers not because they have different interests, but rather because there are procedural differences between the two disciplines. Usually AI researchers have an engineering background, and for them the latest reference is paramount. They do not care much for historical priorities of ideas. Similarly, when a bridge designer wants to look up a particular design, he will refer to the latest handbook of bridge design rather than to Clapeiron, who introduced the basic ideas for constructing bridges centuries ago. After all, if the bridge collapses, it might appear rather ominous to a jury that an ancient design was tried, instead of the most up-to-date one. In this vein, the AI community, with few exceptions, could not care less whose ideas they saw emulated on a monitor. They usually will credit the person whose demonstration taught them a new fact, instead of giving credit to the original inventor or discoverer. Of course, this trend can change. In recent years some of the best physicists (including Paul Cooper and John Hopfield) started to work on neural networks and brought to AI the scientific taste and respect for originality of the theoretical physicist.

B: What about information theory? I recall that you started your scientific career under its spell.

A: Indeed. In my first profession, that of a communication engineer designing microwave relay links, Claude Shannon's insights into the existence of a "channel capacity" (which permitted us to evaluate and compare such systems) were revolutionary. However, when I worked on radar systems, where the initial repertoire of the stimuli to be transmitted (also called the *code* or *a priori probability distribution*) was unknown, Shannon's information theory could not be applied. Such systems for which the code is unknown are called "measurement systems"—in contrast to "communication systems," for which the list of all possible transmittable signals is specified (e.g., the list of the alphanumeric characters). [The only example for which a channel capacity exists for a measurement system was invented by the late John L. Kelly, Jr., a genius at Bell Labs whom we all admired. Kelly (1956) showed that if in a lottery one of the players would have access to a private "communication channel" that would reveal to him the outcome of the winning numbers prior to the event, then for each dollar he played he could win a number of

dollars equal to the channel capacity of his communication link! Indeed, if the private communication channel were noise-free, the player could win by an infinite amount (since the channel capacity of a noiseless system is infinite). On the other hand, if the private channel would transmit occasionally erroneous numbers due to inherent noise, then the player's win in dollars would be equal to Shannon's channel capacity.] Because I arrived to Bell Labs with the knowledge that information theory is almost useless for measurement systems, after my metamorphosis into a psychologist in the early 1960s I was amazed by the excitement of some psychologists who tried to apply information theory to their field. I knew that psychological problems involved measurement systems for which the code is unknown and therefore the sophisticated insights of Shannon's theory (e.g., that if the information to be transmitted is less than the channel capacity then error-free transmission is possible if an adequately sophisticated encoding is used) cannot be applied. Of course, some primitive aspects of information theory—going back to Hartley—can still be used, such as specifying the rate of information in bits per second; however, this is of limited use. So, *scientific bilingualism* again saved me many years of frustration. While it took a decade for several of the smartest psychobiologists to realize the limitations of information theory, I was able to spend my time on more promising psychological problems.

B: I think you are bragging now, fortified by 20/20 hindsight. After all, you entered the international scene by introducing your random-dot stereogram technique at the Fourth London Symposium on Information Theory in 1960 (Julesz

1961). Surrounded by many colleagues whose approval you sought, you were impressed by their mathematical sophistication regardless of whether they applied it toward unattainable goals. As a matter of fact, it seems to me that a similar situation exists now when Bayesian ideas are tried in neurophysiology in the search for a "brain code."

A: I think you are right that using Bayes' axiom in psychobiology is very similar to applying information theory to it. Indeed, Bayes' axiom assumes that all outcomes are equally probable—an assumption that is equivalent, for a measurement system, to believing that its code regards all possible signals as equal in probability. For direct problems this is OK. However, for inverse problems (also called "ill-posed" problems), for which the *a priori* probability distribution (i.e., the "code") has to be known to avoid many false results, the correctness of Bayesian methods is often questioned. Without 20/20 hindsight I leave the problem of the usefulness of Bayesian methodology in psychobiology to the experts!

B: You have spoken about many things that are somewhat tangential to the role mathematics might play in psychology. Could you establish a deeper relationship between psychology and mathematics, rather than regarding mathematics merely as a tool for studying psychobiology?

A: There is a close relationship between pure mathematics and the psychology of the human mind. Both mathematicians and psychologists are studying certain mental concepts (mental objects or primitives) and rules of interactions between these primitives. These interactions between the primitives are themselves mental concepts, and are of primary interest. One of the miracles of our human existence is the fact that these mental concepts "resonate" to some of the important abstractions (invariances) of the real world through millions of years of evolution, yet after coming into being these concepts have gained a life of their own.

Let us start with mathematics. Mathematicians since Euclid have realized that they can discover or invent any primitive as long as they do not ruminate over what it is in itself but instead defined it by rules of interactions with other primitives. *Thus, there is no mathematics with one primitive; there need to be at least two. Mathematicians do not dwell on the problem of what a point or line is in itself; rather, they define a point as the intersection of two lines, or a line as falling on two points.* What the Greek mathematicians discovered was the miraculous ability of the human mind, the ability called *logic*, to inspect the interactions between the primitives and "know" when these were *self-evident* and independent of others. The simplest of these independent rules of interactions were called *axioms*. Any other mental objects and interactions between these axioms were deduced by logic. Sometimes an axiom did not seem as self-evident as the others, and could be tampered with as long as it remained logically consistent with or independent of the other axioms (as Bolyai and Lobachevsky did with the parallel axiom of Euclid). The "primitives" of modern mathematics can be rather elaborate mental concepts, such as "the set of all twin prime numbers," with many unknown properties currently under study. It seems that this network of self-evident mental concepts is rather remote from the real-life invariances that shaped its evolution and enabled it to become an independent entity of its own. Indeed, we know now that we cannot invent just *any* mathematical primitive, only those that are self-consistent. For instance, paradoxes such as the membership in a "set of all sets" demonstrate the limitations of the mathematical mind. Yet within these limits the mathematical mind has the uncanny ability to scrutinize itself and perform mental experiments in order to decide whether mathematical concepts are self-evident or can be derived from axioms whose self-evidence has already been accepted.

The queen of sciences, physics, adopted the Euclidean ideas. Indeed, in Newton's second law, $F = ma$, where F is the force, a is a constant (Galileo's acceleration), and m is the mass, the force and the mass are not defined by themselves, but only as they relate to each other.

In contrast to mathematics, psychological concepts, particularly those concerned with perceptual primitives and the rules of interactions between them, are not governed by "logic." While mathematical objects are either discovered or invented, psychological objects—percepts—are given. These objects are also abstract concepts, evolved over millions of years, able to "resonate" to certain invariances that real-life objects and events possess, and yet are themselves very different from these invariances. The surfaces of a rock reflect light in the visible and in the infrared spectrum, but by themselves they are not "red" or "warm." The qualia (sensations) of color and heat are among the primitives of psychology. The rules of interactions between these primitives are inaccessible to human logic; they are not self-evident through human consciousness. Only the higher percepts emerging from interactions of the primitives are *directly perceived*. One does not have to scrutinize each step by logic to derive a higher percept, as mathematicians laboriously do with their axioms. The higher percepts that we consciously perceive are derived effortlessly, and almost instantaneously and unconsciously from the primitives. In a sense, each normal human being is equivalent to a mathematical prodigy in the area of perception. Any of us can recognize almost instantly a familiar face in a crowd, or perceive effortlessly an utterance as human speech, auditory noise, or a passage of music, and this prodigious ability of form recognition goes beyond vision and audition into smell, taste, and touch (as attested by the blind who can read Braille). [In their ability to perceive form, all members of the human race are "grandmasters." This may explain why perceptual psychologists are not held in high esteem by the layman. The layman takes perceptual skills for granted and does not feel the need for explanation. In contrast, human speech, being more intentional, is somewhere between perceptual and mathematical capabilities, and is mysterious enough to catch the curiosity of the layman. That is why linguists can attain a prominence in the public eye that is usually not granted to experimental psychologists.]

This uncanny ability of the perceiving human mind has intimidated scores of psychologists who believe that the problem of how the neural machinery resonates to the invariances of the flow fields is hopelessly complex and instead study only the mental resonances themselves. Some others, notably James Gibson (1980) and his followers, were so awed by the prodigious feats of the perceiving mind that they assumed mental resonances to be *direct* representations of physical invariances, hoping that studying the physical constraints of the flow fields could reveal the deep structure of the mind. [However, metaphors of "mental resonances,' according to Peter Medwar, as quoted by Ramachandran (1990), are "mere analgesics" that "dull the ache of incomprehension without removing the cause."]

Not wanting to go into a detailed critique of the Gibsonian view here, I will mention only that quite a few psychologists are under its spell. Shimon Ullman (1980), who regards direct perception as identical to a lookup table, notes correctly that whenever the phenomenon is so complex that such a lookup table would become impossible to store one has to do computations instead, and that hence the claim to direct access would fail. [Nowadays even trigonometric and logarithmic tables are not stored in calculators but are generated from their Taylor series at blinding speeds. However, as hardware for memory exponentially increases, workers in AI are starting to again favor the lookup-table approach for simpler problems.] Nevertheless, even if the Gibsonian resonance idea to the environmental invariances is correct, it cannot cope with the many *ad hoc* ways the perceiving mind has evolved to extract these invariances. For instance, as we move around, objects and textures in our environment seem to contract and vanish in a point, but this invariance of perspective geometry does not reveal why our brains use brightness and color sensations, and gradients instead of some other perceptual primitives. These mental primitives do not exist in the inanimate world, but it is through them that the invariances in our environment manifest themselves. To give up interest in the nature of these primitives is to limit psychology to a very narrow scope.

B: I am surprised that you do not speak more positively of Gibson's ideas. After all, in your first and in my opinion your best paper (Julesz 1960), the only psychologist you referred to was Gibson. Furthermore, I know that your interest in texture perception, particularly in textural slant, was greatly influenced by his first monograph (Gibson 1950). So please say a few kind words.

A: I owe a great spiritual debt to James Gibson. He was among the first, if not the first, to try to find the canonical level of complexity that would be needed to make psychology a real science. As I said in the preceding dialogue, molecular biology suddenly became a real science when its practioners found its genuine descriptors (primitives) in proteins, amino acids, and nucleotides. After this epoch-making insight, molecular biologists studied only the interactions of these "primitives." Similarly, Gibson tried to restrict his interest to invariances, particularly to those that the animal could act upon (which he called "affordances"), in the flow field. I accept his view that it is not of primary concern to psychologists how these invariances are ultimately calculated. After all, creative molecular biologists now take the conformation of proteins for granted, and do not care of how the many-body problems of van der Waals forces (governed by nonlinear partial differential equations)—which could explain the folding and unfolding of proteins—are solved. Gibson assumed that when a person moved around (or at least moved his eyes and neck) he would create a genuine flow field as these movements yielded spatial-temporal gradients in the contours and textures of objects. My problem with this basic idea is due to my lifelong preoccupation with stereopsis under retinal stabilization.

When an RDS is briefly presented with eye and head movements prevented, it is not the motion of the observer that creates the flow field; in this case the flow field is created by the binocular disparity gradients that are hidden in the stereograms. Particularly problematic is the case when an RDS is presented as an anaglyph for the Gibsonian flow field concept. Anaglyphs do not exist in real life, since all objects with their surfaces are presented at the same depth, and their different distances are conveyed merely by their different disparities. So, for an RDS in anaglyph format, the only way to extract the depth information is by neural computation! It is a pity that Gibson never commented on this problem, even though he honored me several times by attending my lectures at Cornell. Perhaps one of his students could explain how this situation could be treated by Gibsonian theory.

As a matter of fact, a collaborator of mine, Itzhak Hadani, is working on the passive navigation problem (in which the observer moves only her eyes) and has formulated a very powerful computer model that emulates how the gradients of the retinal image motion are adequate to compute absolute depth from the center of the eye of the observer to the viewed objects. I am even happier that recently we joined forces to study stereopsis and the problem of whether absolute depth can be obtained from an RDS in anaglyph format. Nevertheless, because I am still uncomfortable with the notion that absolute depth can be obtained by the mind, I proposed an alternative hypothesis to Hadani's that seems to me a Gibsonian argument, or a scientific joke, depending on the reader's taste. I was always impressed by the fact that objects at different depths appear to be standing still as we move our heads. After all, objects at a greater dis-

tance move less on our foveal projection than objects closer to us. Hadani and I tried to explain this phenomenon by two very different hypotheses. One assumes that the visual system somehow determines the veridical (absolute) distance of each object and computes the positional constancies with some complex algorithms. However, in our second explanation we do not have to postulate that the visual system can extract absolute depth. Instead, we assume that the mind's eye looks through a telescope. Indeed, a telescope collimates the visual arrays as if objects were at physical infinity, and of course objects at infinity move together when we move our heads. A telescope has two lenses. We proposed that the human eye is one of these lenses, while the cortex (with its cortical mappings) serves as the second lens (Hadani and Julesz 1992). This model is really an isomorphism with the observed facts, and as such does not need further experimentation. It is a thought experiment. Indeed, if one asks how this telescope is moved around, then—in the best Gibsonian tradition—the answer is that the telescope is located at the "ego center" of the observer and thus need not be moved around. Here I only wanted to demonstrate that some very complex models can be substituted with some simpler ones that have heuristic appeal. It also illustrates that in the field of cognition one can build many straw men without being able to knock them down.

So far I have mentioned rather trivial facts, though I may have stretched the analogy between the mathematical mind and the perceiving mind too far. Somehow, I have assumed, percepts can be decomposed into primitives, as in mathematics. Belief in decomposition permeates modern science, from physics to genetics. The properties of chemical elements (molecules) are explained by the interactions of physical elements (atoms), which in turn are decomposed into quarks, and so on. Similarly, strings of DNA molecules form genes, which in turn can be translated into the sequences of nucleic acids that form proteins—the building blocks of living organisms, including their brains. This *structuralist* approach of the sciences might not be gen-

erally true for psychology, as the gestaltist school claimed a generation ago. Looking at figure 4.1, one might notice that Mona Lisa's eyes and mouth have been inverted without affecting the perceived image much. Yet after one rotates the page, the familiar face is strikingly different from the manipulated one, attesting to the gestaltist claim that eyes, mouth, etc., are not just the elements of face recognition but rather engage in enigmatic holistic interactions that render the entire concept of elements (primitives) problematic.

The striking difference between the manipulated Mona Lisa when right-side-up and when upside-down yields an important insight. Obviously,

Figure 4.1

A demonstration of gestalt. The upside-down pictures appear rather similar in spite of the fact that in one picture the eyes and the mouth are inverted. When the page is turned over, the two faces reveal a dramatic difference as a result of gestalt organization. From Julesz 1984, after an idea of Thompson (1980).

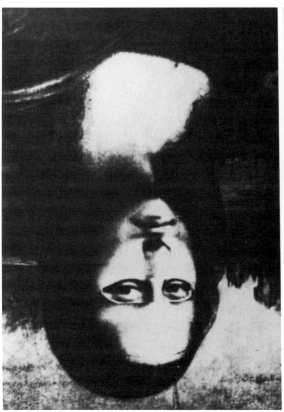
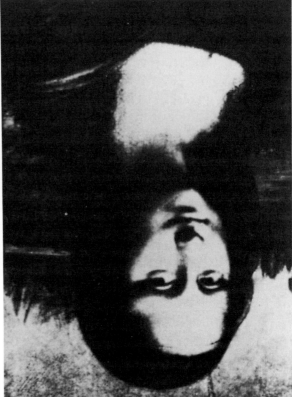

some holistic, "top-down" processes exist that are mainly interested in establishing spatial relations between objects in order to construct some higher percept (e.g, a human face) and are less interested in the objects (e.g. a mouth, or an inverted mouth) themselves. Indeed, some rather primitive objects (lines and ovals) yield the percept of a human face with proper spatial relations, but do not if the spatial relations are scrambled (figure 4.2).

On the other hand, there seem to be some local "bottom-up" processes that ignore the spatial relations between objects in general and detect only specific differences between certain features of nearby objects. I called these conspicuous local features *textons* (Julesz 1980, 1981). Figure 4.3 shows a texture pair in texton equilibrium, where one texture pair consists of a mixture of faces with two eyes and no eyes and the other texture is composed of faces with a single eye. No texture segregation can be experienced, and only detailed scrutiny reveals the different faces that constitute the texture elements (Julesz 1980).

These demonstrations suggest that at least two basic operations are performed in the act of perception. One is a holistic, highly central mode of op-

eration in which complex rules seem to predominate; the other is a more basic mode of operation whose primitives (and their interactions) are much simpler. How could one study this simpler visual system in its pure form without being distracted by the holistic system? It is too early to go into technical details of how to separate experimentally the two modes of operation; here I will only state my belief that the structuralist approach can be applied to the second visual mode, while the holistic mode is too complex for such a quest. Even though the workings of the holistic mode are not consciously perceived, the percepts of this mode (e.g., connectivity of a drawing, or a point's being contained in a drawing, or a drawing's being a human face) are conscious. On the other hand, for the bottom-up processes not even the primitives are consciously perceivable.

Figure 4.3

An iso-second-order texture pair produced by the generalized four-disk method. One texture consists of a mixture of faces with two eyes and no eyes; the other texture is composed of faces with a single eye. No texture segregation can be experienced, and only detailed scrutiny reveals the different faces that constitute the texture elements. From Julesz 1980.

Figure 4.2

A primitive human face and scrambled one.

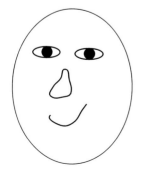 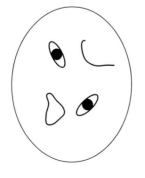

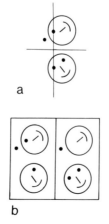

a

b

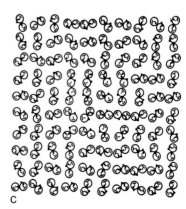

c

I believe that the structuralist approach of mathematics—and of the mature sciences that faithfully adopted it—can be applied to perceptual psychology, if one abandons the requirement that the perceptual primitives be conscious percepts. This is a crucial idea. In mathematics, no one cares what the primitives—numbers, points, lines—are in themselves. That a point can be approximated by an inkblot in the limit as one reduces its size is merely a simile, a crude approximation, perhaps an unconscious percept. As I have already said, the definition of a point emerges out of its relation to another primitive, the line. Similarly, it is a mistake to give a psychological primitive a perceptual existence of its own; instead, one must define it by its relations to other primitives. The belief that psychological percepts could be directly sensed misled psychologists for centuries. Somehow, they thought, psychological primitives must be defined in themselves, and hence must be consciously perceivable entities.

In order to pursue this basic idea further, let us take *trichromacy,* perhaps the only Euclidean theory of psychology. The theory of trichromacy was first stated by George Palmer in 1777, years before Dalton's chemical atom theory, and resurfaced later as the Young-Helmholtz theory of color matching. It states that any color can be decomposed into three basic colors: red, green, and blue. Is this not contrary to what I said before? After all, we take a percept, some perceived color of the range of colors that can be consciously perceived, and we observe that this color can be obtained from a combination of three primitives that are consciously perceivable colors in their own right. It is my contention that the three primitives of trichromacy need not be the consciously perceiv-

able red, green, and blue colors, but instead are more primitive entities, which I will call red, green, and blue textons. If, say, a red texton is presented for an adequate time, so one can scrutinize it with focal attention and thereby bring it into consciousness, then it might become the familiar "red" percept, a highly complex entity. After all, we are far from a true theory of color perception. We have no idea how consciously perceived colors depend on each other in a complex field containing many color patches. (Land's retinex theory is an interesting attempt in this direction, but it is far from complete or able to account for the many nonlinear color phenomena.)

What does the theory of trichromacy really state? It simply claims that if one takes a small blob of some color, then one can place adjacent to it another blob composed of three basic colors and, by varying the amount of these primitives, make discrimination between the two blobs impossible—they appear as a single blob. This criterion really does not require color perception *per se.* One can merely ask for the perceptual dimming or disappearance of the boundary between two patches (or, in the case of color matching by flicker, ask for a sudden change in the flicker threshold for the two superimposed patches). [Here I will not go into technical details, except to state that trichromacy holds only in the foveal center and that, for some colors, one has to place two of the primitives in the comparison blob, and place the third primitive in the test blob together with the selected color and subtract from it, in order to obtain a perfect match.]

We know that Palmer was right when, two centuries ago, he stated a neurophysiological theory of trichromacy. He hypothesized that only three kinds of color receptors exist in the eye, and that these are tuned to the three wavelengths that we sense as red, green, and blue. Only recently, with the advent of microspectrophotometry and the ability to measure the absorption spectra of foveal cones, have scientists verified that only three kinds of color pigments, concentrated in three specific cone types, actually do exist. We also know, particularly from the work of Zeki (1986), that lesions in area V4 of monkey and human cortex can result in cortical color blindness. This type of blindness is very different from the usual color deficiencies, in which one, two, or all three color pigments are non-functional in the retinal receptors. Now, in a normal individual, with three functional color receptor pigments in the retina and an intact color system, a sudden lesion in V4 will lead to cortical color blindness. In this individual, metameric color matching (i.e., trichromacy) is not affected at all, although he is unable to perceive colors. On the other hand, an individual with retinal color blindness could perform metameric matches with two color primitives if one type of color receptor was non-functional. On the basis of this example, fortified by neurophysiological insight, it is my contention that the color textons are extracted by the retinal receptors and early filters before V4, while conscious color—what we usually mean by a color percept—emerges much later in the central nervous system, in V4 or beyond. In this context the exact location of the stages is irrelevant.

What does matter is the insight that primitive features exist, and that they selectively trigger early filters. [I call these primitive features textons, and will define them precisely in dialogue 9.] The extraction of textons occurs at such an early stage in the central nervous system that neither conscious-

ness nor top-down processes can reach them, and thus their primitiveness is preserved. Only to these simplifying conditions, below the level of conscious awareness, can we apply some rules that behave like axioms, and begin to link one texton with another without having to describe what textons are in isolation.

The existence of perceptual primitives, hidden from consciousness and related to the early neural analyzers (tuned to the width and orientation of elongated blobs) discovered by Hubel and Wiesel (1960, 1968) in the cortex of cats and monkeys, has had many adherents among psychophysicists in recent years. These analyzers were revealed mainly by adaptation experiments at threshold, where observers were not asked to report "what" the primitive percept looked like (e.g. a bar-shaped patch, or a sombrero-shaped luminance distribution), but had to indicate that instead of seeing "nothing" they saw suddenly "something." Nevertheless, how the subthreshold primitives contribute to superthreshold (conscious) percepts is still enigmatic.

The logic of trichromacy can be extended beyond color textons to incorporate other perceptual primitives, such as elongated blobs and line segments, Gabor patches, and the spaces between them (which I call *anti-textons*). Any texture or shape will be indistinguishable from a different texture or shape in its vicinity whenever both contain the same textons, provided one refrains (or, better, is prevented) from detailed scrutiny. Let me reiterate that textons by themselves have none of the usual perceptual properties—they are unconscious [or preattentive, to use the term preferred by Neisser (1967)]. In trichromacy, scrutinizing the resonances of retinal color filters evokes in us familiar color percepts. Similarly, in texton theory, as we scrutinize, say, elongated blobs, they become more and more concrete, with distinguishable shapes emerging. However, when we prevent scrutiny by presenting a multitude of elements or by presenting patterns briefly and erasing their afterimages, details of the blobs' shapes have no impact on perception. Only some gross properties—the perceptual primitives of color, length, width, orientation, velocity, stereo depth, and flicker rate—have perceptual significance.

This extension of trichromacy from color matching to the matching of textures and adjacent shapes through the concept of texton equilibrium holds only for scrutiny-free vision. For instance, one could produce from a mixture of elongated blobs of various sizes and orientations a texture that would appear to be that of genuine leather under cursory inspection. However, with scrutiny one would notice the difference between real leather and its texton imitation. On the other hand, no amount of scrutiny could ever tell a genuine yellow from its metamerically matched imitation composed of a mixture of red and green. This fact does not mean that attended color is not richer in its properties than unattended color; it is only that

Figure 4.4

Preattentive (parallel) texture discrimination versus serial scrutiny by focal attention. Whereas the Xs among the Ls pop out effortlessly, finding the Ts among the Ls requires an element-by-element search. From Julesz and Bergen 1983.

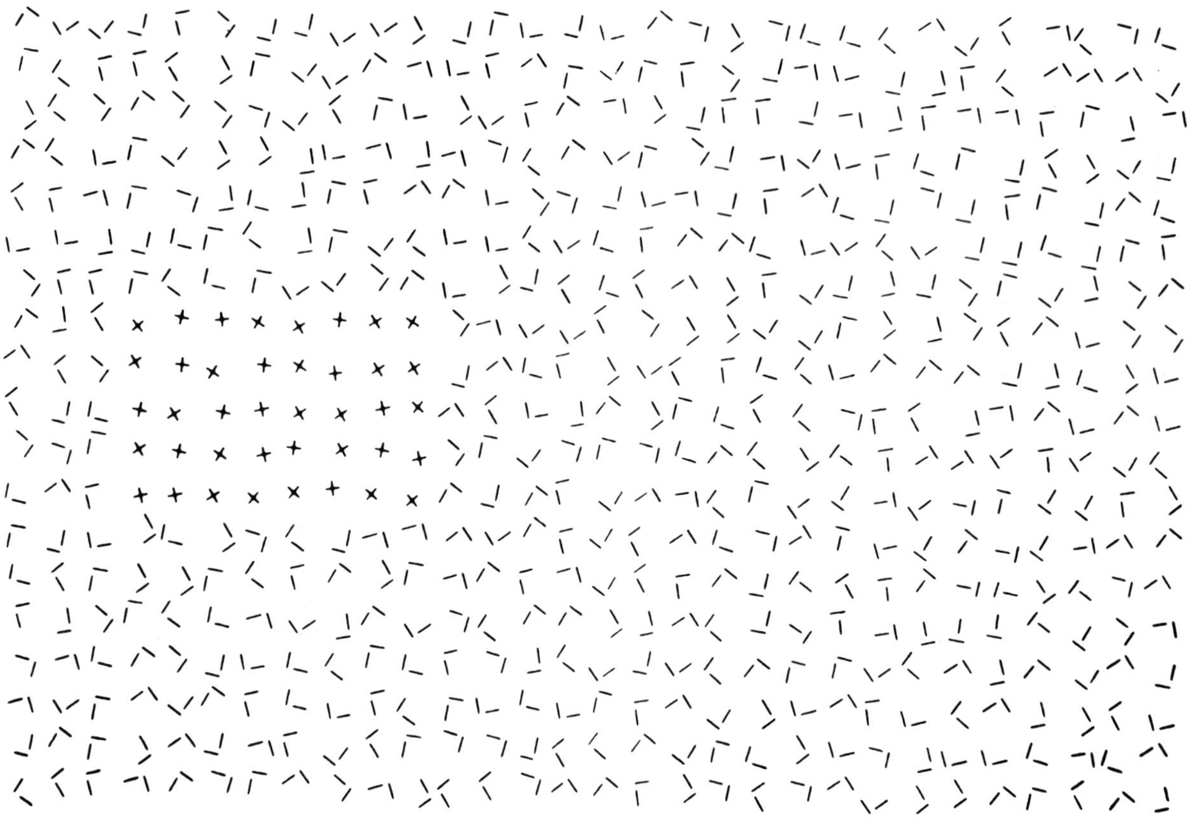

color matching is such a simple process that two different perceptual modes cannot manifest themselves.

Textons have no perceptual significance in themselves, but only with respect to other textons. So, as we view figure 4.4, we can observe that the textons of *crossing* formed by the orthogonal line segments in the area of Xs allow this area to pop out preattentively from the surrounding area of Ls, where the same orthogonal line segments do not cross. On the other hand, the Ts (with small gaps between the orthogonal line segments to avoid crossings) do not form texton gradients with respect to their surrounding L shapes, and therefore do not pop out unless we scrutinize (that is, serially search element by element with focal attention). [This serial shift of attention is entirely neural and occurs much faster than scanning eye movements. The reader could sit in the dark and illuminate figure 4.4 by an electronic flash lasting only microseconds during which no eye movements can be initiated. Yet, the reader could scan at will the *afterimage* of the texture impinged on the retina.] If the observer had not been told to search for the Ts, they would most probably have escaped notice. Similarly, a leather shoe next to its texton imitation might have looked all right, but only if the observer happened not to attend to the imitation. Preattentive vision is thus concerned almost entirely with differences in the number or density of adjacent textons—differences that form texton gradients. It is little concerned with the textons themselves. For adjacent texture or pattern pairs, one can know preattentively whether the pairs agree in their textons or differ. The more they agree, the less they can be told apart in a cursory glance.

Here I will only assure you that textons exist and provide a hint of what they are. They exist in the same way that mathematical primitives or the quarks of physics exist. No physicist is so impatient as to ask what a quark is in the first pages of a physics textbook. The fact that no quark may ever be directly observed does not discourage the worker in physics. The important thing is that quarks act as primitives and all the elementary particles can be deduced from them through elegant theories. Even as quark dimensions proliferate, with color, flavor, charm, strangeness, etc., the theorists keep their faith. A detailed theory that predicts facts can justify the postulation of primitives.

Be patient. Rather than "Do textons exist?" one should ask "How useful would a theory of preattentive vision be?" and "Can the structuralist program outlined here can be extended to higher percepts?" Even though I do not know the answers to these questions, I find it remarkable that the texton theory of preattentive vision can explain the discrimination between many texture pairs examined so far. What is even more important is the emergence of a psychological theory that is adequately precise to be either corroborated or falsified.

B: I would not have believed that an interesting dialogue on the role of mathematics in psychology would end with your texton theory. Perhaps you could add some more interesting thoughts.

A: Of course, I have many ideas about the role mathematics plays in the sciences. Eugen Wigner, a Hungarian-American physicist, published a wonderful paper, "The unreasonable effectiveness of mathematics in the natural sciences" (1960), pondering the enigma of why mathematical ideas and tools are so applicable in physics. It boggles the mind that, millennia ago, some Greek mathematicians cut sand cones on a beach and discovered ellipses, hyperbolas, and parabolas, which turned out to be the trajectories of the heavenly bodies. It is likewise amazing that the distributions and properties of prime numbers, a most abstract branch of mathematics called number theory, would have thousands of useful applications nowadays, from cryptography to the design of concert halls (Schroeder 1986). In many of these cases, the correlation between mathematics and scientific theories of physics and chemistry that are conceived by the human mind are not as surprising as they seem,

since both the natural laws and the laws of human reasoning seem to follow the same underlying principles. Of course, there are many instances when the laws of mathematics and geometry work independently from the workings of the mind.

Congruency is a fundamental aspect of geometry. We all accept that two objects are more congruent when they appear more similar. Of course, there are many definitions of similarity. In a given geometry that has a distance function, the more two objects overlap and thus share the same volume (area), the more similar they are. In 1959 I performed the experiment depicted in figure 4.5 (with the help of Charles Mattke, who built a 100-frame rotating tachistoscope for me). I had noticed earlier that when objects A and B moved along crossed linear trajectories, at the crossing point there was a tendency for both objects to follow their linear paths, A > C and B > D thus had an X-shaped trajectory, provided A was more similar to C than to D, and B was more similar to D than to C. However, it was possible to manipulate the similarities of the two objects so that, instead of crossing, they would bend in a double V shape. To my surprise, the "similarity" was not a geometric similarity, but a rather unexpected kind. (Often the shapes of the objects that bent into the V-shaped path were not similar in a geometrical sense, but would adhere to a dissimilar shape with more contrast.) [Years later, independently and more generally, Paul Kolers and Jim Pomerantz (1971) studied such phenomena. They found that successive targets of very different shapes or colors did appear to move into each other, and that some intermediate shapes and colors could be experienced along the target path.]

Figure 4.5

An experiment on similarity (identity tracking) performed by the author at Bell Labs.

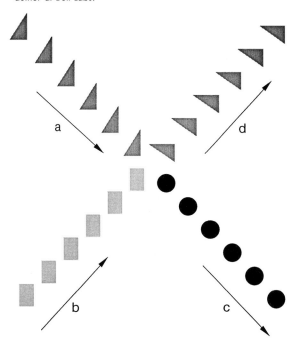

I stopped these experiments in 1960 because I had started to work with random-dot stereograms, which I found more interesting and easier to study. Interestingly, the idea that similarity in stereopsis is quite similar to that in motion perception and differs from the notion of mathematical congruency came to me as I turned to stereoscopic vision. Indeed, I showed in 1960 that an RDS in which one image was altered by removing (say) the diagonal connections [by complementing the black (white) value of a dot to its opposite when the dot had identically colored neighbors along the two diagonals] appeared very different yet could be fused. As figure 4.6 shows, in such an image, the right image contains only horizontally and vertically connected patterns, while the left image remains an array of randomly speckled dots. It turned out that such an operation disturbed the binocular correlation of 16% of the dots and the 84% correlated RDS yielded good fusion. Here was an example where the corresponding patterns (local features) in the RDS were very dissimilar, yet the global binocular correlation was very strong (80%). It was obvious that for stereopsis, increased correlation was the determining factor for similarity at

the expense of feature similarity. Although random-dot stereograms and cinematograms behave quite similarly, particularly for matching corresponding random-dot arrays, I did not study explicitly the role of correlation versus similarity in motion perception. I am very pleased that 30 years later Werkhoven (1990) undertook this problem for motion perception with an ingenious innovation that constitutes a new paradigm.

The demonstration given by figure 4.6, among others, led to the importance of correlation in human stereopsis and motion perception, extending the earlier observations of Werner Reichardt on the motion detectors in the domestic fly (*Musca*). I also observed at this time that blurring both images (by defocusing the projectors) caused the left and right images to appear quite similar. I regarded this observation as a precursor of my later work (Julesz and Miller 1962), showing the importance of spatial-frequency-tuned channels in stereopsis. In the present language, the demonstration of figure 4.6 clearly shows that the high-SF channels can be in rivalry as long as the low-SF channels are binocularly fused.

Whether the deviation of perceptual similarity from geometrical similarity is caused mainly by the dissimilarity of the high-SF information when the low-SF information is identical, or whether the low-SF information could be eliminated altogether and yet correlation would win over geometric similarity for the high-SF information, is an interesting question. As a matter of fact, my iso-second-order texture paradigm is an extension of this problem. In iso-second-order texture pairs, the second-order statistics are identical; hence, the correlation (a simpler parameter, derived from the second-order statistics) must be identical, too. From 1962 till 1976

Figure 4.6

A random-dot stereogram with diagonal connectivity broken in one image and with 84% of the dots correlated (so that the low spatial frequencies are similar). From Julesz 1971.

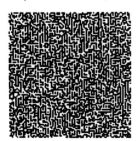 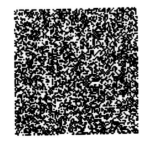

we found no discrimination in such texture pairs, until the discovery of the first textons (Caelli and Julesz 1976). These textons made iso-second-order texture pairs discriminable for the first time, based on some local features. For a while texture pairs with identical second-order statistics (and correlation, hence, the Fourier power spectra) could not be told apart. Indeed, if two stochastic sources were to generate texture pairs side by side one could wait for eons to tell them apart. However, my research with Terry Caelli (1986) sped up this process by creating some local features in these iso-second-order textures that yielded effortless texture discrimination. The pop-out of some textures from others with the same correlation clearly showed that similarity between textures can be based on some local features, but not on any local feature. The local features on which similarity depends must be *conspicuous local features* (texton gradients). Ts and Ls are geometrically dissimilar yet do not yield texture discrimination, while Xs and Ls are geometrically as dissimilar as Ls and Ts; yet the former yield strong texture discrimination and thus are much less similar to each other in texture segmentation.

Charlie Chubb and George Sperling (1992) extended the iso-second-order-texture paradigm for static patterns varying in x and y to motion perception for iso-second-order patterns varying in x and t. They called it *drift-balanced* or *second-order* motion. So far I have not undertaken an adequate effort to find out whether their paradigm is more general than mine, or whether these two paradigms are closely related (as I suspect). I hope that this will be clarified in the foreseeable future.

B: You are back to textons again. While I am impressed by the mathematical sophistication that was required to generate stochastic patterns with prescribed statistics, the texton theory that resulted from these efforts does not seem to me to be adequately relevant to the deep problem of relating mathematics and psychology. I regard the drift balanced stimuli similarly contrived, and wonder how they can be used to illuminate differences between mathematical and perceptual concepts of similarity.

A: Whether one believes in the power of the texton theory or regards it as irrelevant for psychology, the basic motivation that inspired it is of importance to the basic problem raised in this essay. I regard trichromacy as perhaps the only genuine theory of psychology, in the Euclidean sense, and I hope to extend it from color to texture perception. A successful texton theory would be one of the few theories of psychology that might be of interest to mathematicians. Therefore, I continue with my thoughts on perceptual and mathematical similarity, undisturbed by your remarks.

Geometrical similarity (congruence) is a concept that appeals to common sense but has very different meaning in visual perception. In stereopsis one can create texture pairs that locally appear very distinct but yield global stereopsis. In preattentive texture discrimination one can have certain special local features (Julesz 1981) that yield global discrimination. On the other hand, there are local features that are very different from each other and yet do not yield discrimination (since they are in texton equilibrium, as I will explain). The global measures of perceptual similarity are described by correlation (covariance), while the local measures of perceptual similarity are described by texton gradients. For motion and depth perception the global perceptual measure of correlation does predict perceptual similarity. For texture discrimination, global correlation (autocorrelation) predicts discrimination only as long as texton gradients are not formed. So, the deep structure of visual perception is very different from the various geometries that mathematicians created. Perhaps in *visual cognition,* where the shape of an object stays invariant under translation, rotation, and zooming, we are getting closer to mathematical (geometrical) concepts. This is not surprising, since visual cognition yields the final output of the visual system and it is probably at this level where the mathematical mind abstracts its basic concepts.

B: In *FCP* you devoted an entire chapter to Klein's Erlangen program and its relations to mental geometries. Have you changed your views, since you have not referred to these ideas so far in our discussion?

A: Thanks for reminding me. The mathematician Felix Klein proposed a program to study geometries by searching for invariances under given transformations. In *FCP* I mentioned an interesting proposal by William Hoffman (1966) to study visual perception by means of Lie algebras (Lie 1893). In the 25 years since I wrote that chapter, Hoffman (1970) extended his method to infinitesimal Lie transforms, called *Lie germs,* and called it the Lie Transformation Group Model in Neuropsychology (LTG/NP). This model stirred up some interest; the psychologist Peter Dodwell (1983) was under its spell and conducted a detailed study. Unfortunately, these attempts have not succeeded so far. Although I thought Lie germs might be too general to describe the idiosyncrasies of human perception, I performed with Papathomas a benchmark

test on the first generation of a massively parallel machine called the Connection Machine (designed by Danny Hillis). We incorporated in each of its 64,000 processing units the Lie germs of affine geometry in two-dimensional space, nulling all such transformations (Papathomas and Julesz 1982). So, targets undergoing certain selected transformations (or moving along some trajectory) would not appear on the screen. As an AI model and device this generalized "snooperscope" is a useful machine, but I am doubtful that visual perception developed along such lines. It is up to Hoffman and his followers to further advance their ideas. The main support for Hoffman's Lie group theory of human perception is the orthogonal aftereffects of Donald MacKay. If one looks at dynamic noise on a TV monitor and draws concentric circles on the screen with a crayon, the dynamic noise seems to stream as radial lines orthogonally to the concentric circles; radial lines in turn evoke concentric streaming, while parallel gratings evoke orthogonal aftereffects. *Hoffman's theory predicts for binocular vision a series of confocal hyperbolas and their orthogonal set of hyperbolas.* I tried to look at a TV monitor (portraying dynamic noise) at a sharply inclined angle, such that my eyes' centers coincided with the focal points of the hyperbolas I drew on the monitor's screen; alas, I could not see the orthogonal sets of hyperbolas. Whether these experiments were a correct interpretation of Hoffman's ideas or whether a better observer could detect some traces of an orthogonal set of hyperbolas remains to be seen.

In *FCP* (in the chapter on Klein's Erlangen program) I discussed an earlier idea of Hoffman in detail. Hoffman regarded the cortex, with its range of orientationally sensitive neurons, as the isocline (tangential) field of a 2-D differential equation, and its solution depended on the boundary conditions of the perceptual constancies. Thus, an observer possessing size constancy could easily prefer as a solution radial lines (the eigenpatterns for zooming). With rotational constancy the preferred solution might be concentric circles. Gallant et al. (1993) recently found selectivity for polar, hyperbolic, and cartesian gratings in V4 of macaque visual cortex.

Recently, with the inspiration of Ilona Kovacs, we generated a random array of Gabor patches that contained collinear and circular global patches, with large gaps between the constituent Gabor patches. Observers were able to see long lines and closed circles for these select shapes, but they failed to do so for zigzag lines or for not-fully-closed circular lines. Here it is most interesting that a dramatic perceptual change occurs in being able to connect large gaps between adjacent Gabor patches, but only when the global structure suddenly becomes closed. Here is a second instance—the first occurs in the texton theory—where the topological concept of closure has real perceptual significance! After all, visual perception notoriously avoids topological concepts. Indeed, the saying that a topologist is a guy who cannot distinguish between a doughnut and a cup strikes us very funny. Whether we struck on a few exceptional topological phenomena in visual perception, or whether a real hidden topology of vision will eventually emerge, remains to be seen. While this research—using arrays of elements—is closer to my interest in texture perception than to form perception, it is certainly a bridge between the two. I can also envision how Ilona Kovacs will one day be regarded as the founder of a neo-gestaltist school. [For more details, see figures 8.1–8.3 and the accompanying text.]

B: You seem to be carried away with the closure phenomenon. You made sure to test the effect with sharp discontinuities in closed lines, and found that such kinks destroyed the pop-out phenomenon. So the "perceptual closure" is not a topological closure, but merely a "smooth closure."

A: You are perfectly right. A somewhat similar diameter-limited closure concept occurs in the texton theory too, and perhaps mathematicians will develop a differential topology to describe these concepts.

I want to repeat a question which I asked more than two decades ago and which to my knowledge no one has tried to answer. We know now, from the work of the Cambridge School and others, that it is possible to adapt (fatigue) neural analyzers selectively tuned to luminance gratings of given SF and orientation. Since any image can be decomposed into the sum of gratings as shown by Fourier, the existence of neural analyzers that fire for approximately trigonometric functions does not appear very surprising to some colleagues. However, since mathematicians have extended the Fourier decomposition of functions into any set of orthonormal functions, such as Bessel functions, Hankel functions, or prolate spheroidal functions, the obvious question arises as to whether the visual system contains this type of analyzers too, besides trigonometric ones that are related to Fourier analysis. For instance, could one fatigue the visual system with Bessel functions? Although D. H. Kelly (1960) started to use one of the Bessel functions

(J_o), nobody—to my knowledge—has tested the ability of the entire orthonormal set of Bessel functions to adapt the visual system. Until this is done, we have no idea whether the visual system is a special- purpose computer with neural analyzers tuned to sine and cosine waves or a general-purpose computer that contains a great variety of orthonormal neural feature extractors!

[Just before I finished writing this, my colleagues at Caltech (Gallant et al. 1993) finally searched and found neural analyzers tuned selectively for polar, hyperbolic, and cartesian gratings in V4 of the macaque visual cortex. This result is also of importance of finding the affine Lie transformations that result in the many perceptual constancies mentioned in this dialogue. In dialogue 10 I will raise some complex unsolved mathematical questions that I find fundamental for perception. These problems attest to my optimism and belief in the power of mathematics and the ingenuity of mathematicians.]

B: You seem to have missed the opportunity to illustrate the importance of mathematics by the many examples of color and motion theories and by applications using non-parametric multidimensional scaling. Furthermore, your referring to an unpublished experiment of yours (figure 4.1), and not mentioning Burt and Sperling 1981 (which is much more sophisticated than your original idea), is most curious.

A: Because I like to demonstrate by concrete examples, the fact that I could not use color plates or video tapes restricted me to stereoscopic demonstrations. I did not want to follow museum ex-

hibits where the ancient Greek statues are displayed in white marble when originally they were painted in vivid colors. Because I regard readers' participation in experiments as very important and cannot demonstrate motion phenomena in a book, I tried to illustrate concepts of perception with depth and texture phenomena. Furthermore, in *FCP* I discussed hyperbolic geometries and multidimensional scaling, and *Dialogues* is not a textbook. For not mentioning the Burt and Sperling study, my only excuse is my occasional lapses of memory. This is the more curious since I like this study, the authors, and the mathematical theory they used (by János Aczél, who was a schoolmate of mine in Budapest). I am also sorry for omitting the many outstanding recent works that are based on sophisticated mathematics.

DIALOGUE 5
LINKING
PSYCHOLOGY WITH
NEUROPHYSIOLOGY:
THE MIND-BODY
PROBLEM WITHOUT
METAPHYSICS

Suppose that there be a machine, the structure of which produces thinking, feeling, and perceiving; imagine this machine enlarged but preserving the same proportions, so you could enter it as if it were a mill. This being supposed, you might visit inside; but what would you observe there? Nothing but parts which push and move each other, and never anything that could explain perception.

Gottfried Wilhelm Leibniz, *Monadology* (1840)

A: I regard as "scientific psychology" only those subfields of psychology that emulate "statistical thermodynamics" in the sense that higher-level phenomena (of level I) can be explained by lower-level ($I - 1$) phenomena. Similarly to the phenomena (concepts) of temperature, pressure, entropy, and enthalpy that arise from interactions between atoms and molecules as they collide with each other and the wall of the container, I want to define psychological phenomena (percepts) of depth and motion perception, textural segmentation (discrimination), focal attention, etc., as excitatory and inhibitory interactions between pools of neurons tuned to specific features (binocular disparity, motion disparity, texture gradients, etc.). This structuralist (reductionist) quest can be pursued only in vision (and even there within limits), and not in speech perception. Obviously, human speech perception cannot currently be explored by neurophysiological methods. [Although non-invasive methods for studying brain activity already exist, the spatial and temporal resolution of PET scans and MRI techniques are still inadequate. However, MRI methods are rapidly progressing.] Furthermore, the clinical literature on speech defects in stroke victims—though intriguing—by its very nature is more anecdotal than scientific. Because only

Homo sapiens possesses speech, my quest for a scientific psychology can only be pursued in vision, since the monkey visual system is practically identical to the human one and is intensively studied by neurophysiologists and neuroanatomists. Because at present mainly the first stages of the central nervous system of the monkey are studied with microelectrodes, we have to restrict our stimuli so that only the first retinal and cortical input stages (also called "bottom-up" processing stages) are stimulated, thus we have to reduce or eliminate the influence of the higher (and enigmatic) cortical stages of semantic memory and symbolic processing (also called "top-down" stages).

Figure 5.1 depicts such a bottom-up/top-down view of the central nervous system. Of course, both the bottom-up and the top-down processes might have subprocesses with feedback loops, but in general the two main information streams flow as depicted. Focal attention is regarded as a separate mechanism that can inspect

Figure 5.1

Bottom-up versus top-down processes in the visual system and focal attention. From Julesz 1991.

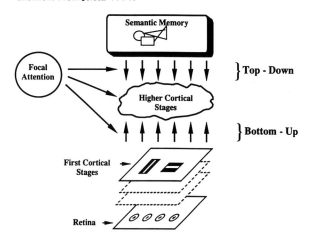

many processing stages at will. Indeed, while ruminating over my last sentence you could easily turn your attention to countless thoughts and then, without effort, return to my next sentence. [One of my reviewers commented that at this particular moment he thought about his lunch and had difficulty returning to my ideas!]

B: Your quest to study the human mind as a thermodynamical system of colliding atoms and molecules is a comical oversimplification. After all, an entire generation of gestalt psychologists demonstrated that a structuralist view of psychology is incorrect, and the whole is more than its parts. You yourself used to demonstrate how in an upside-down image the manipulated eyes and mouth cannot be perceived, while in the normal view, when the gestalt phenomena manifest themselves, the holistic image appears grotesque (figure 4.1). Obviously eyes and mouth are not perceptual atoms and complex global interactions between these entities govern form perception. Furthermore, your figure 5.1 is a bad example of "boxology" (i.e., showing a flow chart and giving the impression that something is explained).

A: Your first point is quite valid, but nevertheless it is counterproductive. I think psychology at present is not yet mature enough to explain holistic phenomena. My point is to restrict research to early vision, for which a structuralist program is possible and productive. I read somewhere that at the time when the Mendeleev (1869) periodic table of chemical elements was invented, some clever chemists already had an inkling of isotopes that seemed to contradict the table—one of the great scientific achievements of the nineteenth century. These guys

were ridiculed, which in hindsight was an injustice; yet, if their premature insight had prevented the triumph of the periodic table, we would regard them now as reactionary wise guys. Similarly, I used to regard gestaltists as very intelligent but "reactionary" psychologists who prematurely drew attention to some enigmatic problems beyond the reach of the scientific tools of their generation. Inasmuch as they helped to destroy the prevalent short-sighted behaviorism of their time, they were progressive; but their ideas were not supported by modern neurophysiology, and their influence was diminished during my active life. Recently, since ideas have become popular that depict emerging global states of neural networks as a flow to attractors of the network dynamics, there has been a revival of gestalt concepts. The only difference between old gestalt notions and ideas of parallel distributed processing is that the emerging holistic parameters are better understood. Even in thermodynamics, the emerging parameters of heat, pressure, and entropy do not exist at the level of colliding molecules, and therefore are holistic entities. In my psychology *à la* thermodynamics, the higher percepts of depth, motion, and texture at level I do not exist at level $I-1$ of neurons with excitatory and inhibitory connections. The only problem with higher cognitive mental parameters is our ignorance of the brain code (that is, the connectivity rules of the participating neural pools). For mental phenomena in early vision, some of these rules can be guessed. Models of early vision abound, such as the probability summations of neural pools, or "winner-take-all" models, or the "pandemonium" model of Selfridge (1958), in which the most sensitive neuron ("the demon that shrieks loudest") determines behavior.

Your other comment on my flow diagram is a matter of taste. I accept people's concern about hierarchical flow charts that ignore the fact that information flow is seldom unidirectional, but many feedback loops exist between all levels. However, in figure 5.1 I wanted to emphasize that there are two main flows of information, one bottom-up and the other top-down; I ignored the fact that in each stream countless feedback loops can exist between cascaded stages. Of course, it could be that many visual centers are not hierarchically connected, but serve some parallel function. I did not dwell on such a possibility, except for focal attention, which I regard as a top-down process and as parallel to the higher semantic stages but whose working I imagine to be very different from the other higher stages.

B: I am still unsatisfied with your reductionist psychology *à la* statistical thermodynamics. You have to be more persuasive to keep psychologists interested in such a "castrated" psychology.

A: Your question is so important to my entire research outlook that I will try to summarize all my arguments here.

First, one can segment objects from their surroundings in most cases without semantics—that is, without any familiarity of the objects. For instance, that the ears of a rabbit do not belong to the background shrubs that they occlude can be guessed by stereopsis, motion perception, and texture discrimination, since the ears of the rabbit must be at similar depth, should move with the same velocity, and have similar texture as the other parts of the rabbit. Because we know—using random-dot textures—that these early processes of stereopsis, motion perception, and texture segmentation are basically bottom-up processes, that early vision could be understood by a thermoynamic-like process is not so far-fetched. Of course, there are some rare cases, when an unusual shadow is cast, in which some top-down process might be evoked. However, what one loses for regarding early vision as mainly bottom-up and permitting focal attention as being the only top-down process is greatly compensated by the reward that there is a possible linking with the current neurophysiological insights already known.

Second, in classical statistical thermodynamics there is only one kind of interaction between the elements (atoms or molecules), and that is collisions. Whether the local law of collisions is governed by Newton's laws or some other rules is immaterial. However, in neural pools the neurons can have two kind of local interactions with their neighbors: excitations and inhibitions. This should increase the emerging states manyfold compared to thermodynamics. Of course, even in physics, as the coupling between the microscopic elements becomes stronger as the elements come closer to each other in liquid and solid states, some more complex interactions form between the elements, including quantum-mechanical rules. These can cause the emergence of very complex macroscopic phenomena, from ferromagnetism to superconductivity.

Third, neurons in the brain also connect with neurons far away. This is not permitted in physics, since every force can only act through near-interaction—even for gravity—and far interaction is regarded by the physicists as just "magic"! This is probably the main reason why brains are much richer in their behavior than physical systems. Furthermore, non-myelinated neurons interact at slower propagation speeds than the much faster myelinated fibers. For nets of non-myelinated neurons that are processing information at some critical speed (at some fraction of the neural propagation speed limit), the myelinated fibers can carry information from remote cortical areas at speeds exceeding their propagation speed limit manyfold. [As if in physics some "tachyons" were to exist that could carry forces at faster speeds than the velocity of light.] Because of these mixed interactions between near and far couplings, studying brains is many times more complex than studying physical systems. However, in early vision we restrict ourselves to systems where we assume that only adjacent systems interact in some nonlinear manner (using inhibition and excitation). Such systems, also called *cooperative systems* in physics, can exhibit multiple stable states, such as solid, liquid, and gaseous phases. Thus, a cooperative system is more complex than the thermodynamics of gases, since for the liquid and solid states the coupling between elements is much stronger. So, my metaphor of studying psycholgy as statistical thermodynamics is an oversimplification. *I regard early vision not as a "mental gas," but rather as a cooperative system that exhibits phenomena similar to or more complex than those that exist in liquids and in condensed matter and beyond.*

Fourth, when in the thermodynamics of gases some higher phenomena emerge (temperature, pressure, entropy, enthalpy, etc.), one should realize that, while these properties have concrete meaning and are observable, there might be some other global properties that did emerge, but they do not appear directly observable to us and therefore we neglect them. Indeed, temperature and pressure are global properties that we can sense directly with our sensory organs, while the propeties of entropy and enthalpy were more abstract global properties that required a century to be discovered and understood. When the early visual (or auditory) system is modeled as a cooperative neural system on level $I - 1$, then the emergent properties on the mental level I are directly sensed as percepts of depth, motion, segregated texture, etc. Some of these mental states might not even reach our conciousness. After all, light intensity changes the aperture of our pupils, or a blink shuts off the gain control of our visual system, without our being aware of it consciously. So, the mental phenomena that control the state of the pupil or the gain control of the blink mechanism are autonomous and hidden from mental awareness. One of my primary interests was the study of texture pairs that would not segregate (thus remaining "ground") while others would pop out (thus becoming "figure"). Again, the processes that decide which areas might reach awereness and which will be skipped over as uninteresting are also unconscious mental processes. Nevertheless, these hidden mental processes determine our sensations, percepts, and behavior and therefore are the very subject matter of psychology, in addition to the sensations, percepts, and behavior. Of course, it is important that in these studies some mental phenomena should enter. For instance, one could measure the diameter of a contracting and dilating pupil as a function of light intensity without asking whether the organism actually can see light as in a decorticated preparation. One could also measure the forces excerted on a hair cell of a Venus flytrap when its flap is triggered. Or one could study the circadian rythm of an animal as a function of day and night duty cycles, or the opening of some glands as a function of some physical stimulus. In these borderline cases we measure neurophysiological phenomena that yield some unconscious behavior. Whether such primitive behavior belongs to mental phenomena is a question of taste. After all, the workings of the kidney or the liver are certainly purely chemico-physiological processes even though their malfunctioning will have a robust effect on our mental state before some fatal poisoning takes place.

One can study only those mental phenomena—either conscious or unconscious—that yield some conscious mental states that can be sensed. [For a similar opinion see Searle 1990.] So, if one studies the dilation of the pupil as a function of light intensity, one had better be interested in how this pupil dilation affects the perceived sensations of brightness. While the unconscious mental phenomena are part of psychology, the conscious percepts enable us to have direct access to those many emerging properties of the brain that otherwise would be hidden as the many global (and, perhaps, important) parameters that were not yet identified by the physicists. Just think of high-temperature superconductivity in some exotic compounds. I regard some subtle mental phenomena we might discover by *direct* scrutiny (e.g. a new aftereffect or illusion) a similar emergent property as the discovery (after decades of searching) of high-temperature superconductivity by the physicists. The only advantage we psychologists have over other scientists is that we have a direct private channel through our perceptual system.

Fifth, as in physics, I do not restrict the study to the linking of level $I - 1$ to level I. Indeed, one can study the temperature or the entropy of two systems as they mix. Perhaps the study of the interaction involving two or more phenomena on the same macroscopic level is more important than the linking of the microscopic with the macroscopic. In my own studies as a psychologist I always tried to formulate relationships involving two or more psychological entities—for instance, how could a finite mix of given textons form a texture that would yield a metameric match to any selected texture? So, the study of psychological entities that interact is the proper study of psychology. However, as in physics, if the underlying microscopic phenomena (neural interactions) can support the mental interactions, then we have gained a deeper understanding.

The leading psychologists can be divided into two main camps. Those who do psychology without any reference to neurophysiology as a geometer study axioms and theorems between geometrical entities without asking what these entities "by themselves" are, those who do psychology as if it were physics by asking what the psychological entities are as they emerge from neurophysiological interactions. Since we do not know the code of the brain, the success of the second camp is limited. Yet, if we learn that global stereopsis of random-dot stereograms can be recorded from the input stages of the visual cortex, that will strengthen the psychological suggestion that stereopsis must be an early process, since semantics is absent in stochastic textures.

Now I return to my original quest to study stereopsis—and psychological phenomena in general—by emulating statistical thermodynamics and, particularly, cooperative models of physics.

In order to explain my concept of emulating cooperative systems in psychology, I will now demonstrate how a few thousand randomly speckled black and white dots in a stereo pair give rise to the global percept of a surface in vivid depth. Of course, it is assumed that these arrays of random dots stimulate a cortical net of neurons of the stereopsis system, which in turn extract any possible global correlation that exists between the left and the right image.

Since you can see the "cyclopean" disks in figure 5.2 after binocular fusion, it becomes apparent that stereopsis is a bottom-up process that must occur before form perception, since the left and right images are devoid of all monocular cues, including shapes and their contours. Furthermore, it can be shown in the laboratory (Julesz 1964; Julesz and Chang 1976), using a masking stimulus 60 msec after the stimulus onset and thus terminating the availability of the stereogram, that one can easily fuse and perceive complex surfaces in vivid depth during such brief presentation provided the maximum binocular disparity is within a limit, called Panum's fusional area. With a dynamic RDS (which nowadays can be easily generated on a personal computer and stored on videotape), each subsequent frame contains uncorrelated random dots (but similar binocularly correlated areas), and these uncorrelated frames erase (mask) the previous frames. Therefore, in addition to the fact that RDSs are devoid of all familiarity cues, quick masking prevents the top-down processes from penetrating down in time and influencing the bottom-up processes of stereopsis.

There are many demonstrations that illustrate that stereopsis of RDSs (to which I often refer as either "global stereopsis" or "cyclopean percep-

tion") must be an early process, based on some correlation-like process prior to object (form) recognition. Here, I only take one example from my monograph (Julesz 1971) that shows that optical illusions must occur after binocular combination of information after several synaptic processing stages in the retina, the lateral geniculate nucleus, and the

Figure 5.2

(a) The classical Ebbinghaus illusion portrayed by luminance gradients. The test figures in the center are actually identical, but because of differences in the inducing figures they appear to differ in size. (b) The same illusion portrayed cyclopeanly by the RDS method. The test and inducing figures are in the same depth plane when binocularly fused, and the perceived illusion is similar to the classical one. (c) Same as b, except that the test and inducing figures are in different depth planes and the perceived illusion is much reduced (if seen at all). From Julesz 1971.

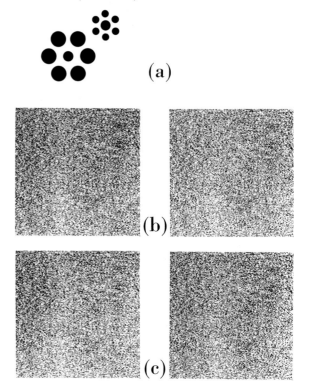

cortex. This technique of process localization without a scalpel, which I called "psychoanatomy," enables us to trace the information flow in the visual system by portraying visual information not with the usual luminance gradients (figure 5.2a), but with binocular disparity gradients (figures 5.2b and 5.2c) using RDSs (Papert 1961; Julesz 1971).

When one inspects the cyclopean version of the classical Ebbinghaus illusion of figure 5.2a by fusing the RDS of figure 5.2b, it is apparent that the illusion (of seeing the identical center disks as having different sizes) is the same as the classical one. Therefore, the many processing stages prior to the "cyclopean retina" (an assumed stage where the binocular correlation is first extracted) do not affect the illusion, and the optical illusion has to arise afterward. With the RDS technique, one gains a new degree of freedom and can portray the center target at a different depth from the inducing figures, as shown in figure 5.2c. When fusing figure 5.2c, one can verify that the illusion is greatly reduced, if not gone. This suggests that if optical illusions are the result of lateral interactions between neural pools tuned to the same binocular disparity, then pools tuned to different disparities do not interact with each other (Julesz 1971).

Thus, the RDS technique, since its inception in 1960, suggested that stereopsis must be an early process and much simpler than form recognition. It was the neurophysiologists who first realized these implications and switched from studying form to explore binocular vision (Hubel and Wiesel 1962, 1970; Barlow, Blakemore, and Pettigrew 1967; Bishop 1969; Blakemore 1969). The perceptual finding of being able to adapt to selected depth planes in an RDS by prolonged viewing and as a result of fatiguing neural pools tuned to the corresponding binocular disparities modify the amount of perceived depth (Blakemore and Julesz 1971) suggested the existence of such neurons. Nevertheless, only in 1984 did Gian Poggio find neurons as early as layer IVB in area V1 (the input stage to the macaque visual cortex) that selectively responded to binocular disparities in dynamic RDSs (Poggio 1984). Since these stereograms are presented at 100 frames/sec, there is no monocular contrast between the correlated areas: therefore, studying these early processing stages can solve the binocular matching problem (figure 2.5) by performing correlation-like processing. While in area V1 only 20% of the probed units are cyclopean, Poggio et al. (1988) found the majority of neurons in areas V2, V3, and V3A to be cyclopean (i.e., to fire for dynamic RDSs).

Poggio's discovery of cyclopean neurons in the input stages of the cortex confirms the psychological predictions that global stereopsis (i.e. stereoscopic depth perception of RDSs) is an early process that neurophysiologically determines the first stages of the "cyclopean retina." That global stereopsis is such an early process has another interesting implication. Since in 3-D there is no camouflage, stereopsis probably evolved in our insectivore primate predecessors (e.g. lemurs), rather late in the evolutionary time scale, in order to counteract the freeze response of insects, which would blend into the foliage at the sign of danger. [That in general there is no camouflage in 3-D is the main insight gained from the RDS. Nevertheless, in a few rare cases insects evolved such that their 3-D shape mimics the 3-D shape of leaves or reliefs of tree branches.] One would expect that such a late development would be relegated to a "mansard room" in some unused area of the cortex. Yet, the emerging mechanisms of stereopsis were important enough to push aside existing machinery and grab the input stages of the visual cortex!

Perhaps the most important aspect of these developments is the linking of a rather complex mental event (global stereopsis) to a neurophysiological event (the firing of neural pools tuned to specific binocular disparities). As I mentioned previously, such a linking was attempted between sensory psychology of color vision and neurophysiology years earlier, but this is the first time in the more complex field of perceptual psychology that such a linking between mind and brain was started.

When it comes to linking hypotheses between mind and brain, different schools of psychobiology have rather different criteria. I found a relevant essay by Davida Teller (1980) most entertaining. Recently, I came across a rather novel linking criterion. Saltzman et al. (1990) applied cortical microstimulation (in addition to visual stimulation by RDS) to an extrastriate area (MT or V5) of the monkey that plays a prominent role in extracting motion information. They used RDCs with decreasing correlation between successive frames and measured the spike histograms of neurons for preferred orientation and direction of motion. The electrical microstimulation biased the animals' perceptual judgments of motion direction. Furthermore, there was large correlation between the neuronal thresholds of certain neurons tuned to the direction of motion and the monkey's behavioral thresholds. This finding implies that physiological events at the neuronal level can be causally linked to a specific aspect of perceptual performance. While the authors used motion in their study, they pointed out that they could have also applied

the same experimental paradigm to color or depth perception.

B: In *FCP* you spent considerable time on the Hermann-Hering grid illusion and its linking to Kuffler units by Günther Baumgartner (1960). You even used this example to point out that these analogies are not very convincing, since the strongest dimming at the intersections of the grid occurs at some strange angle, and not at the orthogonal one. Do you want to comment on the hand-waving nature of linking hypotheses?

A: There are several examples of linking Kuffler units to perceptual phenomena; Baumgartner's idea was among the first. Of course, the idea of linking perceptual aftereffects (particularly the waterfall illusion) to neural adaptation goes back over a century; Wohlgemuth (1911) gives a detailed account of the nineteenth century's explanations of motion aftereffects, including his own. However, before the development of modern cortical neurophysiology all these ideas were just speculations. Davida Teller (1980) used as an example the sensitization effect discovered by Gerald Westheimer for linking this perceptual effect to Kuffler units. The problem was that sensitization only occurs about 0.45 deg arc disk diameter. Since Kuffler units come in all sizes, one has to assume either that the most sensitive Kuffler unit has this diameter or that the average size of pooled neurons with antagonistic receptive fields of the Kuffler kind has an effective diameter of 0.45 deg arc.

Since Baumgartner's idea of linking the Hermann-Hering grid has an immediate perceptual appeal, I want to elaborate on it by proposing a half-baked idea of my own. We know from Eric

Schwartz (1984) that the mapping of the retina to the cortex can be approximated by a conformal mapping, given by the transformation $w = \log(a + z)$. This transform converts polar coordinates to quasi-Cartesian ones (figure 5.3). Neurophysiological studies with deoxyglucose analysis actually confirmed such a mapping in the primate striate cortex (Tootell et al. 1982). Similar transformations exist between higher cortical areas, for example between V1 and V2. Because Ronchi and Bottai (1964) reported that the largest inhibition is perceived when the grid intersects at a 32° angle, I propose that one should look at that stage where the cortical mapping distorts this slanted grid such that it intersects at a perpendicular angle, provided we assume that at this higher cortical stage the receptive fields are such that an orthogonal stimulation would result in maximal inhibition. Here the tacit assumptions that are necessary for linking become more explicit. First, we have to assume that there must be a stage that is adequately isomorphic to the percept to regard it as the place where linking can be attempted and not at an earlier or even higher stage. [This was the hidden assumption of Saltzman et al. (1990), who placed electrodes in the MT and looked for neurons that responded to correlated motion, and who did not search for motion perception in earlier or later cortical stages.] Second, we have to assume that the neurons at higher cortical stages have their own receptive field profiles that are somewhat similar in their behavior to the simple, complex, and hypercomplex neural analyzers found in V1 and V2—a rather bold assumption. Finally, the fact that electrical microstimulation alters the working of these neurons but the same stimulation by itself does not produce "phosphenes of directional motion" is not at all surprising, since this is the essence of Johannes Müller's doctrine of specific nerve energies. These are not the energies in electricity or in electrochemical phenomena. In fact, the *sensation* of motion is *modulated* by these physical energies, but by themselves they are not the stuff that makes up the sensations.

Now I will return to my own work as it relates to the linking hypotheses.

One might ponder whether a computer-generated RDS with rich disparity cues might not be a special case, and top-down processes could still interfere with global stereopsis in natural scenes when higher cognitive cues are present. An example might be depth from shading, noted by astronomers when viewing the craters of the Moon. When viewed upside-down, the concave craters appear to be convex mounds. Such a depth reversal is demonstrated by viewing each of the stereo half-pairs monocularly (figure 5.4), depending on whether the illumination comes from above or below. This "shape from shading" or "monocular depth from shading" might be construed as a top-down phenomenon interfering with the bottom-up processes of stereopsis. Ramachandran (1988) exploited this phenomenon in his study of apparent motion perception, and suggested that this "shape from shading" process operates prior to motion perception. The motion perception studied by Ramachandran is of the "long-range" kind that often disambiguates false matches by higher-order top-down processes, yet it is interesting to note that the bottom-up process of "short-range" motion perception (which occurs for random-dot cinematograms, and particularly for global stereopsis) are also influenced by shape from shading. After all, this

Figure 5.3

A conformal cortical mapping *à la* Schwartz, and its neurophysiological equivalent using dioxyglucose methods. Reproduced, with permission, from Tootell et al. 1982.

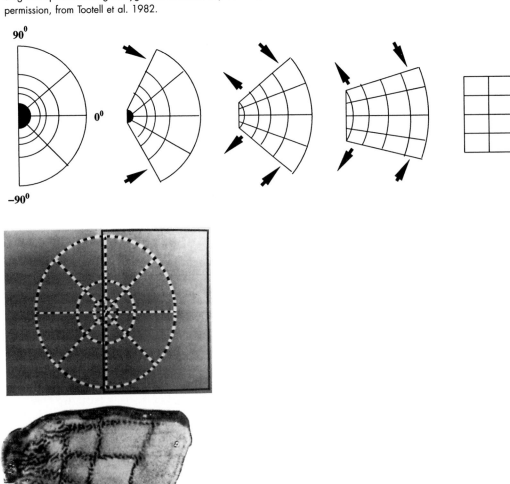

phenomenon must be of a high-level kind, based on the fact that Earth has only one sun that shines from above. If global stereopsis were to utilize such a complex top-down process, based on some learned or genetically inherited information, we would have a counterexample of global stereopsis based on early visual processing alone. In order to test this "counterexample," Jih Jie Chang and I constructed a randomly speckled egg-crate pair portraying the convex (or concave) depth-from-shading phenomenon when viewed monocularly (Chang and Julesz 1990). However, 30% of the egg-crate pair is speckled with an RDS having a crossed disparity (if one views the stereogram with crossed eyes). Whether one views these figures right-side-up or upside-down, it becomes apparent that the convex shape determined by stereopsis will dominate depth from shading. Variations of this experiment, including *ambiguous RDSs* (with two cyclopean shapes at different depth, only one of which can be perceived at a given instant), demonstrate that the monocular cue of depth from shading is rather weak (since observers perceive depth according to their natural bias) and therefore does not influence global stereopsis (Chang and Julesz 1990). In summary, it is most likely that global stereopsis is mediated by early visual processes without top-down influences. It is, in the usage of Fodor and Pylyshyn (1988), a "cognitively impenetrable module."

My original use of "global" stereopsis and motion perception in random-dot stereograms and cimematograms referred to the solving of the false-target problem *globally* (by cross-correlation), since the thousands of individual random dots could be paired in billions of incorrect ways. With increased disparities between the left and right half-pairs in an RDS, or between successive monocular arrays in an RDC, the number of false matches increases. So, for global stereopsis and motion perception, the finding of matches is relatively easy within a short range and rapidly becomes difficult at long range. However, for patterns that can be *locally* identified (by their color, shape, etc., as in a neon sign where a letter jumps back and forth spanning a large distance), the problem of correct matching is virtually independent of disparity, and stereoscopic depth or apparent motion can be obtained at a long range. *Hence, local stereopsis and motion perception are long-range processes, whereas global stereopsis and motion perception are short-range processes.* My use of local versus global was originally given in Julesz 1978 and in Chang and Julesz 1983; on the use of short-range versus long-range motion, see Braddick 1974, 1980 and Snowden and Braddick 1990. For a critical paper evaluating these dichotomies, see Cavanagh and Mather 1989.

Figure 5.4

A monocularly convex (concave) sphere due to depth (shape) shading, in which a random-dot stereogram is mixed in. When binocularly fused, depth from stereopsis dominates perceived depth. When viewed monocularly, depth from shading yields a convex sphere, but appears concave when the page is turned upside-down. Because the RDS has crossed binocular disparity, the binocularly fused image appears strongly convex. From Chang and Julesz 1990.

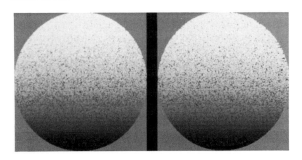

Now I turn to the problem of artificial intelligence models. One could assume that instead of neurophysiology, AI modeling could as well take the role of a level-$(I-1)$ description. While this is a theoretical possibility, it turns out that AI models are too robust—diametrically opposite models can explain equally well perceptual phenomena—and therefore one has to perform psychophysical and neurophysiological control experiments to check the biological plausibility of these models.

Besides the binocular matching problem (or false-target elimination problem), probably first posed by Julesz and Spivack (1967), there are three basic psychological findings of global stereopsis that model builders have to take into account. First, global stereopsis of RDS is *cooperative*, exhibiting multiple stable states, disorder-order transitions, and hysteresis (Julesz 1971, 1978, 1986a, 1990a.] Here I will only mention an experiment with ambiguous RDS where a few-percent bias of unambiguous dots with given binocular disparities can perceptually pull the perceived depth (Julesz 1964, 1978; Julesz and Chang 1976)—a typical cooperative effect. Second, global stereopsis utilizes spatial-frequency-filtered channels (Julesz and Miller 1975). The spatial-frequency spectrum of a left and right stereo half-image pair must overlap to some extent to obtain fusion. And third, binocular disparity gradients are related to fusion, which leads to the postulate that there are "forbidden zones" where fusion cannot occur because the gradient exceeds a critical value. (See Burt and Julesz 1980, where we demonstrated how nearby objects "warp" the disparity space, creating such forbidden zones.)

[In the next few paragraphs, **B** refers to Dr. Bart Anderson, a co-worker whom I invited to join forces with me after I read an influential paper (Anderson 1992) in which he raised some fundamental questions about my notions of cooperativity and drew attention to a paradox about cooperativity. He was kind enough to read a draft of the manuscript and was willing to take the role of **B**. I quote him verbatim here.]

B: Your discussion of your contributions to psychology thus far has focused on the introduction of the RDS as a method for studying stereopsis and the texton theory of texture perception. But this essentially ignores the fact that in addition to the RDS becoming a widely used tool for studying stereopsis, you became the foremost advocate of "cooperative" processing in vision. This idea seemed to be invoked to explain how binocular correspondence was achieved in a perfectly camouflaged stimulus in lieu of all possible "false matches." However, you have suggested that a number of properties may be considered "signatures" of cooperative processing, namely, disorder-order transitions, hysteresis, and multiple stable states. I take this as an interesting possibility, but the connection between these properties and "cooperativity" has never been fully explained. Part of the difficulty comes from understanding what is meant by a cooperative phenomenon. In physics, the term "cooperative" was used extensively by Prigogine, primarily in reference to phenomena that exhibit transformations from a state of atomistic disorder to a state of macroscopic structure (order). Thus disorder-order transitions do seem to be part of the definition of cooperativity in physical systems, at least in the sense used by Prigogine. The core of the insight driving the use of this term seems to be a difference in how the constituents that make up the system are believed to interact. In a noncooperative system, the interactions of the "elements" are not coupled in a way that leads to the formation of new patterns, but more typically, to a more unstructured form (because of entropy). In contrast, in cooperative systems, the elements are strongly coupled, such that their trajectories are no longer independent. Haken termed this effect "slaving," drawing an explicit link to the formation of new "coalitions" between the elements. This also seems to be the essence of how you use the term cooperative.

One characteristic of cooperative systems is that they are energetically open to the flow of energy and/or mass. This is certainly true of the visual system (or any biological system for that matter), and therefore your suggestion that stereopsis is a cooperative process has a large degree of physical appeal. However, it is less clear why a property such as hysteresis should be thought of as a "signature" of a cooperative process. If it could be shown that hysteresis can also occur in the absence of cooperative interactions, then it should not be considered to be, in and of itself, a "signature" of cooperativity, although a specific *form* of hysteresis may be due to cooperative interactions.

For clarity, let me go into this question in detail. In general, hysteresis simply refers to a lag between cause and effect. Perhaps the best-known instance of hysteresis is that found in magnetization curves of ferromagnetic substances. If an unmagnetized ferromagnetic substance is placed in an external magnetic field, the microscopic dipoles will slowly become aligned with the field. Now in one sense, this is a disorder-order transition, since the ferromagnet initially has no macroscopic magnetic field, but upon being placed in the external field, the individual dipoles eventually assume a single orientation, namely, that of the external field. A curve may be drawn that specifies the rate at which the ferromagnetic material becomes aligned with the external field, known as the magnetization curve. However, if the external field is reversed, the magnetization of the ferromagnet changes orientation, but it does not follow the same magnetization curve: the magnetization of the ferromagnetic substance involves some *irreversible* physical processes. The physical theory of the source of this irreversibility (hysteresis) is related to sources of entropy that lead to a degradation of energy. As the individual dipoles in the ferromagnet change orientation, they become "hung up" on some impurities in the material. When sufficient energy builds up, the dipoles snap over the impurities, causing a dissipation of energy in the form of heat and shock waves. This is a physical example where hysteresis is decoupled from cooperativity, even though the material exhibits a disorder-order transition.

Now on to a psychological example. With Chris Tyler, you conducted a number of experiments demonstrating that it was more difficult to effect a transition from disorder to order, than conversely. Now the insight motivating your connection of hysteresis to cooperativity is that there were some interactions that "locked" the state of fusion between the two eyes. Thus, the theoretical role ascribed to cooperativity is that it serves as a persistence mechanism. In the case of binocular fusion, it seems to play the role of maintaining the organization of the fused percept once fusion was obtained. However, this leads to a paradox if you consider the neurontropy (why not neurentropy??) results you obtained with Tyler: It would predict that the correlated RDS should resist being broken; however, you found that it was remarkably easy to detect transitions from order to disorder. More recent cooperative models [including your own with Chang (Julesz and Chang 1976)] have emphasized the role of cooperativity (here, excitation) between similarly tuned disparity mechanisms as a means of achieving and maintaining binocular correspondence. Yet when tested in a similar paradigm as that with Tyler, Anderson (1992) found results similar to that found in the neurontropy studies. He viewed this as a paradox: why did the results of the fusion experiments seem to indicate a cooperative (persistence) mechanism in stereopsis, whereas the Julesz-Tyler and Anderson studies revealed "anti- persistence" of ordered states (i.e., entropy)?

One possible reconciliation of these results was suggested by Anderson (1992), which relied on the experiments by Erkelens (1988) on binocular fusion. Erkelens also found hysteresis, but he measured one additional threshold: the static limit of fusion (i.e., what you keep calling "Panum's fusional limit"). For his patterns, he found this to actually be larger than either of the dynamic thresholds. He suggested that the difference between initial and re-fusion thresholds did not indicate a dynamic expansion of the fusional limit, but rather, represented an interference effect of starting with a stereogram in the state of rivalry (the static limit was found to be much closer to the limit for the increasing disparity stimulus than for the stimulus in which the disparity is slowly reduced). The other studies failed to measure this static limit, which seems to be crucial to interpreting the fusional hysteresis data. Thus, it can be argued that all of the hysteresis effects found to date actually represent entropy-like processes, not cooperative processes. This suggests that we have yet to uncover the contribution of cooperative interactions in stereopsis. This does not mean that such processes may not exist, but that identifying the role of such processes may be "tricky business."

A: You raised several important questions. A few of them I try to clarify. You also raised a paradox that is fundamental in physics as well.

First, the definition of cooperativity predates Prigogine and comes from the theory of ligands, for which "when neighboring molecules interact in a nonlinear fashion then the system is called cooperative." I adopted this definition of cooperativity for brain processes. If the interaction of adjacent processing units (neurons, or aggregates of neurons in cortical columns) is nonlinear (i.e., excitation and inhibition), then I call this neural system cooperative. Of course, in the brain these neurons could interact at greater distance than neighbors, but in physics usually interactions occur mainly between adjacent particles. In order to find analogies between brains and physical systems, I restricted myself to the simplest nonlinear interactions that are similar to structures in physics. Now, in physics we observe that these cooperative phenomena of states of matter and their electromagnetic properties show sudden phase transitions, such as jumps from the solid to the liquid and gaseous states and from magnetic to nonmagnetic properties. Often these jumps exhibit some hysteretic phenomena—for instance, when a supercooled liquid suddenly explodes into a solid state. Whether hysteresis takes place between these phase transitions depends on the coupling constants between the particles and on their number and density. So hysteresis, when experienced, suggests that the underlying system is at least cooperative (or is coupled even more tightly). After all, linear systems do not exhibit hysteresis.

The question of how cooperativity is linked to entropy goes beyond my grasp of physics. I am glad you mentioned the name of Hermann Haken, who invited me twice to contribute to his influential workshops on "synergetics"—a name he used to emphasize the similarities between lasers and biological systems (Julesz 1973, 1990b). It seems that he found my use of cooperativity in stereopsis to his liking, particularly some experiments that we performed. We established experimentally that stereopsis exhibits disorder-order transitions, multiple stable states, and hysteresis (which I regard as the sign of a cooperative system, but you could call it a "nonlinearly coupled" system). Furthermore, we also showed hysteretic differences between the ease of perceiving certain transitions in stereopsis. With Christopher Tyler we defined binocular fusion as an "ordered" state and loss of fusion as a "disordered" state, and observed that it was 10 times easier to detect a change from fusion to loss of fusion than vice versa. This preference for falling into a disordered state over establishing order we named "neural entropy" (Julesz and Tyler 1976; Tyler and Julesz 1976). That we finally named it *neurontropy* (instead of *neurentropy*) was intentional. Since the functions describing the observed transition times were not logarithmic, but instead some odd power function, we wished to avoid any deeper analogy to the concept of physical entropy. [Entropy in thermodynamics is a global parameter that is logarithmically related to the underlying number of micro-states of the system. This number

is determined by combinatorics that uses factorials, which in turn can be approximated (by Sterling's formula) with the logarithm as the numbers get large.]

The paradox you raise in your article about persistence versus nonpersistence in stereopsis goes much deeper than binocular vision. In my youth, physics was under the influence of the Second Law of Thermodynamics, which states that in a closed system the entropy can only increase. That is, a complex system must degrade into an increasingly simpler one (yielding eventually the "heat death" of the universe). Nowadays, physics is preoccupied by the inverse problem: How can complexity increase—and thus entropy decrease—in an *open* system? Indeed, how can ever-more-complex living organisms emerge from the much simpler inorganic matter? Of course, there is no paradox. The subsystem that becomes increasingly complex gains its complexity by reducing the complexity of its surrounding system. Similarly, some perceptual phenomena in stereopsis gain their complexity (increasing their fusional states) at the expense of some lower-level binocular phenomena whose complexity becomes reduced.

In essence, then, there are several entropy-like phenomena in psychobiology that are related to each other, but in ways not yet clear. For instance, it was Leo Szilárd (a scientific hero of my youth) who first pointed out that "negative entropy" was identical to "information." Also, Michael Leyton, in his monograph *Symmetry, Causality, Mind* (1992), defines human memory as an algorithm that tries to reconstruct from a present stimulus an earlier state that had more symmetries and thus higher entropy. Obviously this algorithm evolved in eons by handling a visual environment governed by causality and entropy; it does not reflect the internal organization of the memory system. [Here I stress the difference between "complex" and "complex adaptive" systems. A complex system's inherent structure often can manifest its own structure, whereas a complex *adaptive* system's behavior can emulate almost any behavior (thus it can "lie" about its own internal states). Indeed, general-purpose computers can be programmed to compute functions regardless whether they exist in nature or are forbidden by physical laws.] So, information, complexity, entropy, neurontropy, memory, the emergence of self-adaptability, are concepts that are related to each other in complex ways that require a very detailed understanding of the systems in which they manifest themselves.

Now I turn to cooperative and noncooperative models of stereopsis.

The brief (60 msec) processing time for global stereopsis and its cooperative behavior suggest a *parallel* mechanism. Furthermore, if one of the states of an ambiguous RDS is biased by 4% (in favor of the other state), then a serial search mechanism would often stop at an almost perfect 96% binocular correlation. In fact, the stereopsis mechanism always chooses the perceptual state that yields 100% correlation, suggesting not only that the correlation mechanism is parallel but also that the search mechanism for the best binocular match is parallel too (Julesz and Chang 1976). That perceptual phenomena are based on parallel processing is not a great surprise. In addition to 30 years' neurophysiological evidence, one can easily perform the following thought experiment: It takes about 500 msec or less to perform routine perceptual tasks (e.g., recognize a face in a complex scene or identify a cartoon), and a synaptic event (computation)

requires 2–4 msec. Therefore, the brain might utilize at most 100 stages of computational layers (instructions, or codes)— in striking contrast to the thousands of codes necessary for AI algorithms running on the ubiquitous serial computers, which nevertheless still perform perceptual tasks rather poorly.

My AUTOMAP-1 model was the first computer algorithm that could explain in successive iterations some of the cooperative phenomena of global stereopsis (Julesz 1964). In order to give a better insight into the workings of a model, I intentionally introduced a "spring-coupled-magnetic-dipole model" (Julesz 1971, 1978) that explained the pulling effect and plasticity (i.e., the left image of an RDS can be zoomed by 10% up or down in size with respect to the right without loss of fusion). [On the history of stereopsis models, see Julesz 1990b.] Simultaneously with the development of my cooperative spring-coupled-dipole model, Sperling (1970) proposed an "energy well model" that had a heuristic appeal too. Also, Dev (1974) and Nelson (1975) presented cooperative models based on spreading inhibition between disparity neurons tuned to different disparities, and facilitation between neurons tuned to the same disparity. In addition, Marr and Poggio (1976) published a cooperative model which resembles those of Dev and Nelson, in which inhibition occurs between disparity detectors tuned to different disparities, but these detectors fall on the same lines of sight. [This requirement seems important, since it has a heuristic appeal, but *de facto* it is irrelevant, so the model is very similar to the above-mentioned ones.] Perhaps the contribution of the Marr-Poggio (1976) model is its easy implementation as a computer algorithm, even on PCs. Tomaso

Poggio (1989) implemented a very fast stereo algorithm on the Connection Machine, and Mahowald and Delbrück (1989) designed a 1-D version of the Marr-Poggio (1976) model on a chip that works very fast and solves the false-target problem in milliseconds. Cooperativity underlies even the computation of stereoscopic acuity (which is an order of magnitude finer than visual acuity), as suggested by Westheimer (1979).

While most models of stereopsis are cooperative, David Marr and Tomaso Poggio (1979) developed a second, noncooperative model of stereopsis. Their model is based on the use of SF channels found by Julesz and Miller (1975). According to this model, coarse SF channels in the two retinal projections-which tolerate large disparity searches without false matches—are aligned first by vergence (convergence or divergence) movements of the eyes. This is followed by finer and finer matches of high-SF channels by consecutive vergence movements—under the assumption that increasingly finer image detail has decreasing amount of disparity. Indeed, it seems to me a reasonable assumption that only extended objects protrude in depth (except for thin wires, which we often trip over) and fine surface textures in relief have shallow depth.

Unfortunately, this ingenious scheme is not used by the human visual system. Among others, Mayhew and Frisby (1979) and Mowforth et al. (1981) have shown that a high-SF RDS, with low and medium SFs filtered out, can still elicit large vergence movements and yield fusion at large disparities during a brief flash (when vergence movements are prevented). Regardless of whether the study by Mowforth et al. really disproves the basic assumption of Marr and Poggio (1979) that the noncooperative stereo algorithm based on vergence eye movements is not used by the visual system, this does not mean that a modified version could not be used. One could imagine a model based on neurological couplings such that low-SF channels would monotonically reduce the disparity deviations of the high-SF channels with increasing SF. Nevertheless, such a model could exist despite the fact that it is based on neuronal shifter hierarchy and appears to be much more complicated than a model based on a connected neural net exhibiting cooperative phenomena. For instance, Anderson and Van Essen (1987) proposed models for such neural shifter networks in early stages of the visual cortex, but until now no such shifter nets were found. The fact that we see many objects at different velocities as equally sharp (without using a "shutter" as in a movie camera)—even though we cannot follow simultaneously all these moving objects by eye movement—argues also for a cortical shifter mechanism that can compensate for the displacements of these drifting objects within limits.

B: Although you discussed your use of "cooperativity" as you answered the questions raised by Bart Anderson, I would like to hear your definition again. You discussed some of the behavior a cooperative system might exhibit, such as multiple stable states, disorder-order transitions, and hysteresis. However, you never defined strictly what a cooperative organization is! As a matter of fact, it is difficult to find any hint of cooperativity in the literature of psychobiology.

A: I usually define "cooperativity" at the beginning of my university lectures, and I am surprised that it is not known by my colleagues. I encountered the term in chemistry, in conjunction with ligands. Here the elements (e.g. molecules) can interact only through their nearest neighbors, and the interaction has to be nonlinear. So, mere summation or subtraction of the output of the elements does not result in a cooperative interaction. My earlier discussions on cooperative and noncooperative models of stereopsis should have given you a feel for these concepts.

Of the many AI models of stereopsis, I want to mention the recent one of Sidney Lehky and Terry Sejnowski (1990), mainly because they discuss the interesting debate in brain research between local and distributed representations. Retinal position is locally represented by a very large number of neurons that fire in response to stimulation of specific very narrow SF channels (positions). On the other hand, the many shades of color sensations are not conveyed by thousands of individually tuned neurons, but by the population of some broadly tuned channels of the three principal colors. Global stereopsis contains systems of narrowly and broadly tuned binocular disparity channels (G. Poggio 1984). It happens that Lehky and Sejnowski postulated a model based on the distributed representation of the broad disparity channels. Here again one can see the robustness of AI models, since one could easily imagine that a dual model, based on local representation, might have worked equally well.

B: You have spent considerable time on details. I thought you would focus on the basic mind-body problem, the holy grail of philosophers. Instead, you are talking about global stereopsis and some neurophysiological findings that seem to support it. What is so novel about this? After all, we have known the theory of trichromacy for centuries, and

since the advent of micro-photometry we know that there are indeed three kinds of cones, containing pigments with absorption spectra tuned to short, middle, and long wavelengths. Cones are certainly part of our body, and of our brain. So, we know that somehow cones in the brain and percepts of color of the mind are correlated without making much ado about it. How this miracle comes about is not explained by more and more subtle examples of mind and brain correlation. You only extended this correlation from color to some more complex mental phenomena, such as stereopsis.

A: You are, of course, partly right. In the first paragraph of the introduction to this monograph it is stated that psychobiology is unable to answer its basic questions. However, in my youth "What is life?" was regarded a metaphysical question, and philosophers like Bergson believed in a mysterious *élan vital*. The mystery of "life" evaporated as we learned how proteins and nucleotides fold and unfold in a molecular machine according to the laws of chemistry and physics. This molecular dynamics is then life, and the only secret is how this molecular machinery was put into the proper configuration at the moment of conception. So, the problem of the very nature of life has at least been laid out, and replaced by the problem of how life originated from matter—a tough question, but somehow less enigmatic than the first one. Indeed, one could envision some primitive organism coming into being from some primordial soup in the lucky presence of some catalyst. Similarly, one could envision some special cells, called sensory analyzers, evolving in microscopic organisms for some chemical event and light. With more specialization, neural networks evolved, forming ganglia and brains. A functioning neural net is a machine exhibiting chemical and electrical phenomena, sort of a specialized part of a living organism. As long as these neural phenomena, both local and global, are not sensed, we can easily envision, say, a fly homing on a target emitting light at 540 nanometers. Photons of this light source hit the ommatidia of the fly, and its receptors convert the photon energy into an electric impulse train, which in turn starts complex neural events that regulate flight and leg muscles. So far, the fly is regarded a miniature seeing and flying automaton exhibiting the demystified characteristics of life.

The difficulty starts if we assume that flies can do more than home in on a red target. Do flies perceive the color "red"? My dog yelps when I inadvertently step on her tail; does she do it through some automatic neural process, like a reflex, or does she actually sense "pain" as we humans do? While I do not doubt that dogs probably feel the same pain or sense the same light and sound as we do, I regard this as interesting but irrelevant. What matters is that I can perceive all the known sensations and mental phenomena and assume with certainty that my fellow humans perceive it similarly. There is, then, a rich world of mental phenomena in humans (and almost certainly in monkeys) that are given on their own right and are correlated to neural events that we can measure (in monkeys, and during brain surgery in humans) with microelectrodes, allowing for direct observation of responses of functioning neurons to optical events, using non-invasive methods, such as evoked potentials, PET and MRI scans, and so on.

Most of this neural activity does not reach our consciousness; it belongs to mere reflex activity, occurs under sensory threshold, or takes place in early stages that cannot be scrutinized by focal attention. For instance, that we do not see the world as dark during a blink is a mental phenomenon that borders on a reflex. We are not aware perceptually of how the dimming of vision takes place during a blink, but this does not mean that with ingenious methods this neural gain control mechanism cannot be studied by the psychologists. Indeed, if we could somehow illuminate the eye internally, we would observe that during a blink changes in illumination cannot be detected. It turns out that the upper palate is optically semi-transparent. Volkman et al. (1962) got the creative idea to illuminate the eye sockets through the mouth cavity. Nowadays, from light-emitting diodes to fiber-optics bundles, there are many bright sources that remain adequately cold to be tolerated in the mouth. Volkman et al. measured the muscular current by a myograph (an electronic amplifier attached to the vicinity of the eyelid) and briefly dimmed the internal light source either during or between the blinks. Observers had to press a key when they perceived the dimming. It turned out that the intensity change had to be 10 times more during blinking than between blinks, so the hypothesis that blinking shuts off vision has been proven. The finding is not surprising, yet the way of obtaining it was very elegant and probably could not be done a century ago. I quote this example, among dozens of others, to illustrate that the science of early vision can *indirectly* study the workings of neural mechanisms through finding ways to make conscious some mental phenomena that accompany these neural events!

Another favorite example of mine is trichromacy. It is impossible to tell, say, a single yellow color from a metameric red-green combination. Yet, the impossibility of scrutinizing individual cones, or even some neural circuits in V4 or some other cortical area where color sensations emerge, clearly illustrates the limits and the power of psychology. Psychology cannot study directly the output of a single cone, but it can study the workings of the cone indirectly through cascaded higher stages that have access to our consciousness. An ingenious example of this method was invented by John Krauskopf, who used quantum-mechanical phenomena to illuminate single cones and observe elicited mental phenomena. Since he knew that the poor optics of the eye make it impossible to illuminate only a single cone, he used very low illumination such that only a few quanta would hit one or a few cones. He also knew from the classical experiments of Hecht, Schlaer, and Pirenne (1942) that a few quanta are adequate to trigger the firing of a cone. So, he presented a very dim white light, and watched how often the observer would name the perceived color as red, green, yellow, orange, and so on. If the observer saw pure red, or green, he argued that a *single* cone absorbed the light quanta, while for yellow or orange a *combination* of one red and one green cone, or two red and one green cones, etc., was stimulated according to some Bernoulli distribution (Krauskopf and Srebro 1965). This example shows, again, that one can indirectly study the workings of the brain by making conscious some mental phenomena.

The essence of my comments is that *we take for granted that some neural activity must be conscious, without having to know the very nature of what consciousness is*. If we were to deny the existence of consciousness in a brain , then the brain would be similar to a kidney or a liver—a rather absurd assertion (Searle 1990). [For comments on Searle's treatise, see Julesz 1993) and the open peer reviews in *Behavioral Brain Research* (1990, 1993).]

B: If I understand you, it is your contention that psychology can operate by using conscious mental phenomena, without having to know the very essence of consciousness. Shall I assume that you are not inconvenienced by this fundamental ignorance in your daily work?

A: I can assure you that neither I nor any practicing psychologist I know is hampered by the meta-scientific state of the mind-body problem, or by its final manifestation, the enigmatic nature of consciousness. It is usually philosophers and some Nobel laureates above 60 who are concerned with this problem. Nevertheless, I have to confess that, in my early youth, when I decided to become a psychologist, this problem affected the choice of my research projects. Indeed, it was annoying that I found no way to assert that green to me was not another person's red! On the other hand, if I asked an observer to trace with her fingers the surface of a spiral portrayed by an RDS, she would trace it the same way as I saw it, and the only "solipsistic" difference between me and her could be that she saw the spiral as concave, while it appeared convex to me. That much noncommunicable uncertainty I could easily tolerate, and so I decided to work on stereopsis, motion, texture, and similar topics, where I am quite sure that if one sees something moving from left to right and shows this direction with her finger, or points correctly to a single pixel in a dense array of a stereogram where I produced binocular rivalry, then there is no ambiguity in the communication between experimenter and observer. I digressed into this personal story because I am convinced that my esteemed colleagues who work in color vision—the Queen of Psychophysics—carry on their work without ever thinking of the "my red/your green" problem.

To sum up what I have said: I believe that neurophysiological phenomena are unconscious, or are conscious, and to the extent they are brought into consciousness they can be studied by the methods of psychophysics. If they cannot be made conscious, as pupillary dilations or movements of head-eye coordination cannot, these neural phenomena that govern muscles belong to the provinces of neuroanatomy and neurophysiology, in the same way that the opening of glands that squirt hormones and neuropeptides into our bloodstream belong to neuro-endocrinology. However, in many cases of such phenomena one can study the accompanying mental events thus bringing them into the field of psychology.

B: Here is a rare opportunity to speculate about the nature of consciousness without being taken too seriously, and you are still reluctant to do so!

A: If you provoke me, I can speculate on a few aspects of consciousness, since, indeed, I am well over 60 and follow the lead of some of my heroes in psychobiology—to name a few, Penfield, Eccles, Sperry, and Crick. First, let me state that I consider psychology without consciousness as boring as mathematics without infinity! As you know, the mathematicians called intuitionists tried to extirpate infinity in order to avoid the many newly discovered paradoxes that threatened the foundations of mathematics. Although in this "finite mathematics" all applied mathematical tools still

functioned well, and the paradoxes were removed, no self-respecting mathematician was interested in such a castrated discipline. I hope that the discovery of the brain code will include an explanation of how consciousness emerges, and I only regret that I may not live to witness this greatest moment in the history of mankind. I have no doubt that consciousness is closely related to memory, another mysterious neurophysiological and psychological phenomenon. I am quite sure that Crick and Koch (1990, 1991) are right when they claim that a person without long-term memory, but with short-term memory intact, still appears as a conscious human being. This connection between short-term memory and consciousness is not clear, but there must be some minimal storage to be able to have some plan for action, or logical reasoning, not necessarily related to language. I always felt that the speechless hemisphere of *Homo sapiens* might be still conscious, but cannot share this experience with others through speech. By the way, after my car accident, while under sedation, I had difficulty speaking German, though I could speak Hungarian and English fluently. This is the more curious since I learned Hungarian and German as an infant, while English later at ten. It seemed to me that suddenly the noun and verb in German drifted too far away and my shrunken working memory could not hold them both. So, if one were to play the Turing imitation game to fool a judge whether he is conscious with a very brief memory span, then Germans might have more difficulty than others.

B: I must warn your readers of your anecdotes. As we were waiting to die, it was my least priority to try to speak German to myself. However, I have to admit that I am mainly residing in your speechless hemisphere that has very limited linguistic abilities, and therefore your linguistic experiments remained hidden from me. However, consciousness interests me and if you have something to say, then continue.

For me consciousness is not as mysterious as the mental states of sensations (qualia). I would like to see some split-brain experiments where the left hemisphere is asked to do psychophysical tasks, such as metameric color matches, and compare these matches with the right (speechless) hemisphere. Will these matches be identical? Could somehow the speechless hemisphere report sensations? Does a person with his dominant hemisphere under deep anesthesia still feel pain? Answers to some of these questions are probably known, and I regard the split-brain paradigm a royal road to the mind-body problem, but I could be wrong, and it could be that some of these complex states are beyond the grasp of the human brain, much as some complex questions in mathematics have proven undecidable.

DIALOGUE 6
METASCIENTIFIC
PROBLEMS

Si tacuisses philosophus mansisses. [Had I remained silent I had stayed wise.]

Latin proverb

A: I have claimed that brain research—and particularly my own specialty, visual perception—is in the same state that physics was in prior to Galileo, or biochemistry prior to Watson and Crick. Obviously, the physicists and chemists have to be reminded that the human visual cortex, the most complex structure in the known universe, is many orders of magnitude more complex than the atoms and molecules they usually study, and it is no surprise that psychobiology is in such a premature state. Of course, my colleagues in experimental psychology and neurophysiology know the fragmentation of our field in the absence of some fundamental insights yet to come. One of the basic and unanswerable questions is whether there is a really strategic problem in brain research—similar to the DNA double helix—or whether brains evolved in *ad hoc* ways and, as a result, operate by using "a bag of tricks" (Ramachandran 1985). Since I regard this as beyond our present scientific understanding, I classify it as a metascientific question.

B: May I take it for granted that you will not propose "a bag of questions" but good ones?

A: I think you misunderstood me. I did not argue with the quality of Ramachandran's questions. He usually works on questions I regard as fundamental. I merely argued about the metascientific question Ramachandran raised: whether there is some grand design underlying the workings of the brain, or whether the brain processes are *ad hoc* solutions using many available "tricks" to cope with environmental pressures.

So, I regard the following questions—perhaps among the most interesting problems of mankind—as unsolvable at present, even though some famous scientists think otherwise:

Why do higher organisms sleep?

Why do most sleeping organisms dream?

What are the mechanisms of short- and long-term memory?

Is there free will?

What is the essence of the state called consciousness?

Obviously these metascientific questions are not equally complex. Perhaps the riddle of short- and long-term memory will be solved in the not-too-distant future. However, it could be that "consciousness" belongs to a Gödel-like problem, that might exclude brains and neural nets to inspect (solve) certain complex states of their own. [Whether the human brain is equivalent to or more powerful than a Universal Turing Machine (UTM) is another metascientific problem, although Penrose (1989) thinks he can discuss it scientifically. The fact that the relatively simple "halting problem" cannot be solved (computed) by a UTM should caution us about ever having the mental power to answer the really tough metascientific problems of our mental states.]

B: Until now, the only question you raised of scientific interest is the problem whether the human brain is equivalent to a Universal Turing

Machine. If I am not mistaken, Penrose claims that his mathematical insights, particularly his ingenious novel tessellations of the plane by nonregular tiles, were conceived through some mathematical processes that were not algorithmic. If his statement is true, then mathematical insights are beyond algorithmic processes, and therefore the human brain might be more complex than a UTM. Do you believe that?

A: While I find the problem of the brain's being a UTM much less interesting than the other metascientific problems listed above, I think that while I do not have the mathematical sophistication of a Penrose I can also accept his view that there are mathematical processes working in us that are beyond algorithms. Let us take, for example, *mathematical induction*—the remarkable ability of the human mind to accept that if a statement is true for N, and is also true for $N+1$, then it is true for all N (that is for an infinite set of Ns). This insight is one of the cornerstones of mathematics and is regarded as self-evident. It is obviously non-algorithmic, since it is not going step by step to ever-increasing N numbers, but instead invokes in us an actually infinite set consisting of all N. Whether this insight is really true or is merely a "delusion of grandeur" on our part is another metascientific (metamathematical) question, and I leave it to better-qualified minds. So, as I see it, *if mathematical induction, and thus our ability to grasp actual infinity, is a delusion of grandeur, then our brain is a faulty computer, not even a Turing machine. On the other hand, if we indeed can grasp actual infinity, then our brains are non-algorithmic, and thus better than a Turing machine, since such machines can only handle potential infinity and suffer from the halting problem.*

B: I recall that you used a half-baked idea about the extension of Turing machines to torment your mathematician friends. Usually I protest when you put forward half-baked ideas, but in this case I think you have a chance to find out whether your problem makes some sense or is just silly!

A: With hesitation I accept your challenge. I mentioned before that I regard mathematical induction, our ability to imagine *actual* infinity beyond *potential* infinity, as crucial. If this ability of ours is really true, then we are better than a UTM; however, if it turns out that our belief in this ability is merely a delusion of grandeur, then we are not more than a Turing machine or are a strange machine with some logical bugs in our system. On the other hand, if, indeed, the human brain is able to grasp actual infinity, so the insight of mathematical induction is correct, then the brain is more than an algorithmic device and therefore our brains are more complex than a UTM! So, it occurred to me that perhaps one could construct a more general machine than a UTM having some 3-D structure of an exploding polymer. Let us call this bomb-like machine BM and assume that it could be as powerful as a UTM. [Indeed, I like to play Conway's game of LIFE on my computers. This game, which performs as a powerful cellular automaton as well, can be regarded as a general-purpose computer.] Now, if a statement would turn out to be true, like a proof based on mathematical induction, then this BM would explode in the infinite space of numbers, and one could see that this explosion should continue forever, reaching all numbers without a halt.

However, there is a metascientific question that interests me much more than UTMs or even consciousness. This is the problem of "sensations" (also called "qualia"). Wherever the neurophysiologists probe the brain with their microelectrodes, they seem to record similar histograms of neural spike activity, regardless of whether the corresponding sensations are brightness, color, pitch, itch, temperature, pain, pleasure, anxiety, hunger, or contentment. Similarly, the synaptic connectivities with their neurotransmitter sites are of a rich variety, yet are rather similar in their organization throughout the central nervous system. So, the secret of sensations does not rest in spike activity or in synaptic connectivity, at least not at the coarse level at which we are now able to observe them. Johannes Müller (1844), in his doctrine of "specific nerve energies," already was aware of the problem of sensations, and stated that *specific sensations arise in specific brain areas.* While this doctrine might seem somewhat vacuous, I challenge any philosopher or brain researcher to say more with certainty at present than Müller said 150 years ago. [For a debate between John Searle and the author, see Julesz 1993.]

The problem of sensations raises several related metascientific questions:

(F1) Are the known laws of physics an adequate basis on which to understand the emergence of "sensations (qualia)" in functioning brains, or are there some unknown forces (laws) of physics acting?

(F2) Is the mind-brain problem identical to F1, or is it different?

(F3) Is the brain equivalent to or more powerful than a Universal Turing Machine? [discussed above]

Physics has similar metascientific (in this case metaphysical) problems: What was the universe like (and its physical laws) before the Big Bang? Why do elementary particles obey probabilistic laws? Why should all forces of Nature be unified into one super theory? Why should there be some ultimate particles that could not be further reduced *ad infinitum*?

I do not regard metascientific problems as ridiculous or useless. Indeed, many problems that were considered metaphysical at the time of my birth have become respectable, and some have been solved. The origin and age of the universe as revealed by the 3°K background radiation, the real meaning of $E = mc^2$ as revealed by nuclear fusion and fission, and unification theories from quarks to superstrings have become scientific problems and, according to the epistemologist Karl Popper, are now falsifiable.

Let me repeat some points I raised in my debate with the philosopher John Searle, which I alluded to earlier while discussing Johannes Müller's specific nerve energies: "In every scientific field there are tacit assumptions used unquestioningly and 'taboo' problems that workers in the field tend to avoid. Most of these taboo problems are avoided not because they are messy and not well formulated, but rather because our ignorance of these issues does not seem to impede progress. Indeed, these 'luxury problems,' whether solved or not, do not affect the daily routine of a scientific enterprise. For instance, "are mathematical structures and theorems (e.g. the Mandelbrot set, with its striking self-similarities, or analytical functions with their amazing properties, or twin-prime numbers and their distributions) discovered or invented?" (Julesz 1993)

Such a luxury question is usually asked by a layman, while a professional mathematician goes on creating new structures and proving theorems. I doubt that a creative mathematician ever pondered while solving a tough problem, whether he followed some logical steps ingrained in his brain or stumbled on some eternal truth. Of course, the philosopher could argue that the structure of the human brain evolved under the evolutionary pressures of the environment, which in turn obeys the laws of physics, so it is no wonder that the structure of the mathematical mind reflects some of the laws of the universe. Again, whether such a statement is true or not has no effect on the practicing mathematician! I do not regard this problem as trivial. After all, there is a qualitative difference between asking whether mankind might have stumbled eventually on, say, the four-color problem, or could have created the six Brandenburg Concerti without a J. S. Bach. This problem of understanding the difference between scientific and artistic activities may be rather deep; nevertheless, for the active mathematician it is a luxury problem. Similar luxury problems occur in almost any scientific discipline, but these are so well known to the specialists that I will not dwell on them further. While I admit that these luxury problems can be quite interesting, amusing, and thought-provoking in their own rights; nevertheless, they are usually orthogonal to the fundamental problems of the field they address and therefore I regard them metascientific.

While luxury problems belong to the class of metascientific problems, not all metascientific problems are luxury problems. For instance, Darwin's theory of evolution, perhaps the greatest of scientific insights, was a metascientific theory in his time, since the carriers of evolutionary change—recombination and mutation of genes—were unknown (even though some of Mendel's experiments could have been known, but were not). In spite of that, the best scientists of that period immediately understood the significance of Darwin's theory. Thus, whether a theory or problem is metascientific and important or whether it is metascientific and of the luxury kind depends on how the scientists receive it. A luxury problem (theory) is a problem that good scientists disregard almost by instinct, because it does not help them in their research.

B: Listening to you, I became quite pessimistic, realizing the premature state of psychobiology. If the most fundamental questions—questions usually asked by the general public—turn out to be metascientific, then what is the point of working in this field rather than in physics or molecular biology?

A: Even though I started in physics and engineering, and have been impressed by the ten-decimal-point precision of these disciplines, I nevertheless felt a great elation when I first encountered psychology. It was a strange metamorphosis of getting out of a team of thousands of colleagues working on well-defined projects and onto the frontiers of human knowledge, into the real *terra incognita,* where everyone's idea could be tried and it was possible for an individual to make some lasting contribution. I am not claiming that, say, in physics a single genius cannot invent a fundamentally new concept; this has been done from relativity theory to quarks to superstrings. I am claiming that the experimental testing of the more sophisticated concepts is getting increasingly difficult. [For example, I am told that testing the tenets of superstring theory is not possible at present.] On the other hand, some concepts of psychobiology at their very introduction yielded convincing experimental verification. Let me refer to George Palmer's concept of trichromacy—the first scientific atom theory, proposed years before Dalton's atom theory for chemistry. It was suspected by painters in the eighteenth century that one could produce the gamut of colors with a finite number of colors. Nevertheless, it was the theory of trichromacy—stated by Palmer in 1777 and rediscovered in 1802 by Thomas Young [whose publications are reprinted in MacAdam 1970 and referred to in Barlow and Mollon 1982]—that any color can be matched perceptually to a combination of three primary color "atoms" of given weights. So, even though my introduction seems somewhat pessimistic, it is easy for me to switch to a more optimistic tone. After all, I was an eyewitness to the monumental discoveries in psychobiology that took place in the last 30 years. There are now many exciting questions in vision research that can be attacked with existing scientific tools.

B: You have not listed a single metascientific question in vision research. Why do you expect me to believe that vision research is more mature than brain research in general?

A: Obviously the metascientific questions of psychobiology I listed above apply to vision research as well as to any other branch of psychobiology. Some of these are even more crucial to vision research than, say, to the study of heat perception. Indeed, since I regard the problem of sensations as one of the deepest of the enigmas, I view heat sensation as just a monotonic function of physical temperature. Of course, why this temperature is felt

as "warm" above some subjective threshold and as "cold" below it, and the subjective quality of these sensations, are fundamental riddles of the mind. For vision this mystery is even deeper, because the sensations are multidimensional. The range of color, brightness, motion, flicker, and depth percepts that by themselves do not exist in the physical world raises some fundamental questions. Are these "qualia" universal codes that evolve in organisms with ancestries similar to ours, or are there creatures in our world that have sensations different from ours? There are some vertebrates with more than three color pigments. Do these animals experience a richer repertoire of color sensations than humans? Is my red sensation different from yours—might you sense green instead? Obviously, these are two different problems. One is the very nature of the quality of subjective sensations; the other is our inability to communicate this quality to others. In the case of another qualia question (Do we sense absolute depth, or only relative depth?), the problem of the sensation of plasticity is as impenetrable as the essence of the sensation of "color"—these qualia questions are of the Kantian *Ding an sich* (thing in itself) kind. However, in the case of depth the problem of absolute versus relative can be easily communicated to others. Each time one can quickly hit a distant nail with her finger (thus without any visual-motoric feedback), the question of her seeing it at the same absolute depth as her companion is answered in the affirmative. Perhaps this explains why I was drawn to study spatial object perception instead of color perception.

DIALOGUE 7
MATURATIONAL
WINDOWS AND
CORTICAL
PLASTICITY

Author: Why did I get such a small salary increase this year?

Supervisor: Because you turned from an engineer into a psychologist. And, as you know, psychology has no A-bombs!

Author: That is not quite true. Psychologists are discovering maturational windows, which are more important to mankind than nuclear energy.

Supervisor: If you will find out what to do with these windows, I will give you a large raise.

A: We all have heard of "wolf children" who were raised without a language and who, beyond a critical age (say, 5 years), never learned to speak well. In recent years an entire book was devoted to the rehabilitation of "Genie," who was raised in a cellar in Los Angeles by sadistic parents without being spoken to, and was liberated when she was 12. Even at 20, she could only use three-word sentences. It is also known that a child whose dominant (speech) hemisphere has to be removed because of a brain tumor will not suffer permanent loss of speech if the surgery occurs while the child is very young. This neural plasticity for speech vanishes a few years after birth. So, we have a "maturational window" for speech acquisition, provided hemispheric plasticity cannot work. It is less well known that in visual perception there are similar maturational windows, measured not in years but in months. For instance, if severe astigmatism is not corrected a few months after birth, at a later age there will be a deficit at the given angle, even after the astigmatism is corrected with the proper cylindrical lenses.

B: I did not know that you were interested in developmental psychology, or that your work was somehow related to maturational windows.

A: I am not surprised that you do not know about my quest for a way to diagnose and prevent stereo blindness in human infants, or of my efforts to find practical ways to measure evoked potentials in monkeys and human infants in order to test stereopsis. However, since without a medical degree I was not permitted to study stereo-blind patients directly, I was at the mercy of ophthalmologists who were less interested in long-range research problems than in healing. I never discussed this with you.

Let me start with the fact that 2% of humans are stereo blind and 4–6% are stereo deficient, as revealed by the random-dot stereogram test plates in *Foundations of Cyclopean Perception*. Interestingly, there were a few stereo-blind subjects who did not know about their handicap before they tried in vain to fuse an RDS. Of course, motion parallax and the many other monocular familiarity cues of depth give us adequate plasticity of real-life scenes when we use only one eye. This explains why there were one-eyed flying aces in World War I. However, there are professions in which stereo deficiencies cannot be tolerated. For instance, in stereo x-ray fluoroscopy the catheterization of the heart requires the viewing of an x-ray stereogram presented in anaglyph format, so that the physician can guide the catheter from the arm into the heart. It was in the x-ray department at Temple University that RDSs were first used to weed out applicants. From astronauts to truck drivers and forest dwellers, there are professions and lifestyles for which the lack of stereopsis is a great handicap.

A patent of mine contributed to better quality control of silicon chips, which are routinely inspected with stereo microscopes. It turned out that, besides the usual 4% incidence of stereo-deficient individuals the among inspectors, most of the microscopes were inadequately aligned. Inserting tiny stereograms with a hidden cyclopean message in order to test the inspectors' performance improved the yield dramatically.

In the last two decades my colleagues and I developed methods that surrounded human infants and monkeys with dynamic RDSs and measured their evoked potentials with electrodes attached on their scalps. We have observed the sudden onset of functional binocularity in normal human infants at 3.5 months after birth. We still do not know the limit of the maturational window of stereopsis, but it is probably close to this early onset. Indeed, surgery to correct for strabismus in esotropes (whose strabismus causes their eyes to be crossed in the nasal direction) by operating on their eye muscles is merely a cosmetic intervention at age 1 or 2. Similarly, "lazy eye" (amblyopia ex anopsia), in which the non-dominant eye is shut off by the visual system as long as the dominant eye is open, will not be alleviated if the surgical intervention occurs too late. Interestingly, exotropes (who squint in the temporalward direction) can often regain stereopsis even when surgery for their cross-eyedness is performed rather late in life. When these patients' eye muscles become fatigued, for some brief periods the two eyes may become parallel when corresponding areas in them are aligned. It appears as if a sporadic time of correct stimulation of the stereoscopic system during the critical period would be sufficient to keep stereopsis intact.

In spite of the fact that we developed techniques that permit a quick and unfakeable determination of stereopsis in humans and monkeys we still do not know for how long the maturational windows are open after 3.5 months. Our evoked potential techniques with dynamic RDSs are mainly used by neurophysiologists. After all, training monkeys to steadily fixate on a marker during experiments is a cumbersome business, and it is troublesome to find out later that the selected monkey happened to be stereo blind.

In fairness to clinical neurologists, nobody knows at present whether stereo blindness is always caused by strabismus or whether strabismus is the result of a poorly functioning neural system. However, Hubel and Wiesel (among others) firmly established that artificially inducing squinting in kittens and infant monkeys rewired their brains. Neurons that normally would fire for binocular stimulation became monocular and would fire only for stimulation by one eye. This condition became permanent unless the duration of the maturational window had been artificially extended by the application of some neurotransmitter (e.g. dopa) to the striate cortex (Pettigrew 1974, 1990). So, it is most frustrating that in these many years I could not find clinicians who were interested in our techniques. At least they could try to operate on cross-eyed babies at the earliest age (a rather routine procedure now) and find out whether their patients' recovery rate of stereopsis improved.

B: So far your story about maturational windows has been rather pessimistic. It seems as if the genetic information is inadequate to fine-tune the nervous system. At birth we have laid down the "deep structure" for certain skills, such as being able to learn a language. However, it is the environment that fine-tunes this existing deep structure by almost automatically filling it with the knowledge of, say, English or Chinese in a very brief time. To learn these languages later from scratch requires great effort. If I understood you correctly, this fine-tuning has to occur at an early stage after birth, and if it is missed then some irreversible damage is done.

Someone told me during the Soviet occupation of Hungary that he could sometimes identify Russian soldiers in civilian clothes. When I asked him how, he told me that most of them came from farms, where it was still the custom to bundle infants tightly in swaddling clothes while the parents worked in the fields. This early deprivation of free locomotion later resulted in strange gaits. Are there examples when instead of deprivation one could *enrich* an infant's environment so that the child would become more skillful?

A: While I do not know how true the story about the swaddling clothes may be, several studies on infant animals have shown that suturing eyes or immobilizing legs during the critical period resulted in permanent neurological damage. So your comment that the main function of maturational windows is to permit the rapid matching of fine details to the environment is correct.

Your question of enriching an infant's environment in order to improve the complexity of the child's brain is a difficult question. Most middle-class infants in the United States probably receive adequately rich stimulation. Whether babies raised in the ghetto get adequate stimulation during their maturational windows is an important but difficult research topic. [Indeed, it is hard to establish whether in a particular case some neural damage is due to the impoverished surroundings or to lead poisoning from licking old paint.] So far I do not know of any evidence of unusual perceptual skills that were due to enriched stimulation during infancy. Nevertheless, I have some comments that will please you, since they convey an optimistic story.

Let me start with the observation that there is a fundamental difference between incorrect stimulation and the lack of stimulation. For instance, with a mirror stereoscope (haploscope) and special optics I can stimulate nearby areas, occluded by my nose, that can be seen only by one eye. So, here is a cortical area that, although never binocularly stimulated, yields normal plasticity after the first presentation of a stereo image. This finding attests to my maxim that virgin cortical areas are different from incorrectly stimulated areas, particularly if the wrong stimulation occurs within the maturational window after birth. In experiments in which adult observers were presented with brief RDSs (so that they could not make convergence movements), my co-workers and I found that after a few thousand trials, as we slowly increased the binocular disparity, the original Panum's fusional area was extended by an order of magnitude, as if neurons that had never been stimulated before would arborize to great distances. [See "Cortical plasticity for stereopsis" in the index.] We also found evidence that this slow but robust perceptual learning is most prevalent after the observer has had a good sleep. This neural plasticity is a robust learning phenomenon and fits well with very recent evidence. I will summarize these new findings briefly, relying on a recent paper by Vilayanur Ramachandran (1993) and on some talks by Michael Merzenich.

When Ramachandran (1982) poked the left cheek of a 17-year-old boy who had recently lost his left arm with a cotton swab, the patient felt tingling both on the cheek and on the phantom limb (hand and arm). Poking the right cheek did not elicit tingling in the phantom limb. Dribbling warm water down the left cheek evoked the sensation of water running down his arm. Up to this point it was thought that brain cells would die when the body part they were connected to was amputated, and that the tingling of the phantom limb was attributable to the stimulation of nerves near the missing limb's stump. Now it seems that there is a capability of reorganization and rewiring over incredibly large distances.

That such a rapid change is a property of healthy and injured adult brains was shown by Charles Gilbert. Vision scotomas (e.g. in diabetics) are filled in by adjacent areas, and therefore these blind spots are not seen. Laser-induced tiny lesions of the retina within minutes are not "silenced," but begin sharing with neighboring cortical neurons. This change might occur in seconds, allowing adaptation to the changing environment. This activation by neighboring cells might also explain optical illusions.

Michael Merzenich and Jon Kaas, using monkeys, amputated one finger and found that, instead of one gap, adjacent fingers could activate the same cortical locus. However, when two adjacent fingers were amputated the "filling in" phenomenon was absent, so they believed that the cells rewire only over very short distances. They were wrong. Tim Pons examined monkeys whose arms were paralyzed 12 years earlier by cutting nerve connections to the brain. The neural aggregates that used to serve the limb were not only alive, but responded to the face. Merzenich's human patients have observed that cochlear implants with crude electrode spacing first sounded mechanical and impractical, but after a few months' use began to sound natural and distinctive.

In the sensory homunculus, fingers and face, eyes, nose have a cortical map adjacent to each other. Genitals and toes are also adjacent to each other. Monkeys trained to pick up small pallets develop expanded brain areas for fingers, and Braille readers have increased neural maps for their index fingers.

After a stroke, recovery occurs as neighboring areas take over functions. This finding leads to new strategies for rehabilitation of stroke victims. A patient with weak fingers but strong arms should use his fingers and not further strengthen his arms. In a patient with spinal injuries, new sprouting is necessary but not adequate. It will require special training that will prevent changes in cortical maps by adjacent brain tissues that serve some unrelated body parts.

I find these new findings of great importance to psychobiology:

• Neural plasticity occurs mainly between adjacent cortical sites that occupy almost instantly the neighboring areas when they become inactive

• Globality is achieved by scrambling the neural representation of sites that belong to distant body parts. Perhaps this scrambling is not *ad hoc*, but reveals the evolutionary history of a species as damage to injuries was minimized by proper mixing of functionally related body parts.

• The brain remains active throughout life, and new ways of learning through neural plasticity can now be envisioned.

• Micro-lesions begin to be filled in by neighboring neurons after a few seconds of inactivity.

• Scotomas (like the blind spot) may not be perceived because the adjacent areas fill in their former function.

The last point explains how one can perceive textured information in the site of a scotoma. Since textures have a certain stochastic regularity, at the site of the damaged cortical representation a percept is "hallucinated" with the help of the newly acquired neighboring neurons that grabbed the site of the scotoma. After all, these nearby neurons have almost the same stimulus information as the scotoma would have received!

[Several of the above-mentioned researchers participated in a workshop on maturational windows and cortical plasticity, held at the Santa Fe Institute in May of 1993, which I organized. I am in the process of editing the proceedings of this unusually informative meeting. For a brief summary of recent work on learning, see Polat and Sagi 1993.]

Darian-Smith and Gilbert (1994) showed evidence for axonal sprouting in the striate cortex of the adult cat—a revolutionary finding!

B: These findings are rather interesting, but I still do not see how they are relevant to my questions. You have not given any example of how our potential mental skills can be enriched by the proper use of the maturational windows! It is good for both of us that you became a tenured professor at Rutgers; at Bell Labs, you might have had to wait a long time for a raise.

EPILOGUE

A young reporter, being interviewed for a job by a famous newspaper tycoon, acts rather timidly. After a few minutes of silence the tycoon loses his temper and shouts "How dare you be modest when you have nothing to be modest about!"

A: I regard myself as linking two generations of scientists, two cultures, and two disciplines. When I suddenly appeared in the United States in 1956, after the abortive Hungarian Revolution, I did not know that I would play this role. I had spent my first 28 years in Hungary under oppressive fascist and communist regimes. Johnny (János) von Neumann, Dennis (Dénes) Gábor, Leo Szilárd, Georg (György) von Békésy, Albert Szentgyörgyi, Abraham Wald, and Eugen (Jenö) Wigner, who had all escaped to the free democracies before World War II or shortly after, were merely legends for me. Besides these geniuses of Hungarian origin, I had my other living heroes: Claude Shannon, Alan Turing, Kurt Gödel, Harry Nyquist, and Norbert Wiener, to name a few. I never dreamed that I would meet any of them. My secret longing to talk to these idols was not based on snobbery; rather, I felt that they carried the torch of the previous generation and knew many things even beyond science that were suppressed during my youth under dictatorship—things that, for me, might be lost forever.

B: How did you come up with such a varied list of scientific heroes, with backgrounds in engineering, physics, and mathematics?

A: In fact, most of the idols of my youth had physics or engineering backgrounds. I started with a similar background. It seemed unlikely that, as a communication engineer, I could ever achieve anything that would be of interest or of intellectual value to these geniuses. Abraham Wald was a mathematician, but my first scientific interest was the "ideal observer," and the fact that Wald's paper on sequential analysis was perhaps the only classified mathematical paper during the war added some mystique to his surprising insights. I first learned of the mathematical work of Gödel and Turing from Rózsa Péter, and I found the feat of proving that certain mathematical problems were undecidable a fantastic achievement of the human mind. Thus, all my heroes ventured beyond routine mathematics, quantum physics, and relativity theory into revolutionary new areas that caught my fancy, such as the foundation of digital computers, the limits of human thought processes, holography, biology, cellular and self-reproducing automata, information theory, consciousness, models of learning, and stochastic processes.

It was my good fortune that I wound up, a few weeks after my arrival in the United States, at Bell Laboratories in Murray Hill, New Jersey, as a member of the technical research staff. I would occasionally see Nyquist, already retired, from a distance in the library, or talk and lunch with Claude Shannon. Then, I had another break: I arrived almost simultaneously with the first mainframe computers. This coincidence fostered the invention of the computer-generated stereograms, cinematograms, and textures, which together with my work in auditory (echoic) memory catapulted me into another career. I metamorphosed from a communication engineer into an experimental psychologist. Slowly I drifted into the field of physiological psychology, influenced by the epoch-making discoveries of the neurophysiologists.

B: I am surprised that you have not mentioned the many other distinguished colleagues you met at Bell Labs just after your arrival: Willem van Bergeijk, Ed David, Ed Gilbert, Newman Guttman, Leon Harmon, John Kelly, Rudi Kompfner, Max Mathews, John Pierce, Manfred Schroeder, Roger Shepard, David Slepian, and many others, each of whom had a lasting impact on you.

A: Obviously, my mentor, John Pierce, my boss's boss at Bell Labs— inventor of the traveling-wave tube, the Echo satellite, and a musical scale—was more influential in my life, than, say, Claude Shannon (whose information theory cannot be used so far in psychology, since the code of the brain is still an enigma). Indeed, I used to ponder on how the role my early heroes played in my scientific life might have changed had I remained in Hungary as an engineer.

Closely related to this thought is your question about why I have mentioned so many names instead of my own work. In our century, knowledge is so vast that a single mind cannot absorb more than a tiny fraction of it. It was mainly the work of my selected heroes—and only a certain subset of it—that influenced my scientific work, both consciously and unconsciously, and helped me to become an experimental psychologist in my own way. Without their influence, I could not have achieved much. For instance, throughout my work— from my thesis on reducing perceivable information in TV signals to iso-second-order texture-pair discrimination—I used correlation techniques learned from Norbert Wiener. (For example, for black and white images the second-order statistics is the auto-correlation function.)

My psychological "creations" got me invited to some prestigious conferences, where I met Dennis Gabor and Georg von Békésy.[1,2] I also recall a week in Versailles, at one of the Institute de la Vie Symposia, where I sat at the breakfast table together with Mark Kac (who had invited me to this meeting), Eugen Wigner, Albert Szentgyörgyi, and Stanislaw Ulam. It was a great moment to hear them discuss daily events and verify that, in spite of my different background, I shared their values, and we were able to laugh at each other's jokes. Furthermore, I was fascinated how some of my intellectual heroes had had to cope with the same problems of cultural differences that I now faced, and I was greatly reassured that they had not only learned the ropes but had also enriched American culture. Unfortunately, Alan Turing was already dead, and Abraham Wald, John von Neumann, and Leo Szilárd[3] died before I had a chance to meet them. I did not have the nerve to meet Kurt Gödel.

B: So far your story reminds me of funny inscriptions on old hotels announcing that GEORGE WASHINGTON never SLEPT HERE! What is the point of listing the names of famous people whom you never saw, since they died before you could meet with them? I find your naive quest of mingling with a few select geniuses somewhat irritating. After all, we routinely stumble into Nobel laureates and famous colleagues at our workplace, or at scientific meetings, and often are on friendly terms with them. Why is meeting, say, Dennis Gabor such a big deal?

A: If one is not familiar with his work, it isn't. But if one is acquainted with the incredible creativity and insight of my heroes (as I became through their published works), and if one has been deprived of the freedom to travel for a decade (as I was), then my longing to meet with them has another dimension. Although I had several interesting discussions later on visual perception with the best minds in America, from Richard Feynman to Max Delbrück, these outstanding and charismatic individuals were not the mysterious idols of my youth. That I was able to have intellectual contact as a psychologist with some of my early heroes gives me great satisfaction.

B: What was so special about the work of Gabor?

A: Most people think of him as the inventor of holography, a rather esoteric technique that was practically useless before lasers provided coherent light. While Gabor had many other original ideas—from searching for best sampling functions to novel nonlinear system analysis—most people assume that if lasers had not been invented during his lifetime he might not have received the Nobel Prize. However, for Gabor, holography was merely one of the means to achieve his quest, which was the creation of a genuine million-power microscope. [See Gabor 1948.] He had the ingenious idea that between light and ultrasound there is a wavelength difference of a million. If the hologram is created by light but is then read out by ultrasonic wave, a magnification of a million is achieved without any loss of detail. I am glad that Gabor lived to see a cover picture of the journal *Nature* showing an atom surrounded by electrons. That was achieved by making a hologram by electron waves and retrieving it by a proton beam. Gabor's magnification idea worked again. Obviously, the same idea works in reverse, and great reduction in pic-

ture size can be achieved. I can imagine that in the twenty-first century VLSI chips will be manufactured by this technique of hyperreduction. Furthermore, Fourier-transform holograms in such miniature size could be used for optical pattern recognition.

Of course, in my new profession of psychobiology I met several great scientists, and became good friends with some, but that is another matter. Here I was not a link anymore; I belonged to them.

B: Being a part of you, I understand your romantic attachment to the heroes of your youth. At the same time I know how pleased you were with the long chats you had on epistemological questions with Max Delbrück and Murray Gell-Mann, or participating in the Helmholtz Club meetings of Francis Crick during your winter semesters at Caltech. I also know that you enjoyed many years of consultation on perceptual problems, particularly on stereopsis, with Salvador Dali. Perhaps you could say a few words about your interaction with these charismatic individuals.

A: My early encounters with Jerry Lettvin, David Hubel, and Torsten Wiesel shifted my interest into physiological psychology just at the beginning of my career. I am also proud that random-dot stereograms shifted Hubel and Wiesel's interest from form to problems of binocular vision. Furthermore, my acquintance with Gell-Mann drew me to the Santa Fe Institute, a powerful think tank for work on complex adaptive systems. I learned a lot from its members, and I hope to pay back my debt by bringing psychobiological ideas to them. Similarly, I am greatly indebted to another Nobelist, Gerald Edelman, and to Neuroscience

Associates (which he now heads). My nine years with him, and with some of the best minds in brain research, as an associate, opened my biological vista manyfold. Francis Crick read and liked a precursor of these dialogues, my 1991 article in *Reviews of Modern Physics*. I spent three winter semesters (1979–1981) as a Fairchild Distinguished Scholar at Caltech. I am particularly grateful to the anonymous talent scouts who recommended my work to the MacArthur Foundation for their prestigious award in 1983. This enabled me, from 1984 until now, to spend an additional nine consecutive winter semesters at Caltech. A joint grant with David Van Essen to study texture discrimination in monkeys and humans brought me to Caltech. I worked with John Allman on non-evasive methods of studying stereopsis in monkeys, and I enjoyed my frequent talks with Derek Fender, John Hopfield, Carver Mead, and Christof Koch and my occasional visits with Seymour Benzer and Roger Sperry.[4]

I also had several encounters with artists. In June 1965 I took part in the very first "computer art" exhibit (with another engineer colleague from Bell Labs, Mike Noll) in the Howard Wise Gallery in New York. Although there was a disclaimer below my computer-generated stereograms and textures that these were merely the results of scientific experiments, and that their creator did not regard them as pieces of art, the newspapers disregarded it. I have many clippings with headlines such as "Cold computer art!" and "Computers take over arts!" To my further amazement, there were "artists" who used several of my images in collages. When Salvador Dali invited me to his studio and showed me his recent work, I was honored. There was a picture of Christ nailed on a cross made of the DNA double helix. At the feet of Christ were

two cascaded silk scarfs, giving rise to a moiré effect, and around the head was a stereo viewer and a cutout of an RDS portraying a torus from my *Scientific American* article (Julesz 1965). This torus, after fusion, served as a halo on the crucified Jesus. I knew immediately that I finally "made it."[5]

After this first encounter with Dali, he asked my advice several times, particularly as he painted some large stereo pairs at an angle with a half-silvered mirror between them. He also asked me to supply him with some random-dot stereograms so he could modify them according to his taste.[6] [See figures E.1 and E.2.] I mention this episode merely to illustrate that the impact of the RDS even permeated art. Because I was impressed by Dali's perceptual knowledge during our conversations, I feel that he paid tribute to the RDS not only as an artist but also as a colleague well versed in my specialty. I should also note that several times I was invited to artistic gatherings by Op artists. While I was always proud of my affiliation with Dali, I did not care much for Op art. I always felt that artists should be revolutionary thinkers, decades ahead of the rest of mankind (including perceptual psychologists), as Albers, Escher, Kandinsky, and Klee were.

I really do not mind what an artist "borrows" from a scientist's work, if the artist is creative and genuine. Whether in such cases the artist should give credit to the scientist depends on many factors. In my case, I can easily imagine that centuries later not a single copy of my books and articles might survive, and of course no one would recall my name, yet in a church or a museum the cyclopean halo on Dali's painting might still enchant some curious viewers.

That I met some of my scientific heroes of the previous generation, that I metamorphosed from an engineer into a psychologist, and that I found refuge in the United States—each of these is a personal happenstance of minor interest to most people. However, that I belong to the generation that attempted the first successful linking of perceptual phenomena to neurophysiological findings should be of primary interest.

B: Throughout this epilogue I have heard you praise Bell Labs and Caltech, two world-famous institutions you were lucky to join during your most creative years. Yet for over five years now you have been at Rutgers University. I find it strange that you have not mentioned your experiences there.

Figure E.2

Dali's *Cybernetic Odalisque*, 1978 (oil on canvas, 78.75 × 78.75 inches; private collection). The original legend reads: "This work started with an anaglyph diagram of Bela Julesz, an American scientist who successfully did research on visual perception." This painting is reproduced in color on page 413 of Robert Descharnes's book *Salvador Dali: The Work, the Man* (Abrams, 1989).

Figure E.1

Salvador Dali "improving" on a 32 × 32-pixel random-dot stereogram (in anaglyph form) from *Foundations of Cyclopean Perception*.

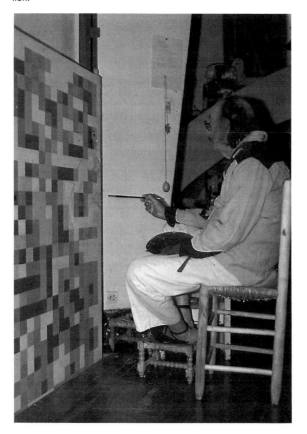

A: Obviously five years at a new place are difficult to compare with my most formative years. After all, I spent 32 years at Bell Labs and over a dozen at Caltech. Yet institutions, however famous, do change. After the divestiture of the Bell System, AT&T Bell Labs could not afford psychobiological research. Caltech is too small to support a group of visual perception experts, at least so far. So, when I was invited with my group to Rutgers University in January 1989 as one of the newly established institutes of excellence this was much more than a lucky break. After all, I could have found myself a good place at most universities, and so could my talented colleagues. But to stay together with my co-workers, and be able to remain in our familiar environments and devote full time to research and teaching, was and still is a happy break. That I can invite to my own laboratory anyone I like, have several talented postdocs, and can and do collaborate with many specialists is a wonderful experience.[7,8]

Notes to Epilogue

1. Just to hint at the extraordinary character of Békésy, I tell you the following episode. As member of the Colloquium Committee of Bell Labs I invited Békésy to give an Auditorium talk at his convenience. As usual, he was very cordial to me, but hedged to give a definite date. Just a few weeks later I read an article by him on the changes of receptive field sizes of touch receptors after nembutal anaesthesia. There were two curves given, taken at different times with the same observer. In small print it was mentioned that these two curves where measured in the recovery room on his own arm by GvB at his first, and somewhat later, at his second colotomy as the anaesthesia slowly wore off. So, I suddenly found out why he did not accept my invitation, and soon after he died. How many scientists do my readers know who would use their own surgeries to report their scientific swan song?

2. In a somewhat similar episode, I recommended my other hero, Dennis Gabor, for an Auditorium talk, and in early 1973 I picked him up from Grand Central Station in New York City to drive him to Murray Hill. [He often visited his old friend Peter Goldmark (the inventor of the LP record and grandson of the famous opera composer Karl Goldmark) at the CBS laboratory in Connecticut.] During the hour ride he wanted to know whether researchers at Bell Labs really wanted to hear a talk on holography, since he rather wished to give us a talk about a much more relevant topic. I asked him what this was about. He said that, according to his estimates, within 3 months the citizens of the US and Europe would queue up in long lines for a few drops of gasoline, and he had some ideas on what to do about it. I politely assured him that we were certainly more interested in his holograms than in such an unlikely event. I certainly goofed!

3. Szilárd is pronounced as "Silard"—the Hungarian sz sounds as the English s, whereas the Hungarian s is pronounced as sh. For this reason the younger brother of Leo Szilard, Bela Silard, changed his name to preserve its proper pronunciation. (My own name, pronounced as "You-less," is usually not mastered by my postdocs, who call me by my first name.)

While writing this epilogue I read an excellent book, *Genius in the Shadows: A Biography of Leo Szilárd: The Man Behind The Bomb*, written by William Lanouette with Bela Silard (1992), that reminded me of a long-forgotten episode. In the early 1960s I received a postcard from Dr. Albert Korodi, a former department head of mine at the Telecommunications Research Institute in Budapest, while visiting relatives in the US. The postcard was signed with several other names, one of them Leo Szilárd. I did not pay attention to this signature, because I thought it unlikely that it was signed by my hero. This is quite curious, since I vaguely knew that Dr. Korodi lived for a while in the West, and worked in the Philips Labs in Eindhoven. As I was reading this biography of Szilard I read about the close friendship between Szilárd and Albert Kornfeld. At that very moment, I had a sudden hint and looked up Kornfeld in the name index.

Indeed, Kornfeld changed his name to Korodi. So, after all, Leo Szilárd signed the postcard, and most likely Korodi must have mentioned me to him. The terror under Stalin's rule was so total that Korodi never dared to tell even to his closest co-workers about his friendship with Leo Szilárd.

4. During my yearly Caltech visits, I used to pay my respects to Professor Sperry, whose work on split brains was the very first scientific breakthrough related to some aspect of consciousness. [For an up-to-date review on hemispheric localization, see Gazzaniga 1989.] [I would also meet Joe Bogen, who used to perform split-brain surgery on epileptic patients—a procedure seldom used nowadays.] When I learned that Gian Poggio and I were to receive the 1989 Karl Spencer Lashley Award from the Philosophical Society in Philadelphia, I visited Sperry, since I remembered that he knew Lashley. It turned out that Lashley had a great influence on Sperry, who worked hard to disprove equipotentiality, an idea of Lashley's that the engram of memory is over the entire brain. So, Lashley was a "great" scientist not because his idea proved to be right but rather because he posed a strategic problem that was within the reach of scientific scrutiny; and its falsification would earn Sperry the Nobel Prize.

5. Later, during the student revolt in 1969, while I was on sabbatical at MIT, students often praised my work as being peaceful and without political impact. I always told them that they were wrong. The crucified Christ with the RDS halo was soon to be sent to Spain, where some innocent Spanish farmer would view it in a church. And lo and behold, a miracle would happen. Out of nothing a halo would slowly emerge, and Generalissimo Franco's power would be strengthened by this divine miracle!

6. After this first encounter, Dali asked my advice several times, particularly as he painted some large stereo pairs at an angle with a half-silvered mirror between them. He also asked me to supply him with some random-dot stereograms for him to paint in colors according to his taste.

7. The entire dialogue 12 is devoted to our activities and findings while at Rutgers.

8. While the reader can understand why von Békésy, Von Neumann, Gabor, and even Wigner were included here, others, particularly Szilárd, seem an enigma. Indeed, Békésy worked on the cochlea and the role of lateral inhibition in the brain, and Von Neumann pioneered the digital computer, all quite relevant to my work. Furthermore, Pennington and I were among the few, if not the first, to draw an analogy between memory storage in brains and Gábor's holograms (Julesz and Pennington 1965). Even Wigner, who speculated on the role that human consciousness might play in quantum-mechanical states when the Schrödinger equations were solved, had something to do with psychology.

So, let me explain to the reader the role Szilárd played in my life. As a teenager I felt incredible shame and frustration as the Nazis slaughtered innocent and defenseless people around me. I felt great pride and elation, when years later, the secrecy was lifted and I discovered the role played by Von Neumann, Wigner, Edward Teller, and especially Szilárd in ensuring that the atom bomb would not fall into Hitler's hands, and consequently helping the United States and the Free World to withstand Stalin's blackmail. These scientific and politically omniscient geniuses, who lived within walking distance of me in Budapest when I was a child, were not idle. Indeed, they expended a great amount of energy (mc^2) to protect all of us, and their deeds shortened the war. Of course, we were greatly indebted to the non-Hungarian geniuses as well, from Enrico Fermi to Stanislaw Ulam, who participated in the Manhattan Project. But at the same time they also helped to unleash frightening forces that could wipe out our civilization. Szilárd was keenly aware of the moral consequences of his quest. Few people know that, just before Szilárd and Einstein sent their letter to President Roosevelt that initiated the Manhattan Project, Szilárd formulated his own version of the Ten Commandments:

1. Recognize the connections of things and the laws of conduct of men so that you may know what you are doing.

2. Let your acts be directed toward a worthy goal but do not ask if they will reach it; they are to be models and examples, not means to an end.

3. Speak to all men as you do to yourself, with no concern for the effect you make, so that you do not shut them out from your world, lest in isolation the meaning of life slips out of sight and you lose the belief in the perfection of the creation.

4. Do not destroy what you cannot create.

5. Touch no dish except when you are hungry.

6. Do not covet what you cannot have.

7. Do not lie without need.

8. Honor children. Listen reverently to their words and speak to them with infinite love.

9. Do your work for six years; but in the seventh, go into solitude or among strangers so that the memory of your friends does not hinder you from being what you have become.

10. Lead your life with a gentle hand and be ready to leave whenever you are called.

(August 4, 1939. Translated from the original German by Jacob Bronowski.)

II
DIALOGUES ON SPECIFIC TOPICS

DIALOGUE 8
SOME STRATEGIC
QUESTIONS ABOUT
VISUAL PERCEPTION

Problems arise in a variety of ways, and it is often worthwhile to list the forms that they may take. Thus we can distinguish the following:

1. The classical problem, which has had much effort expended upon it, but without any acceptable solution.
2. The premature problem, which often is poorly formulated, or is not susceptible to attack.
3. The strategic problem, which seeks data on which a choice may be made between two or more basic assumptions or principles.
4. The stimulating problem, which may lead to a reexamination of accepted principles and may open up new areas for exploration.
5. The statistical question, which may be only a survey of possibilities.
6. The unimportant problem, which is easy to formulate and easy to solve.
7. The embarrassing question, commonly arising at meetings in the discussion of a paper, and rarely serving any useful purpose.
8. The pseudo problem, usually the consequence of different definitions or methods of approach. Another form of pseudo problem is a statement made in the form of a question. It is often the result of discussions in meetings.

It is frequently helpful to attempt to place a given problem in this array of possibilities, for such a classification may provide a hint as to the problem's significance, the difficulties involved in its attack, and the sort of solution that may be expected.

Georg von Békésy (1960)

A: In the following dialogues I will skip all the metascientific problems and leave them to Nobel laureates (but not to students in search of Ph.D. thesis topics), and turn to the more tractable ones that I regard as strategic in visual perception. I call them "Hilbert-like problems." My reference to David Hilbert, a famous German mathematician, is not immodesty on my part, but rather an allusion to the well-known strategic (meaning fundamental) questions he raised at the turn of the twentieth century. Many of these questions were proven to be undecidable by Kurt Gödel, Alonzo Church, and Allen Turing in the 1930s, when Hilbert was still living. Indeed, it is ironic that his famous problems were proven undecidable already during his lifetime. Among his "strategic problems," the most celebrated ones were concerned with proving the consistency of several subfields of mathematics whose very foundations were shaken by the paradoxes that showed up in set theory. Unexpectedly, Gödel, among others, proved an epoch-making theorem (known as the incompleteness theorem) that there exist mathematical problems that are undecidable. So, most of the fundamental problems of Hilbert were preempted by Gödel, Church, and Turing, who proved that some rather simple mathematical problems could not be proven to be right or wrong, or in algorithmic form could not be computed. It is in this spirit that I pose my Hilbert-like problems in vision research, and I would be the happiest person if some unexpected insights might preempt this list during my lifetime! Of course, in psychology we cannot prove that some of my questions are undecidable (except, perhaps, for the emergence of "consciousness" in the highly complex neural nets called brains). But in the next years new insights might be gained in brain function that will yield questions much more strategic than the ones I pose.

Here is my list of strategic questions in vision research, with emphasis on early vision. These problems are given in random order, as they came into my mind, without any hierarchical order of importance or inherent structure, but I will single out my favorite ones. I urge the reader to go over the entire list. Some questions will appear clear, some others obscure. I will try to give my associations to many of these problems afterwards. However, I do not dwell on them in great detail, because I want to be merely a catalyst, and wish to encourage the reader to interpret the questions or add some new ones to the list.

1. How, when, and where (in time and processing stages) do retinotopic coordinates convert into environmental (or egocentric) ones? This question is discussed in this dialogue.

2. Is the "cortical magnification factor" already compensated internally? That is, could we perceive better if the stimulus were increased in size with increased eccentricity? This question is discussed in this dialogue.

3. How is motion blur avoided without a "shutter"? That is, how do we perceive objects moving with different velocities as sharp? Could it be that cortical shifter circuits are used? This question is discussed in this dialogue.

4. Why do certain feature conjunctions (i.e., color and orientation; color and motion) usually require scrutiny, while others (i.e., color and stereopsis; stereopsis and motion) pop out? This question is related to the interesting finding of Treisman (1985) that color and orientation (or color and motion) appear to be mapped independently since elements defined by the conjunction of these two attributes do not pop out but require serial search.

This is a rather surprising finding, since most neurological feature extractors are triggered by multiple attributes. Indeed, when in addition to these two a third attribute is presented (say, binocular disparity), then, as Nakayama (1990), and Nakayama and Silverman (1986) have shown, search becomes parallel and the target defined by triple conjunction usually pops out. The reason why I did not go into details is my ignorance as to what a double conjunction really means. For instance, Dov Sagi (1988) has an interesting demonstration of the double conjunction of orientation and spatial frequency (figure 8.1). Since I regard Treisman's discovery of the independence of orientation and color and Sagi's finding that orientation and spatial frequency are coupled as important in-

Figure 8.1

This figure demonstrates target pop-out, even though its detection requires conjoining the spatial frequencies and the orientations of the individual Gabor patches that generate each texture element. From Sagi 1988.

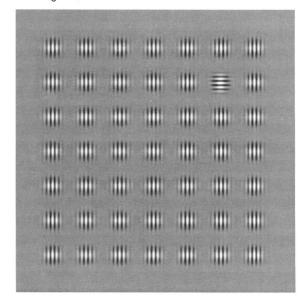

sights in perception, I have two possible reactions: Either it is not true in general that color and form are independent attributes, or orientation is more like form than SF is. Whatever is the case, the story becomes much more complex than is believed in the cognition community, and I would rather wait until the dust settles.

5. Is the preattentive/attentive dichotomy real, or does it merely apply to the extremes of a continuous scale? This question is discussed in this dialogue.

6. How is fast search (i.e., scanning by scrutiny) at rates from 10 to 60 msec/item possible, when cuing locks focal attention to a place over 100 msec duration? This question is discussed in this dialogue.

7. Items in a crowded array do not pop out. It seems that lateral inhibition by neighboring elements reduces visibility. Is focal attention preventing this inhibition within its aperture? This question is self-explanatory. The reason why I did not want to go into details is the large literature devoted to this problem. At the same time, I do not believe that the essence of this inhibition is clarified–the more so, since the neurophysiological mechanisms should be further explored. When the aperture of focal attention was measured, the detection of a faint target was found to be enhanced within this aperture (Sagi and Julesz 1986). Now, is this enhancement in the aperture the same mechanism as the reduction of inhibition by neighbors outside the aperture?

8. Under what conditions is "where" parallel while "what" is serial, as Sagi and Julesz (1985) found in textures? This question is discussed in this dialogue.

9. What is the role of figure-ground separation in texture segmentation? Before we clarified the asym-metry effect of texture discrimination (Williams and Julesz 1991) by assuming that illusory contours close the gap (figure 9.10), I thought this effect was based on some complex figure-ground phenomenon. Now I see that bottom-up processes can explain it, because illusory contours can extracted by V2 in the monkey (von der Heydt, Peterhans, and Baumgartner 1988). I also noted that when one of the discriminated texture pair becomes the ground the high-SF components appear to dominate (Julesz 1977). So, besides texture segregation there must be another effect of perceiving one of the texture pair as the figure.

10. Is the asymmetry for "same"/"different" judgments the same for a few items presented transiently as for many items (forming texture-like aggregates) presented in a stationary way (due to lateral inhibition of nearby items)? This is a rather obscure question. Egeth and Blecker (1971) studied *single* patterns briefly presented and asked whether "same"/"different" judgment was mediated by different search mechanisms. For quasi-stationary *texture*s, the many items inhibit each other; thus, one can view them somewhat longer. Is there some similarity between these two paradigms? Egeth seemed taken aback when we raised the problem of "where" and "what" in vision (Sagi and Julesz 1985), which seemed to contradict his concepts. Recently, Egeth seems to have come to grips with our paradigm (Egeth and Dagenbach 1991). Again, I do not wish to dwell on differences between cognitive and perceptual interpretations of perceptual phenomena, and I only hope that the gap between these two disciplines will narrow as non-invasive methods will make some of the human thought processes directly visible.

11. Can nonlinear spatial filters explain filling-in effects, such as subjective-contours, and can they explain gap-completion effects too? In dialogue 9 I discuss the differences between the Rubenstein-Sagi (1990) and Williams-Julesz (1991) interpretations of the asymmetry effect of texture discrimination.

12. Is there only one searchlight of attention, or are there two or perhaps seven? This question is discussed in this dialogue.

13. Are there pre-cues of attention that can be (voluntarily) ignored in perception? This is an interesting problem with some practical consequences. Are there some powerful stimuli that capture our attention against our own will? Obviously some sudden moving target, as it enters our visual field, will elicit an almost reflexive shift to it; however, in a laboratory setup, could a relaxed observer be instructed to ignore a sudden cue? While this has been studied (Kröse and Julesz 1989), the problem has not been solved.

14. Does aperture size of focal attention scale (similarly to eccentricity) with other factors (e.g. element size)? This is another straightforward but difficult question. We have shown (Bergen and Julesz 1983) that texture discrimination scales with element size (and thus follows the Aubert-Foerster law). We have also shown (Sagi and Julesz 1986) that the size of focal attention scales with eccentricity. Whether the aperture size will also scale with the average element size in a texture is an interesting question that, to my knowledge, has not yet been solved.

15. What is the mechanism and where is the locus of focal attention? This question is discussed in this dialogue.

16. Is there learning in early vision (e.g., slowly getting better in discriminating an array of Ts from Ls)? Is this learning retinotopic (Karni and Sagi 1990)? Where is its locus? This question is, at the moment, close to a metaphysical problem, even though Karni and Sagi (1990) have shown that some of their learning phenomena do not transfer binocularly. Whether this lack of transfer always means some early visual process is another interesting problem whose outcome I do not know.

17. Are 3-D and shape-from-shading cues texton-like? For instance, is texture segregation between an array of small 2-D cubes that appear as convex or concave an early visual process? This question is discussed in this dialogue.

18. What kind of feature differences (texton gradients) can be detected preattentively (that is, when focal attention is engaged in some identification task)? This question is discussed in this dialogue.

19. Are there features that can be recognized (identified) preattentively? A large portion of dialogue 11 is devoted to this problem.

20. Is binocular hysteresis (Fender and Julesz 1967) due to fusional or binocular-matching (label-preserving) mechanisms? This highly specialized problem is discussed in dialogue 14.

21. Is color utilized by the magnocellular system (e.g., for motion or stereopsis) at iso-luminance, and can such neurophysiological problems be decided by psychological methods? This question is now solved. In dialogue 11 I will discuss recent findings under metaisoluminance (Kovacs and Julesz 1993; Gorea et al. 1993).

22. Are there processes in early vision that are not bottom-up but depend on top-down (semantic-memory-like) processes (e.g. the object-superiority

effect)? Do some segmentation processes that work on objects and their cast shadows require sophisticated semantics, thus top-down information? This question is discussed in great detail, in several places, in conjunction with the work of Jochen Braun.

23. At what stage, and how, do color, form (orientation), movement, and stereopsis begin to interact? This question is closely related to question 4, and the answer is not known.

24. In spite of a two-diopter difference between blue and red color resolution, due to the poor optics of the human eye (caused by the high chromatic aberration of the lens), why do we see both colors sharply when they are simultaneously presented? This problem is discussed in detail in dialogue 12, but without satisfactory solution.

25. Can one attend to scale (coarse versus fine detail, or low versus high spatial frequencies) the same way as to spatial location? This problem is related to question 14. Some research has been done (Julesz and Papathomas 1984), but the answer is controversial.

26. If a brain has N working neurons (each with two states), then the brain can be in $M = 2^N$ states. Thus, an additional $M - N$ retrieving neurons are needed to "sense" each state of the brain. These retrieving neurons can be regarded as the "grandmother cells." What other retrieval principles could those who do not accept such cells propose instead? This question is discussed in this dialogue.

27. How can seemingly similar spike histograms of aggregates neurons give rise to unique sensations, such as color, pitch, itch, and pain? Is it that some important neural parameter of activity has been overlooked, or is it that the brain areas that are stimulated determine the qualities of sensations (as Johannes Müller assumed in his doctrine of specific nerve energies)? Does any theory exist that would be more specific than Johannes Müller's concept formulated generations ago? This question is discussed in this dialogue. However, question 37 has some bearing on this problem.

28. If rapid search is limited to scanning rates of about 10–60 msec/item, how can observers perceive a large number of items in a complex image presented, say, for only 150 msec (Biederman 1985)? This question is discussed in this dialogue.

29. When is strabismus the cause of stereo blindness, and when does binocular neural disfunction cause strabismus? My most important quest is the diagnosis and possible prevention of stereo blindness. Unfortunately, the answer to this fundamental clinical question is not known. Parts of dialogue 7 are devoted to this problem. See also dialogue 14.

30. Are the "maturational windows (critical periods)" in early vision merely serving the need of fine tuning to the environment, or are there some sophisticated perceptual skills that can be acquired only within the critical period (similar to language acquisition)? I discussed this problem, to some extent, in dialogue 7.

31. Does the McCollough effect belong to early vision, or to some higher-level cortical stages? The famous McCollough effect is quite enigmatic. If the reader does adapt to alternate red-vertical and green-horizontal gratings for about 4 minutes, then black-and-white test patterns with horizontal and vertical stripes will appear to have the complementary colors of the adapting gratings. The effect does not seem to transfer binocularly and is rather retinotopic (thus it suggests some early processing), yet when one eye is patched (to prevent new

stimulation) the effect lasts for several days. The latter indicates some higher-level processes at work. This long-lasting aftereffect sets the McCollough effect apart from the many other contingent after-effects. For the latter, Barlow (1990) gives a plausible explanation based on modifiable inhibitory synapses (an extension of the modifiable excitatory synapses by Hebb (1949)). According to Barlow, in the McCollough effect the "redness" neurons and the "verticality" neurons are excited simultaneously, so the strength of mutual inhibition between them increases. When a vertical white grating is shown, this inhibits the redness neurons, so the lack of redness biases the output of the color system toward the green. This arguments seems to explain in general contingent aftereffects (say, between color and direction of movement) that last for a few seconds after adaptation, yet the real explanation of why the McCollough effect can last for days is still a mystery.

32. What is the difference between perceptual mechanisms that process "projections onto the retinae" and those that "project out in space"? This question is discussed in this dialogue.

33. Does stereopsis provide only relative depth, or do some overlooked parameters, such as convergence of the eye, contribute to absolute depth judgment? After all, it is believed that one can hit a nail with a long ruler more accurately when using both eyes; if this is true, how does it come about? This problem is addressed in detail in dialogue 12, where I discuss recent work by Hadani and Julesz (1992) and some neurophysiological findings by Trotter et al. (1992) that indicate that neurons exist in V1 that extract absolute depth information from extraretinal factors, probably accommodation and convergence.

34. Often correspondence, say, in stroboscopic (apparent) motion between successive patterns is based not on some obvious "similarity" but on some more complex features that enhance the cross-correlation between the corresponding patterns. Is it always the principle of maximum correlation that governs perceptual correspondence, or does some more complex function than correlation underlie perceptual behavior? This question is discussed in this dialogue.

35. Can we establish a relationship between the extrema of curvatures of 3-D objects and the extrema (or some other geometrical singularity) of their 2-D projections? Solving this important problem would extend the scope of the segmentation studies by Hoffman and Richards (1988). In visual cognition Hoffman and Richard (1988) showed that the extrema of curvature can help in figure-ground segmentation. Unfortunately this is extracted from the 2-D projection of object contours, and we still do not know how the original 3-D object contours' extrema relate to the extrema of their 2-D projections.

36. In noise-free systems where a function has many derivatives, a Taylor expansion at a local point defines the function globally. Are there examples in visual perception where local knowledge helps to restore the stimulus in its entirety? This question is discussed in this dialogue.

37. Is it possible to elicit color percepts in rods by temporal-spatial manipulations (Benham's top)? This is a question often asked (e.g. by Christof von Capenhausen) but not yet answered. In 1971 Charles Stromeyer III and I tried to elicit the usual Benham colors with temporally modulated stripes after we adapted observers in the dark and made sure that they were at their cone-break threshold,

so that only rods were functioning. Unfortunately we could not agree on the outcome, and this problem is still unsolved. If it were possible to elicit color sensations in rods by spatio-temporal modulation, we might be perhaps closer to a "code of the brain." In this unlikely event, the concept of the specific nerve energy would be extended to include, in addition to the neural site, a specific temporal code.

38. Can psychologists give neurophysiologists a hint as to what a cortical area's main function is? For instance, what is the main function of V1? This is a tricky question, but I can give a hint. We found (Kovacs and Julesz 1993; see also text related to figures 8.4 and 8.5) that closed curves made of Gabor patches (needles) pop out from an aggregate of needles, and this does not transfer to the other eye. If punctiform mapping of needles' position and orientation together with monocularity are indicators of V1 function in the monkey cortex, then is it the function of V1 to search for global closure?

39. With aging, it seems to me, the unit of time gets increasingly shorter. Does this mean a reduced perception of detail too, or is it merely a reduced sensation of duration? I recall vividly how, at parties 20 years ago, the late Rudi Kompfner (the inventor of the traveling-wave tube and a pioneer of the acoustical microscope) would ask his younger colleagues about their "Doppler shift" of time. Indeed, I recall in my childhood the boringly long Sunday afternoons, and now that I am over 60 time flies at a rapid pace as months rush by. If the sampling of time were as dense as that of spatial detail in a high-quality photograph, we could enlarge the image manyfold without loss in detail. However, as it is the case with digitally stored photographs of limited resolution, any zooming up will keep the stored resolution constant and will result in a coarse image. Thus, is this reduced time scale resulting in a loss of perceived quality of detail, or just a more economical way of storing things (as a 35-mm film might store very fine detail that can yield magnified images orders of magnitude larger)? Of course, such a question is much more complex than those related to early vision, and I pose it merely to encourage the reader to extend this list.

B: That is quite a list! While I like some of your questions, I am not convinced that some other more interesting ones could not be posed. I also find the order of your questions rather idiosyncratic. However, I like the challenge you give us with the strategic questions that are still "in the bag" (i.e., not explained in detail). I am sure that the challenge of taking them out of the bag will help the field to develop. Looking at the metascientific questions you listed in dialogue 6, a few of your colleagues will recognize the most important ones at first glance; some will single out the strictly experimental questions. However, for most of your readers the list looks like a big, big bag. Of course, they should read the entire book first, then the questions. But still, I think they would appreciate some clues about where you actually answer a question or elaborate on it. Or they might like some more explicit categorization of the questions–for example: Questions 5, 6, 7, 8, 12, 13, 14, 15, 18, 19, 25, and 28 are related to attention; questions 5, 12, 14, and 15 are more general ones asking about the existence, mechanism, locus, size, or number of attentional windows. Questions 18 and 19 are concerned with preattentive mechanisms, questions 6 and 28 with speed of attention; question 7 is more specific on the mechanism of attention. Finally, questions 13, 15 and 39 are explicitly unrelated to the others. You could also give a task to find the "odd men" from the whole selection; these might be specially interesting, since they are not related to the rest, and they might be the best candidates for new discoveries (e.g., question 31).

I also find some questions relating to new mathematical tools lacking.

A: This list of questions [first posed in Paris, at the ECVP Conference; see Julesz 1990a] was intended to inspire my esteemed colleagues to add their own. Obviously, some of the questions might turn out to be more strategic than others, and therefore a rank ordering is impossible. With respect to questions relating to mathematical tools, I will now list a few mathematical questions, but I emphasize that answering some of the 39 questions I raised above will probably require novel mathematical tools.

1*. Is it possible to extend the group concept so that it would be valid only within an interval, and not outside of it? (E.g., this could explain why a rotated face appears familiar within a certain angle but cannot be recognized beyond this angle.)

2*. The aperture problem of motion perception: What mathematical constraints would disambiguate the orientation of perceived motion in an aperture?

3*. Under what conditions can the 3-D shape of objects be determined from their 2-D projections (e.g. shape from shading)?

4*. Extrema of curvature of 2-D projections of 3-D objects seem useful in perceptual segmentation (Hoffman and Richards 1984). Can one establish a relationship between the extrema of curvatures of

3-D objects and the extrema (or some other geometrical singularity) of their 2-D projections?

5*. Further research on iso-second-order and iso-third-order texture pairs. For instance, can one create iso-fourth-order texture pairs that perceptually segregate? Regarding this question, I seem to share Hilbert's fate, since recently Yellott (1993) proved that textures with iso-third-order statistics are all identical. Even though my definition of textures differs from Yellott's [for a critique of Yellott's ideas see Victor et al. (in press)], it is clear that increasing the order of the statistical constraints makes the textures themselves more and more identical. In the light of my fallen iso-second-order texture conjecture (which led to the textons and showed that texture segregation is not a statistical problem), the search for iso-higher-order stochastic textures seems of limited value. However, the criticism of Yellot by Victor brings up the question whether an organism evolves for actually seen images or for an ensemble of stochastic processes that can generate them. In the latter case the study of stochastic textures with increasing order of constraints might still have some value.

6*. What kind of perturbations of objects can be perceived as one manipulates an object's shadow?

B: I notice that you have not listed several problems that you and your collaborators have worked on in great detail. Do you think that these are less important, or do you believe that you have already solved them? Furthermore, many of your listed questions are not novel, and I remember some articles in which others attacked them!

A: First, I will answer your last question. Obviously I do not claim that my questions are original or that I chose the most strategic ones! In this dialogue I merely list questions I regard as strategic, whether or not they were have been worked on. What these questions have in common–besides being strategic in my opinion–is that I regard them as still unsolved. Furthermore, I raised most of these questions three years ago, and I am glad that some of them are now being worked on by colleagues not affiliated with my laboratory.

With respect to your second question: Indeed, there are some unlisted problems that became paradigms in the last three decades and which therefore should be treated separately. Perhaps I should turn to these before I turn my attention to the listed questions.

One of these questions that I did not list, since I found it so strategic that I devoted much of my scientific life to it, is this: "How can the visual system reconstruct the best possible 3-D representation of the environment from two 2-D retinal projections?" Variants of this question (for example: How can the visual system reconstruct a 3-D relief from a single 2-D retinal projection containing the reflectance distributions of Lambertian surfaces from a specified light source?) have been successfully attacked by Horn and Brooks (1985), Pentland (1986), and Bülthoff and Mallot (1990), among others. The first question led to the introduction of random-dot stereograms and random-dot cinematograms into psychology (Julesz 1960); their impact on brain research is reviewed in Julesz 1986 and in Julesz 1991b. In essence, computer-generated random-dot stereograms and cinematograms showed that—contrary to common belief—stereopsis and motion perception are *global* processes, based on some cross-correlation kind of operation, and do not require the enigmatic cues

of semantics and gestalt. This insight permitted global stereopsis and short-range motion perception to be linked to the neurophysiology of the input stages to the cortex. That is why nowadays I use the term "early visual perception" instead of "cyclopean perception."

The second strategic problem that I did not list for similar reasons was my 1962 question: What statistical parameters underlie preattentive texture discrimination? This led to many mathematical inventions that produced stochastic texture pairs with identical second- and third-order statistics. The surprising outcome of this paradigm was the realization that–contrary to common belief– preattentive human texture discrimination was not governed by global (statistical) parameters, but was based on the density of *quasi-local* features, which I called textons. Recently Fogel and Sagi (1989) and, independently, Malik and Perona (1990) developed texture-segmentation algorithms based on local spatial filters (the former used oriented Gabor filters, the latter difference of Gaussian filters) followed by a quasi-local nonlinear operation (simple squaring by Fogel and Sagi, some inhibition between neighboring elements by Malik and Perona) and a second spatial filter for final segmentation. I will return to these models and their implications when I discuss figure 9.9.

In summary, I think that these two problems I raised in my youth were proven "strategic" and became paradigms, as attested by my many colleagues who devoted their efforts to render the strategic problems paradigms.

A third problem that preoccupied me during the last decade is focal attention and the role it plays in early vision. In more general terms, this problem is related to the preattentive/attentive dichotomy of vision. In 1962, when I started to work on effortless texture discrimination (that is, discrimination without scrutiny), I was more interested in discrimination than in the process of scrutiny. Later I even adopted Ulrich Neisser's term "preattentive" for "effortless," "instantaneous," and "automatic," which I had used previously. It was only in 1979 that I became actively interested in focal attention. My first paper on textons and asymmetries in texture perception (Julesz 1981) attests to this new focus. First with Peter Burt and then with Jim Bergen, I developed a technique of presenting a target element among an array of distractors followed by a masking array with variable delays (SOA). This backward masking proved to be quite effective, and correct responses as a function of SOA gave interesting insights into some properties of focal attention. Our work differs from the influential work of Anne Treisman basically in presenting targets and distractors as a dense array, so that they formed textures, as we were less concerned with sporadic targets and distractors that are widely scattered. Furthermore, even though masking is a tricky business, I trust the direct SOA findings in the 16–120-msec range more than the indirect measurements of the slopes of reaction-time (RT) curves, where the RTs are typically in the 1000-msec range.

B: For a change, let me pose a question; you may list it as question 40 if you accept it as strategic. You regarded your elimination of false target matches as the fundamental problem of stereopsis. As a matter of fact, you called the stereopsis of the RDS "global stereopsis," to emphasize that no local tokens exist that might help the elimination of "false-target noise." However, recently some re-searchers have defined higher-order local primitives (Jones and Malik 1992; Anderson and Nakayama 1994). If you select adequately complex primitives, does the false target-problem seem to evaporate?

A: I discuss your question in detail in the chapter on global stereopsis in Julesz 1978. For instance, I have several examples of RDSs in which each even row (column) portrays one depth surface, while each odd row (column) portrays another surface, and one can perceive two transparent surfaces in vivid depth. How could an algorithm find these odd-even horizontal vectors? Of course, real-life images contain unique features that reduce the matching noise problem. However, transparent random-element stereograms, when fused, are the existence proof of what the visual system ultimately can cope with.

As a matter of fact these new developments remind me of my youth, when I wrote AUTOMAP-1, the first computer algorithm on a digital computer (Julesz 1962). At the time automatic stereo-contour-map plotters existed, driven by analog computers that helped mapmakers who sat at stereo comparators and tried to fuse stereo pairs of the terrain and drew contours in depth. If the selected aperture was small, many false targets were generated. On the other hand, a large aperture led to inaccurate localization and, worse, too many irrelevant half-occluded features diminished the correlation in the left and right apertures. AUTOMAP-1 was my answer to this dilemma. I started with the smallest pixel size, and then a relaxational (cooperative) process swelled the aperture size, but such that it tried to emulate the shape of the target to be fused! In the present approaches a large aperture size is selected [with appropriately complex primitives (vectors)], and then the aperture might be narrowed as the result of finding unrelated half-occlusions. Whether my approach of swelling and their ideas of narrowing the aperture do converge to the same solution remains to be seen.

The entire field of automating depth perception reminds me of the field of automatic speech generation and recognition, where the thousand times less information just barely permits the "concatenation" of phonemes and syllables in real time. Speech sounds very different depending on how a unit of speech is surrounded by others, and recently an "encyclopedia" of such rules has been published by Olive et al. (1993). I can predict a similar trend in machine vision. As memory size will further grow, one could concatenate patches of visible and half-occluded areas where the texture and color of these adjacent patches might have their probabilities stored that in turn help to eliminate false matches.

I turn now to some other problems that are on my list. Since work on focal attention is not as advanced as that on the other two paradigms discussed above, I will continue with questions from the list related to attention, and evaluate their present status. I start with question 6. This question is a very profound one and concerns the paradox that it seems to take considerable time to shift attention to a cue, and even more time to disengage attention from this cue (Nakayama and Mackeben 1989), and therefore it is not clear how one can shift attention rapidly from item to item. These serial shifts of focal attention underlying scrutiny can take place rapidly without eye move-

ment. The answer probably is based on confusion about the term "focal attention."

Focal attention was first mentioned by Helmholtz (1896). However the speed of Helmholtz's searchlight of attention shifts is not clearly stated. Helmholtz presented his stimuli in a brief flash to avoid eye movements, but before the onset of the stimulus he steadily fixated on a mark and simultaneously placed his attention to a focus that was remote from the fixation spot. He observed that attention helped him greatly to perceive items around this focus. He did not mention how much time it would take to place his focal attention to the desired focus. This might take 150 msec or longer (Posner 1978). On the other hand, many authors (including me) used focal attention to connotate a rapid search process. Sperling et al. (1973) achieved 40 msec/4 items = 10 msec/item scanning rates. This rapid "reading" rate was only made possible by avoiding changes in focal attention and eye movements by placing in the same aperture, by electronic means, an array of 4×1 characters at 25 frames/sec.

So, the many experimental results that are interpreted by the metaphor of the "searchlight of attention" scanning with a speed of about 10–60 msec/item (Sternberg 1966; Weichselgartner and Sperling 1987; Treisman and Gelade 1980; Bergen and Julesz 1983) should be called "rapid scanning." Jukka Saarinen and I measured the scanning speed of focal attention directly by briefly presenting (with masking) 2–4 numbers at random locations, and though observers made mistakes in reporting the order in the sequence, they could follow and identify as many as four consecutive numbers at 30 msec/item with few errors. Recently, however, we presented the same 2–4 numbers in parallel followed by a mask 16 and 32 msec later (Hung et al., submitted for publication) and found better performance than in the serial study by Saarinen and Julesz (1991). We presented our items (numbers) at *different* random locations (on a circle around a fixation point) such that subsequent numbers were placed far from each other to avoid lateral inhibition (crowding), which had been observed years earlier (Sagi and Julesz 1986). So it seems that if items are presented at some distance to avoid lateral inhibition, one can achieve the rapid scanning observed both by RT slopes and masking techniques.

The question of why during rapid search one can avoid the locking of attention to a given cue position is because of this confusing use of the terminology of "focal attention." If we avoid to use rapid scanning to mean focal attention and use it for the slower process, then in situations when a marker is presented in the vicinity of an already presented item, as practiced by Nakayama and Mackeben (1989) and Kröse and Julesz (1989), one cannot dislodge the cue for over 100 msec. As long as the experimenter shows items in this captured aperture, without having to dislodge it from the cue, the obserever can read out items at 40 msec/4 items = 10 msec/item. However, one cannot move the aperture of focal attention from the cue for about 100–150 msec duration to a new position.

B: How could researchers misconstrue "rapid scanning" and "shifts of focal attention"?

A: This is the result of the preattentive-attentive theories of Treisman and Gelade (1980) and Julesz (1962,1981). Certain items (disjunctions or strong texton gradients, respectively) pop out, while others (conjunctions or weak texton gradients) require time- consuming element-by-element scrutiny. The pop-out is regarded as an almost instantaneous (parallel) process, while scrutiny is a serial search. [See figure 4.4.] It is this serial search that both Treisman and Julesz called attentive search. To call it "shifts of focal attention" might have been a mistake; "rapid search" might have been a better description. Nevertheless, because this scrutiny is attentive (as opposed to preattentive), and does not require eye movements, the metaphor of the shifting searchlight is justified even though misleading.

At the same time that nearby items inhibit each other, it is interesting that when observers identify a target by attending on it, this mental operation "lights up" the vicinity of the attended item and the detection of a dim test flash is much enhanced in this vicinity (Sagi and Julesz 1986). As we see, many problems of the rapid scanning of attention are not solved. Question 12 [the number of searchlights] is related to focal versus divided attention. Is there only one searc light, or are there more? If there are more that act simultaneously, are these discrete searchlights equivalent to the resource metaphor of divided attention? According to an interesting paradigm by Pylyshyn (1991), observers can simultaneously track at least four object among many randomly moving ones. Thus, which of the various metaphors of attention (searchlight, divided resources, bottleneck, filters, and so on) is valid is another important unsolved question.

Here I turn to the related questions 5, 8, and 18: whether the preattentive/attentive dichotomy is real as posed by Treisman and her collaborators (Treisman and Gelade 1980; Julesz and Bergen 1983), or whether it is just a metaphor pointing to the two extrema of a continuous scale of attention strength (as we found in experiments where the responses varied with the positional accuracy of the texton gradients (Bergen and Julesz 1983). Interestingly, the problem of preattentive/attentive dichotomy can be further refined. The first step in this direction was the finding by Sagi and Julesz (1985) that detecting the position of a texton-gradient could be accomplished in parallel (independent of the number of distractors), while identifying the actual orientation or color of an element at·the location of the texton gradient required element-by-element scrutiny (which monotonically increased with the number of distractors). Unfortunately, in this study the question of detection versus identification is blurred. After all, the detection of a very fine positional variation is similar to pattern recognition, and the coarse identification of a blurred pattern might permit the estimation of its position. Therefore, a recent refinement of an experimental procedure by Braun and Sagi (1990) deserves special mention. They made the "two-visual-system" concept even stronger by showing that while loading attention (by asking the observer to identify a letter) it was possible to carry out simultaneously the detection of texture gradients without interfering with the identification task, but, surprisingly, perceptual grouping affected identification. Jochen Braun and I are now searching systematically for perceptual tasks that can be performed without interfering with the identification task. Of course, it is crucial that focal attention is engaged during the entire identification task, so it cannot quickly inspect the surround for further identification. That is one reason why in our masking paradigm it is so crucial to determine the highest search speeds. Regardless of the outcome of

these studies, the existence of two visual systems that operate simultaneously, such that one can perceive certain features in the environment without attention is a most interesting insight in brain research. [For additional comments on the work of Braun and Julesz, see dialogue 11.]

B: I do not understand the rationale of the Saarinen-Julesz (1991) experiment. There is solid evidence over a generation that vision is a parallel process. Therefore it is immaterial whether one scans a few items in 200 msec, in 32 msec, or even in 1 msec. The only result of erasing the stimulus at increasingly briefer times is to reduce the signal/noise ratio, thus decreasing performance. In my opinion there should be no difference between your rapid step-by-step presentation and presenting all the items simultaneously and masking them with an SOA of 16 msec!

A: Your comments are based on the findings of several investigators (Eriksen and Spencer 1969; Shiffrin and Gardner 1972; Shiffrin et al. 1973) that performance was essentially the same between simultaneous target presentation and sequential presentations at different rates, based on 50 msec/item scanning rates with masking. From this finding it was concluded that the bottleneck must be the limitation of short-term memory. However, using three-times-faster rates, we found (Hung et al., in preparation) that, in contrast to previous findings, the percentage of correct responses was better for simultaneous than for sequential presentation. Also, for both the simultaneous and sequential presentations, performance declined as the presentation rate increased. In particular, performance dropped much more for the serial presentation than for the simultaneous case. These results indicate that some of the informational bottleneck ("the magic number of 7 ± 2") might be due to the perceptual strategies observer's use to read in information into the short-term memory. For simultaneous presentation these strategies are better matched to the input mechanisms of short-term memory, while for the serial presentation at a random order the scanning rules violate the structure of these mechanisms. We found, confirming the findings of Saarinen and Julesz (1991), that it is still possible to report four sequentially presented characters at acceptable accuracy if temporal order is not required, and it can be done at 16.7 msec/character rates.

Schiffrin and his collaborators did not speculate about this bottleneck, but instead concluded that the identity of serial versus parallel performance at 50 msec/item must hold at even much faster rates and therefore no shifts in focal attention are necessary for this process. Having established that at faster than 50 msec/item scanning rates serial performance deteriorates much faster than parallel performance, we do not know how they would interpret these results. We have nothing to say about whether this bottleneneck is related to focal attention or merely reflects a mismatch between our serial scanning routine and the rules of the input mechanism.

Furthermore, it has been shown (Sagi and Julesz 1985) that *detecting* the position of a texton gradient, or *counting* the number of such gradients, could be accomplished in parallel (independent of the number of distractors), while *identifying* the actual orientation or color of an element at the location of the texton gradient required element-by-element scrutiny (which monotonically in-

creased with the number of distractors). So your original hypothesis that the recognition of alphanumeric characters is a parallel process is only true for nonattentive tasks, such as localizing a texton gradient in a dense array, while identifying the target at this location requires serial scrutiny (usually requiring a cue; that is, a texton gradient) to find the spot to be scrutinized. Whether this serial process is due to shifts of focal attention or to some other bottleneck in the processing of complex forms is another question and cannot be decided on at present.

B: I am still not satisfied with the way serial and parallel processing are defined. The idea of Sternberg, Treisman, Sperling, you, and your co-workers to define parallel processing as independent of the item (distractor) number, while parallel processing increases with item number, is not very convincing to me. Townsend (1972) created stochastic processes that could not be identified as parallel or serial by this criterion. (You used to quote George Sperling's quip about the serial/parallel dichotomy: "Is rain a serial or parallel process?" At first approximation people would regard rain a parallel process, but sitting on individual raindrops one could change his opinion.)

A: For me this definition is quite convincing. I am rather worried about not knowing whether the serial search process is, indeed, due to the need to scrutinize the complex items by focal attention, or whether it is only some processing bottleneck that takes time to recognize items in memory. The problem of parallel versus serial search is further complicated by the dichotomy between texture segregation and finding a target among a number of distractors. Preattentive versus attentive texture discrimination refers to textures that I define as an array of elements so dense that the elements are within a critical distance, about twice the average element size (Julesz 1996b). Texture pairs defined this way either appear as two distinct entities or require element-by-element scrutiny. Research in cognition, particularly by Shiffrin and Schneider (1977) and by Treisman and her collaborators, uses a target among distractors, and if the RT increases with the number of distractors for finding a target, then the search is called serial. When the target is present, the slope (of RT/distractor number) appears half of the slope when the target is absent. This finding is regarded as an indication of a terminable search process. For conspicuous targets the slope is almost parallel, a finding that in cognition is called a "parallel search." *Because in the cognitive literature the spatial density between targets and distractors is usually larger than the critical size to form a texture, one cannot compare texture discrimination with target search in sparse arrays.* [The reader might find a comparison between these two processes by Jeremy Wolfe (1992) of interest.] In dialogue 3 I discussed some of these problems in more detail. Now I turn to the problem of neurophysiological findings of attention.

This renaissance of attentional studies by cognitive and perceptual psychologists is paralleled by the neurophysiologists. Robert Desimone and his collaborators (Moran and Desimone 1985; Desimone and Ungerleider 1989) found neurons in V4 whose firing for certain trigger features changed in accordance with the focal attention of the monkey. I highly recommend that my psychologist colleagues study these important papers carefully. Obviously, no speculation can answer question 15, and the neurophysiologist can work on this question only by using some of the sophisticated techniques of the psychophysicist. Whether some of the novel non-invasive techniques (such as PET scans) might have adequate spatio-temporal resolution to permit psychologists to work on locus questions, without the help of physiologists, is an important technical question that only time can answer. [As the reader might have noticed, I did not list any of the crucial technical breakthroughs in the making by phrasing them in question form, such as "Would it be possible to perform microsurgery by ablating specific brain tissues with monoclonal antibodies?" or "Could the direct-optical-inspection-of-brain-activity method pioneered by Grinvald and his collaborators (Ts'o et al. 1990) be further improved such that brains with many sulci can be studied *in vivo?*"]

The interesting question 17 stems from the work of Enns (1986), who made up arrays of little Necker cubes with targets (cubes) favoring one kind of 3-D depth organization amidst cubes biased in the dual 3-D organization. This depth from 3-D perspective cues yields preattentive texture segmentation ("pop-out"), with the implication that, in addition to the textons of brightness, color, orientation and aspect ratio of elongated blobs, flicker, motion, and stereopsis, even perceived depth in 2-D perspective drawings might act as a texton. Accordingly, some primitive 3-D processing of depth based on mechanisms processing shape (depth) from shading and occlusion might belong to early vision. Recently, Jennifer Sun and Pietro Perona (1993) extended Enns's study. They found that some tasks involving shaded elements (that yield 3-D interpretations) can be performed in parallel for durations as short as 50 msec. However, unshaded line targets of the similar shapes are processed serially, so SOA increases with number of distractors. Only shapes with familiar configurations and lighting conditions may be perceived preattentively. They suggest that preattentive processing of shape may depend upon local calculations that focus on salient 3-D cues like shaded Y-junctions, and is generally unaffected by high-level cues like context information.

Of course, the second possibility is that early vision cannot be solely bottom-up but must include (besides focal attention) some top-down processes too! This is question 22, a fundamental problem in brain research. Indeed if we can demonstrate that most of the perceptual processes in global stereopsis, motion perception, and texture discrimination are essentially bottom-up, their linking to present neurophysiological results obtained in early cortical areas of V1, V2, V3, V4, or MT is now possible. This is also in agreement with David Marr's view of computational vision as basically bottom-up. However, Roger Watt (1988) argues for algorithms in early vision that are under the control of high-level processes as well as memory. This is an unsettled problem. For example, Jih Jie Chang and I (Chang and Julesz 1990) showed that depth from shape-from-shading processes yields a monocularly strong percept; this depth is completely dominated by global stereopsis. This would argue again that global stereopsis is a bottom-up process that overrides many top-down processes or operates independently of them. On the other hand, there are many perceptual phenomena that depend on high-level processes, including semantic memory. A well-known example in cognition is the word-superiority effect, which denotes the fact that the recognition of certain letters is superior when

contained in an English word than when contained in a nonsense word. This makes a lot of sense, since recognition of letters and words is surely a high-level semantic process. However, as Naomi Weisstein and Charlie Harris (1974) have shown, the same phenomenon exists in visual perception; they named it the object-superiority effect. The detection of a line segment of certain orientation was greatly improved if the segment belonged to a line drawing that portrayed a 3-D object, deteriorated if the segment belonged to a random line drawing, and was the worst if the line segment was shown in isolation.

Of course, object and form recognition are enigmatic, high-level processes in which semantics and gestalt organization play prominent roles. Therefore, the experiments by Gorea and Julesz (1990) are of special interest. We converted the object-superiority effect from an identification paradigm into a detection paradigm as follows. We presented an array of oblique line segments into which three horizontal and one vertical line segments were inserted as shown in figure 8.2. These four non-oblique line segments were clumped in a random fashion or organized to represent a primitive human face (two vertical lines representing the eyes, the vertical line segment between the eyes representing the nose, and the bottom horizontal line segment portraying the mouth). Observers were not aware that occasionally a face was presented, and were asked only to detect any line segment that was not oblique. Surprisingly, observers detected the horizontal and vertical line segments better when they belonged to the faces than when they belonged to the random clump (or to a symmetric four-line-segment symmetric pattern that was not a face). I always had assumed that the detection of a line segment in a texture [based on a texture (texton) gradient between adjacent orientation differences] was a simple parallel bottom-up process. And here is a case where even such a simple perceptual task might depend on top-down processing! I say "might" because the effect is very small (though statistically significant) and only four observers were tested. Because of the importance of this experiment, I would like others to repeat this study with more observers, perhaps inventing some other experimental designs.

Next I will take up question 28. This question is related to the interesting experiments by Biederman (1988), who flashed a complex image briefly and reported that his observers could correctly identify many objects and scenes contained in the image. This finding always puzzled me, since observers could at most capture only 4–9 items. If

these items are objects in a real-life scene, then these items are meaningful chunks with well-known relations between them. Now, we know from the work of Chase and Simon (1973) that a grandmaster of chess can reconstruct a briefly presented chess board from 5–7 chunks, but only if the board configuration resulted from a real game. If the board configuration was random, grandmasters' recall was no better than that of beginners. Since real-life scenes are rich in thousands of semantic cues that relate objects to one another, and since many subset of objects that relate to each other form a chunk, it is not so surprising that Biederman's observers do well with briefly presented TV frames. After all, every human who is not legally blind is a grandmaster of visual perception.

B: I am disappointed that you spent much time on your favorite questions but did not clarify some of your other questions that I find quite interesting even though I only guess their meanings.

A: Time does not permit me to dwell on each of the many questions I listed. Most of them are self-explanatory, at least to the experts, and this essay is written for the experts. Furthermore, I hope that each question evokes rather different associations for my colleagues, and I do not want to interfere with this creative process. I am also convinced that many of my colleagues would add other questions to my list and remove several existing ones. Indeed, it is this lack of consensus in psychobiology that reminds me of the fragmentation of molecular biologists before the discovery of the structure and role of DNA. As a matter of fact, each time I read my own list some new questions come to my mind, and I am surprised that I did not think of them

Figure 8.2

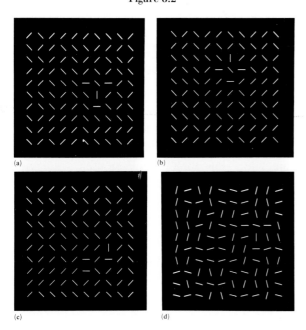

(a)

(b)

(c)

(d)

before. I would be grateful if my colleagues, particularly those who believe in my paradigms, would add their strategic questions to this list.

Just to illustrate what I mean by free associations about these problems, let me discuss question 1 [on retinotopic versus environmental coordinates], which I regard as fundamental but which I did not work on directly (except for an interesting collaborative effort with Bruno Breitmeyer, which was inconclusive because of technical difficulties with the afterglow of phosphors in video monitors—see Breitmeyer et al. 1982). If a worker in AI ponders this question, David Marr's three-level hierarchy of "primal sketch," "2.5-D sketch," and "stick figures" (1982) will come to mind. My own first thought is related to Emmert's Law, and my first demonstrations of it were to my introductory psychology classes. I "burned" a bright spot on the retina of my students with a flash whose afterimage could last for several seconds and ask them to "project" this afterimage on actual surfaces in the classroom at different distances from them. Since the size of the afterimage perceptually zooms in inverse fashion (to achieve size constancy) with physical distance, one can appreciate that the problem of the relationship between retinal coordinates and environmental coordinates is intimately coupled in early vision. [Recently, instead, I mount a tiny monitor on a spectacle frame together with a half-silvered mirror and portray a text on the screen. Depending on whether the observer looks through the transparent mirror at a nearby or a far surface, the letters in the text shrink or expand, respectively. I have many other associations in mind, and I leave the rest to my readers.]

Here is another example to illustrate my free association to question 3 (How is motion blur avoided without a "shutter"? Could it be that cortical shifter circuits are used?): From early youth I was intrigued that we can perceive stroboscopic (apparent) motion from a sequence of still pictures in a movie. It was obvious that a quickly presented frame would exponentially fade and somehow would be interpolated into the next frame. Much of the echoic memory experiments by George Sperling and his followers supported this view. Leo Ganz, and his student Bruno Breitmeyer (who worked with me as my second postdoc), believed that backward masking by metacontrast was a way to ensure apparent motion perception by preventing the previous frame from lingering. However, both echoic storage and metacontrast masking might have time constant too long in duration for the best apparent motion rates. I was also impressed by the work of David Burr (1980), who explicitly raised this problem in recent times. I was even more illuminated by the discovery of Vincent Di Lollo (1978, 1980), who showed a sequence of dots randomly displayed on the surface of a monitor, say, at 20 msec/dot. Observer would see at any time only six dots having equal brightness. The "oldest" dot appeared as bright as the "youngest" one. Yet, after an additional 20 msec the oldest dot died (disappeared) and a new dot appeared. When the presentation rate was decreased to 40 msec/dot, only three dots were seen simultaneously. This finding indicated that there was a "stack memory" with a 120-msec time window without any exponential decay. As the most recent item entered the stack, the oldest would be pushed out. Furthermore, with brighter dots the memory span was reduced to, say, 100 msec. So, here again the memory span is too long for the best apparent motion perception, which occurs around 16–32 msec/frame. Of course, the possibility exists that apparent movement is processed in MT (V4) or higher and not in the earliest cortical stages. I usually stressed that when one is viewing a dynamic RDS the individual dots appear in random walk, but never cross a depth boundary. I always interpreted this robust observation to mean that first depth is processed by stereopsis mechanism and only then are the nearest dots in depth identified as belonging to each other in successive time frames. So, I assume that the interpolation between two successive still pictures (in order to perceive apparent motion) might occur at some cortical stage where adequate computational power is available to process the images rapidly.

Of course, my associations might be all wrong. Apparent motion could be just an epiphenomenon of motion constancy. As objects move or we move (both with our body and eyes), the world outside appears stable to us, even though its retinal projection moves around. This perceptual stabilization must occur very early in the processing link where the spatial representation of the retinal image is still precisely preserved. For instance, David Van Essen believes that some of the many neurons in the input layers of V1 might be shift registers that compensate for rapid shifts of the retinal projections of moving objects. Maybe apparent motion perception is just a special case of motion compensation and should occur in V1. Since stereopsis of RDS is also processed as early as the first layers of V1, my observation that motion must be processed after stereopsis is neurophysiologically possible. Also my thinking of a hierarchy of processing stages might be all wrong. Most likely there might be complex feedback loops between various specialized modules that extract stereopsis, depth from motion,

motion, motion constancy, compensation for occlusion, auditory stereo, etc., and it depends on their priorities how the perceptual system evaluates them. Hanspeter Oswald and I showed how motion from cyclopean depth (without monocular cues) and monocular motion (based on moving luminance contours) is combined by probability summation at some higher perceptual stage (Julesz and Oswald 1978). I am quite sure that the reader has very different associations to this questions, and this is the reason why I am hesitant to continue.

For further illustration, let me elaborate on question 2* [on the orientation of perceived motion in an aperture]. When a grating or a single line is moving behind an aperture such that the terminators of the line are hidden, the direction of the motion is ambiguous. Without additional cues, usually one perceives motion at right angles to the moving gratings. Adelson and Movshon (1982) and Hildreth (1984) have studied this problem in detail. However, it was Reichardt and Egelhaaf (1988) who pointed out mathematically that, contrary to common belief, the ambiguity of motion in an aperture, called "the aperture problem" by Wallach and O'Connel (1953), can be locally solved by two correlation-type motion detectors. Recently, Ramachandran (1990) made contributions to this problem by showing that the aperture problem could be solved for drifting plaid patterns as long as the plaids were not transparent. However, if one grating of the plaid pattern appeared transparent, so that the other grating was perceived as being behind the first, the two gratings would drift independently from each other in ambiguous directions. This demonstration serves to illustrate Ramachandran's view of the many bags of tricks the visual system uses in trying to disambiguate ill-posed problems. On the other hand, Werner Reichardt and his collaborators have looked for some general mathematical principles that are necessary and sufficient to solve the aperture problem. I think both approaches are useful in vision research.

It is not by error that I included question 27 [neural spike histograms and sensation] in my list in spite of calling it a metascientific problem in dialogue 6. Somehow it is my feeling that with luck we can add a little more to Johannes Müller's doctrine of specific nerve energies. One thing that comes to my mind is optokinetic movement perception. In 1976, during my sabbatical year in Günther Baumgartner's neurological laboratory at the University of Zürich, I watched some experiments by the neurophysiologist Volker Henn and his collaborators. They would probe with a single microelectrode some vestibular neurons in a monkey's cortex, while the chair of the monkey was rotated or an optical cylinder with vertical stripes was rotated around the monkey. Similar to humans, both stimuli induced the percept of self-movement, or circular vection, (similar to the ambiguity of not knowing whether one's train started to move or a nearby train has started to leave the platform). The novelty in Henn's experiments was that he was recording from a neuron one synapse away from the vestibular organ, and this neuron responded the same way for mechanical acceleration of the chair or for optical acceleration of the grating. Although Johannes Müller (1844) emphasized in his *Handbook of Human Physiology* (which I read in German recently, translating into English some relevant paragraphs; see Julesz 1992b) that the same visual percepts (sensations) can be evoked either by visual stimulation or by producing me-chanical or electrical phosphenes (e.g. by pressing slightly against the eyeball), the situation here is slightly different. If, for instance, the vestibular neurons that are tuned to mechanical acceleration, or the visual neurons that are tuned to temporal acceleration of spatial gratings, are very close in the brain to the neurons that respond equally to both, then there are two possibilities: Either this neuron is merely combining the two modalities and transmitting them to a further stage where the "specific nerve energy for perceiving self-motion" resides, or this neuron belongs to the neural structure that elicits the percept of circular vection. It might take decades to probe the brain in order to find out whether there are some higher centers that give rise to circular vection in addition to the ones already found. However, if one is convinced that no higher center exists (a rather difficult claim to make), then there is some hope of elucidating the mysteries of qualia. Of course, arguments can be made similar to that for V4 as the earliest brain structure that gives rise to the sensation of color, but I believe that the vestibular neurons belong to a simpler system that is more appropriate for probing the doctrine of specific nerve energies.

B: I still think that, while some of your listed questions are adequately understood, some others are still rather obscure. For instance, the psychological questions 2 and 32 might not be obvious to me.

A: Let me dwell then on question 2. Many colleagues believe that the poorer resolution in the periphery can be compensated for by presenting, say, letters with increased sizes at larger and larger eccentricities. [This is the famous Aubert-Foester law, often quoted by Helmholtz (1896).] However, this is not always the case. In a classic paper, Sperling and Melchner (1978) showed that when such stimuli are shown (i.e., stimuli compensated by the cortical magnification factor) these cannot be focally attended as well as arrays of letters with equal sizes (provided the most peripheral letters can be still resolved). However, Farrel and Pelli (1993) found that for identification one can attend to different scales simultaneously as well as to a single scale.

Similarly, question 32 might require further elucidation. We often take for granted that 3-D stimuli that cast their 2-D projections on our retinae are perceived as being actually "projected out" in the environment at some x, y, z position. That the latter is not an ability to be taken for granted is clearly demonstrated by Békésy (1960), who would stimulate two distant areas of the skin and search for the observer's perceived position in between, and even ask whether one could learn to sense the position projected outside of the skin surface.

B: I have difficulty even with some of your questions that are spelled out in detail, yet I am unsure what you really are after. For instance, could you elaborate on question 34 [on perceptual shape correspondence for motion]? I also have great difficulty with question 26, particularly with the fashionable question of the existence of "pontifical" or "grandmother" neurons!

A: I am glad you asked for clarification of question 34, which has preoccupied me since my first psychological paper (Julesz 1960) until now, when it has become quite fashionable again. I discussed it at length in dialogues 2 and 8. In figure 4.6 I

showed from my 1960 article an RDS in which I broke the diagonal connectivities in one of the stereo images, and, as the reader can attest, the two images appear very dissimilar. However, since the binocular correlation is still as high as 84%, the two images can be easily fused. Indeed, when one defocuses the two images, they appear very similar; since the low-SF spectrum is identical and only the high-SF spectra (which can be removed by blurring) differ. Here the notions of "similar" and "dissimilar" are based on some "common sense" concept of geometrical congruency which we might call "folk similarity." So, the notion that for stereopsis it is the similarity based on binocular correlation (a global statistical measure) that gives rise to binocular fusion, instead of local folk similarity, was firmly established in 1960. The same stimulus, when shown as an RDC, yields motion too. After all, the concept of correlation is of basic importance both for stereopsis and for motion perception. However, the fact that for these stimuli the low-SF spectra agree and in turn can be noticed in the blurred image makes the distinction between psychological similarity and folk similarity not very dramatic. What I am asking is this: Would it be possible to create images that have no low-SF spectra, thus differing only in their high-SF spectra, and would appear very different when the two arrays are compared (have no folk similarity), yet would yield stereopsis or motion, based on some global measure (perhaps some generalization of correlation)?

Question 26 is composed of two questions. First I pondered how the brain can "sense" its own states. This is partly a metascientific question, but it also has a more tractable side. The reader probably has seen or used relays. These are magnetic switches with many contacts that were used in telephone exchanges in my youth. Now, say, a memory circuit composed of 10 relays [where each relay can be on or off] can store 2^{10}=1024 states. The many contacts of these relays can uniquely be connected to 1024 output wires indicating all the states the circuit happens to be in. However, these are contacts and not relays. If relays had only one contact, one would need 1024 more relays to be able to read out the number of states the original circuit with 10 relays could be in. If in place of the relays one substitutes N neurons in the brain, then this brain can be in 2^N states (if we assume that a neuron has only two states). Again the question arises: What other device (corresponding to "contacts") reads out the state of the ensemble of neurons? Does the brain consists of merely $M = \log N$ storage neurons, and does the rest merely read out the states of these M neurons? Or does the brain use all its N neurons for storage and reads out the 2^N states by some huge chemical machinery? Perhaps, when the brain is sensing any of its states, then this is the direct read out by chemical molecules whose fine structure we directly sense?

B: Your argument sounds silly. Brains do not have to read out their states. They have the ability to sense their states directly! Psychologists should not bother with how this sensing is achieved. It is one of the hidden assumptions, perhaps one of the fundamental axioms of psychobiology, *that brains do sense their mental states, and this is the very essence of thinking!* I hope you will have more sense when you discuss grandmother detectors, introduced by Horace Barlow and others.

A: Grandmother cells are closely related to the problem of how the 2^N states of the brain can be read out. As I suggested in my previous paragraph, one could have state-sensing neurons that are the final mental thoughts or percepts, including our image of grandmother. Since there are not enough neurons to encode (represent) this enormous number of states (percepts, thoughts), the idea of such grandmother neurons is not well received by psychobiologists. I used to tell my students that these pontifical cells did not have to be single neurons. After all, a single dot's Fourier spectrum is uniformly distributed noise and the two descriptions are isomorphic. So, if the brain would store the Fourier transform of a Dirac function (an infinitesimal dot) that is uniform white noise, or the Fourier (or some similar) transform of grandmother's face, it would be stored by a large number of distributed neurons, instead of a few or even one.

However, until recently I did not think of the ingenious alternative that is suggested by the findings of the neurophysiologists Kuniyoshi Sakai and Yasushi Miyashita (1991). They found association units in the inferotemporal (IT) cortex in great abundance that formed long-lasting correlations between any two patterns (A and B) of the most complex designs (made of fractals) that were presented within a brief temporal window. After a few trials, when pattern A was presented to a trained unit it would not fire for any other complex shape, except for B. Since there probably exist billions of such association units in IT, the concept of a grandmother unit is unnecessary. After all, one such unit will fire for a face seen in profile and from front view. Grandma's spectacles will be associated with her hair and her smile. So thousand of such association units will form *at random*, describing every possible coincidence an object might have with other objects in the environment. They will fire in unison when one's grandmother appears or is imagined.

This is a typical illustration of why I refrain from interpreting the listed questions. When I presented this list three years ago, I did not comment on this question (Julesz 1990a). Now I am glad that I did not, in the light of these revealing findings.

Furthermore, Ilona Kovacs has recently discovered some unique perceptual phenomena that permit me to illustrate question 36 in an unexpected way. In dialogue 4 I alluded to a finding of ours that line segments with gaps became visible when the they suddenly became closed (Kovacs and Julesz 1993). In order to understand the significance of this finding, I have to explain the Glass effect, which is shown in figure 8.2 as first reported (Glass 1969). Glass took two identical transparencies of the same random array of black and white dots and overlaid them after shifting, expanding, or rotating one with respect to the other. The resulting pattern contained global structures of gratings, radial lines, or concentric circles, respectively.

In the lower image of figure 8.3 the pattern is rotated with respect to its identical dual, and the resulting pattern shows a global structure of concentric circular lines. It is easy to show that this is not merely a moiré effect, but has some global component, since restricting the field with a small aperture affects the visibility of the circular structure. There is also a perceptual limit to the maximal displacement for all three kinds of operations. I will call this the *coherence limit* (λ). Kovacs and I became interested in the global extent of this coherence limit λ, so we embedded in an array of

Figure 8.3

Two images of achromatic Glass patterns. It is easy to identify the radial transformation in the upper image and the circular transformation in the lower one. After Glass 1969.

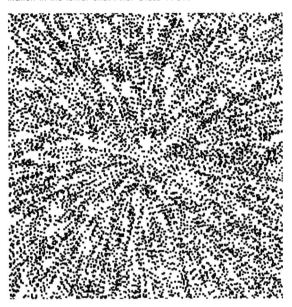

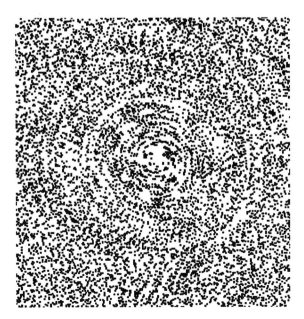

randomly oriented line segments (actually Gabor patches, as shown in figure 8.4) some quasi-collinear Gabor patches with gaps that appeared as "snakes" as shown in the inset.

The snake cannot be detected in a brief flash (T~180 msec) provided the gap between its con-

Figure 8.4

This figure illustrates the superiority of closed curves to open ones. Above: two contours embedded in the background of randomly oriented elements. Below: the same contours, highlighted for didactic reasons. In A, a non-closed contour composed of aligned Gabor patches (GPs) is only barely visible against the background. In B, a closed contour with the same angular difference and distance between elements is perceivable against the background. Closed contours are perceived best when presentations are brief. When the presentation exceeds 180 msec, the observer starts to scrutinize other global structures at the expense of the primordial closed contour. Inset: One GP. Wavelength (λ) was 0.12 arc deg; Gaussian envelope size was equal to λ; GP amplitude was 24% of mean luminance (30 cd/m^2). From Kovacs and Julesz 1993.

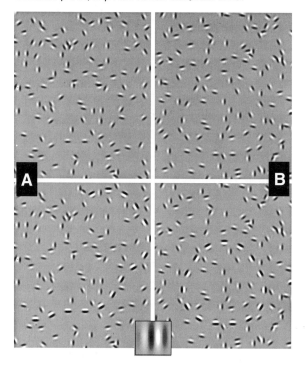

stituent Gabor patches is above a critical size. However, if the snake "bites its tail" (that is, the target suddenly becomes closed) the closed loop pops out from the clutter (Kovacs and Julesz 1993). This remarkable phenomenon is depicted by figure 8.4. These closed stacked curves cannot posses kinks, that is, adjacent line segments (Gabor patches) must be quasi-collinear (within 30 degree orientation) for this robust pop-out effect. Also this perception of closure is the best for brief presentations. For $T\gg180$ msec the observer starts to scrutinize some other global structures at the expense of the primordial closed structure. So the reader will see a stronger effect when looking very briefly at figure 8.4. Of course, among these zigzag shaped snakes a long quasi-collinear line pops out the best. Figure 8.5 and its caption describe the psychophysics in detail.

It seems that long lines, large circles, and relatively smooth closed loops are easily extracted by the early visual system when embedded in a noisy background. It seem logical that this type of early segmentation might have served our arboreal ancestors well in dense foliage. Without the need of recognizing a leopard, a snake, or some pray lurking behind the leaves and branches, a line or closed contour detector can quickly segment the environment into figures and ground.

Gestalt psychologists, particularly Kurt Koffka (1935), were fascinated with closure phenomena and talked much about "good gestalt" and *Prägnanz*. These concepts, however, were difficult to quantify with classical line drawings. It is only in texture perception of random elements—for which the geometry and the statistics of the texture and targets are under computer control—that these gestalt concepts gain some concrete meaning. For details see Julesz 1993.

Now, it turns out that the visibility of a patch within the closed curve depends on the periphery, as illustrated by the psychophysical results shown in

figure 8.6. [The mathematically sophisticated reader is reminded of a Green function, for which integrating an analytical function on a peripheral curve determines its values in the inside! Analytical functions have infinite order of derivatives, which

Figure 8.5

Closed versus open curves, continued: psychophysical results corresponding to figure 8.3. Percent correct performance for the detection of curved contours was measured as a function of distance between neighboring elements in a two-alternate-forced-choice paradigm. Results of three observers (triangles, circles, and squares) are shown. Targets were presented on a 16 × 16-arc deg field containing 2000 randomly placed and oriented Gabor patches. Target curves were built up from 19–23 GPs (giving rise to the maximal length of the field with all different displacements) of the same parameters as the background, having ±30 arc deg relative angular difference between neighbors. The center of gravity of the lines was randomized around the center of the field in a range of 1 arc deg. Stimulus duration was 160 msec. Detection of the stacked line at 75% correct response was defined. Δ_o was 3.3 times the wavelength of the patches (open symbols). Δ_c (closed contour) was 6 times the wavelength (closed symbols). Insets: Δ_o and Δ_c separation. From Kovacs and Julesz 1993.

Figure 8.6

Threshold elevation presented for the detection of a single GB as a function of distance from the surrounding line (closed circle). From Kovacs and Julesz 1993.

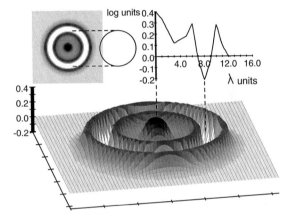

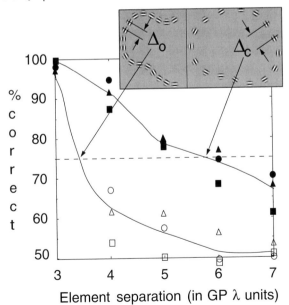

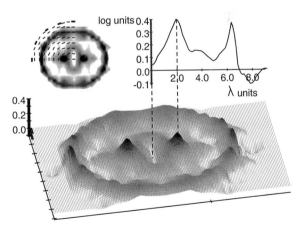

explains why a linear operator (taking the integral over a curve) can yield all values of the function within the curve.] For highly nonlinear sytems, such as visual perception, the determination of the field inside these closed curves is a very difficult problem and requires very sophisticated neural models.

Going back to complex function theory, analytical continuation (when a function has derivatives of infinite order and thus can be expanded in its Taylor series precisely at any given point) permits the global knowledge of an entire function from knowledge at a single local point. In a noise-free system that is not really magic, since each derivative means the knowledge of an $f(x)$ function at a distance $dx, 2dx, \ldots ndx$ from x, thus as $n \to \infty$, the higher-order differences scan the function at an infinite distance. So, in mathematics local and global often cannot be separated. However, in real life there is always internal noise, and *the amount of noise tells us how much we can extrapolate from local information to obtain global information.* Indeed, as you drive your car you can scan the road, and for a few meters (or a few seconds) you can extrapolate safe passage, but moments later a fallen log or a jumping deer could interfere with your assumed predictions.

I am quite sure that in the near future much research will be directed to estimate the influence of internal and external noise on optimal prediction in perception. Here again, knowledge accumulates so rapidly that it is better to raise questions without prematurely trying to interpret them.

While our research is in an early stage, this dependence of closed curves on the curve's inside reminds me of some exciting work by my late friend Harry Blum (1967, 1973). He set up a "brush fire"

simultaneously on the circumference of an ellipse, circle, triangle, or any closed line and determined the shape of the last "surviving" grass. For a circle it was the center point, for an ellipse a line between the focal points. Blum claimed that these "skeletons" were an important invariant for shape recognition. It seems that we are also finding some coupling between the circumference's shape and its skeleton inside. It seems that we are at the beginning of a novel field theory of vision that the gestaltists were searching for in vain. [Figure 8.6 shows the skeleton of a center point for a closed circle, but we obtained two displaced points for ellipses as well.] It seems to me that this visual field is "carried" by the dense needles (Gabor patches) that act as if they were the "gluons" of these field effects. I can also envision how these psychophysically determined fields could be found by MRI techniques and by the direct optical mapping techniques of Grinewald and others.

B: I liked the findings with Ilona Kovacs on the enhanced visibility of long lines and closed lines, but I was annoyed by your half-baked ideas on "gluons." I also dislike your teleological interpretation of "seeing the contours of closed objects partially obstructed by the trees in a forest." After all, a snake usually appears neither as a long line nor as a closed loop. You could have also said that, since birds build their nests in circular shapes, circle detection must be built into their nervous systems at birth. It seems to me that in the natural sciences you learned that teleological arguments are a crime, and after your metamorphosis into psychobiology you made teleological statements with a vengeance.

Turning back to your Hilbertian questions, I can see how all of us could interpret your questions in very different ways, and I am glad that you encourage us to have our own interpretations. I also have many questions that did not occur to you, or were not regarded by you as strategic. Since *de gustibus non est disputandum,* I'll just ask you to sum up this dialogue.

A: I listed some questions that I regard as strategic for vision research. Most of my questions are concerned with early vision, a subfield of visual perception that is devoted mainly to the study of bottom-up processes except for focal attention, which is clearly a top-down process. This emphasis on early vision is brought about by the present state of brain research, where recent advances in neurophysiology opened up the study of early processing stages in the monkey cortex. I hinted at some questions related to form recognition and gestalt organization that are based on higher mental functions. I touched upon some "taboo" questions, such as speculations about the nature of "consciousness," since it is my belief that psychology without consciousness is as boring as mathematics without the concept of infinity. [Of course, some areas of finite mathematics, particularly combinatorics, are not only useful but also beautiful.]

According to my friend and former mentor John Pierce, a good scientist is one who works not on problems he would like to solve but on problems which he thinks can be solved but which are so complex that their solution requires the utmost concentration and devotion. It is in this spirit that I pose my questions, hoping that they will inspire some colleagues searching for a topic. I hope that many other questions will be raised by my colleagues to expand my list in order to enhance the progress of vision research.

DIALOGUE 9
PERCEPTUAL ATOMS:
THE TEXTON THEORY
REVISITED

Q: When is a needle seen in a haystack?

A: When the needle is composed of different textons than the hay.

A: In dialogue 4 I mentioned some aspects of my texton theory, but here I start from scratch. In 1962 I asked a combined mathematical and psychological question that has kept many mathematicians and psychologists busy ever since (Julesz 1962). Because I knew that texture pairs that differed in their first-order statistics would be effortlessly segregated (on the basis of differences in tonal quality) and assumed that differences in second-order statistics could be distinguished from one another (on the basis of differences in granularity), I wanted to study textures with identical Nth-order statistics but different $(N+1)$th-order statistics. (Here I define Nth-order statistics as the probability that the vertices of an N-gon thrown randomly on a texture fall on certain N colors.) I wanted to determine the highest N that still yielded texture segmentation, and I wanted to know what perceptual quality would accompany such discrimi-

nation. For example, would texture pairs with identical second-order statistics (hence identical first-order statistics, and identical Fourier power spectra) be discriminable, and what would the perceptual difference be called? Surprisingly, at that time mathematicians did not know how to create such constrained stochastic textures, but from 1962 to 1975 David Slepian, Mark Rosenblatt, Ed Gilbert, Larry Shepp, and Harry Frisch were instrumental in creating iso-second-order random texture pairs whose elements in isolation appear conspicuously different, yet as textures they cannot be separated. The indiscriminable texture pairs depicted in figures 9.1 and 9.3 were obtained by these efforts. It seemed that iso-second-order textures were so severely constrained globally that the visual system could not tell them apart.

Figure 9.1

An iso-second-order texture pair composed of Rs and their mirror-image duals. In isolation (a) the elements are discriminable; in an array (b) they appear indistinguishable. From Julesz 1981.

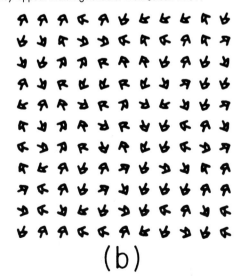

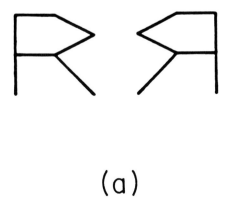

(a)

(b)

Figure 9.2

The four-disk method. From Julesz 1975.

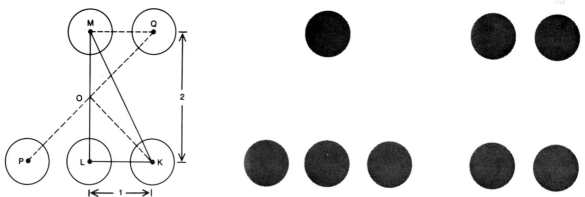

Figure 9.3

An indiscriminable texture pair.

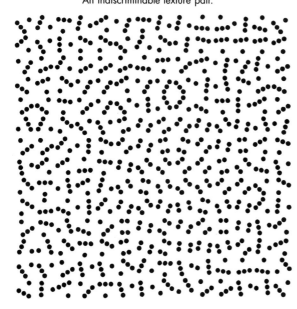

However, in 1977 and 1978 Terry Caelli, Ed Gilbert, and Jonathan Victor helped me to invent stochastic texture pairs with global constraints of identical second-order (and even identical third-order) statistics that yielded preattentive texture discrimination based on some local conspicuous features which I later called textons. Luckily, now that we know what textons are and their role in vision has been clarified, the reader need not take the tortuous mathematical path that led to their discovery. (For details see Julesz 1981, 1984; Caelli et al. 1978a; Julesz et al. 1978.) [It can be mathematically proven that the four-disk method of Caelli et al. (1978a) is the only one using identical disks that can generate iso-second-order texture pairs in the Euclidean plane, thus permitting a thorough search for dual elements whose aggregates might pop out. Indeed, figure 9.5 demonstrates the first iso-second-order discriminable texture pair we found, using the four-disk method. This, together with figures 9.6 and 9.7, which were generated with the help of the "generalized 4-disk method" (where the disks are replaced one by one by specific

Figure 9.4

The generalized four-disk method. From Caelli, Julesz, and Gilbert 1978.

(a)

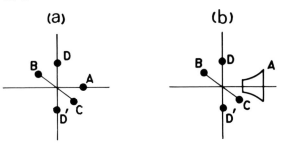

(b)

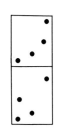

(C)

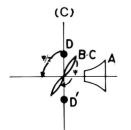

(d)

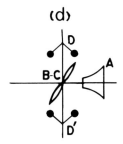

(e)

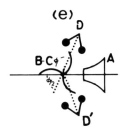

Figure 9.5

An iso-second-order texture pair (generated by the four-disk method) that is discriminable owing to the local conspicuous feature (texton) of "quasi-collinearity."

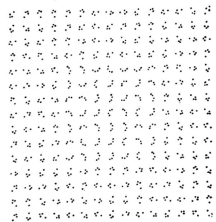

Figure 9.6

An iso-second-order texture pair (generated by the generalized four-disk method) that is discriminable owing to the local conspicuous feature (texton) of "corner."

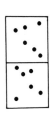

symmetric shapes), depicts some iso-second-order texture pairs that are preattentively discriminable on the basis of the local features that might be named "quasi-collinearity," "corner," and "closure" (Caelli et al. 1978a). However, as mentioned all over, these are just names, without a real geometrical connotation, similarly to "strangeness," "beauty," "charm," etc., given by physicists to the various quarks. Indeed, quasi-collinearity also results in more empty space between the elements, so the real texton properties are a combination of many factors. This comment is particularly relevant for "closure." In some of my later papers I wanted to use another name, since "closure" is a topological concept rather useless for vision, and therefore I renamed this textonal property "zero terminator number." This new name was a particularly bad choice, since several authors took it literally and started to count terminators in an array that were

spread far from each other. Perhaps "local closure" might be a better name for this textonal property, but these names serve merely as mnemotechnique.

Figure 9.8 shows iso-third-order textures (Julesz, Gilbert, and Victor 1978) with the property that any triangle thrown on these textures has the same probability that the vertices of the triangles will fall on the same colors (however the vertices of probing 4-gons will have different probabilities). As the reader can verify, discrimination is effortless and is obviously not due to computing differences in fourth-order statistics, but rather due to elongated blobs with different orientation, width, and length.

What textons really are is hard to define. For instance, in figure 9.1, besides quasi-collinearity, there are also more white gaps between these elements, giving rise to anti-textons. As I pointed out (Julesz 1986), it is not only the black (white) tex-

---

Figure 9.7

An iso-second-order texture pair (generated by the generalized four disk method) that is discriminable owing to the local conspicuous feature (texton) of "closure." From Caelli, Julesz, and Gilbert 1978.

Figure 9.8

An iso-third-order texture pair that is discriminable owing to the local conspicuous feature (texton) of "elongated blobs of specific orientation, width, and length." From Julesz, Gilbert, and Victor 1978.

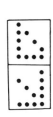

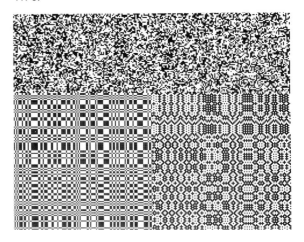

tons whose gradients yield texture discrimination but the white (black) space between them that act as textons too (see also dialogue 10). When Mendel postulated that certain genes were the units of some hereditary traits, he just gave a name for some readily observable morphological properties, and it required almost a century of research to give finer details and to decipher slowly the nucleotide code of a few genes, a job still not completed.

In essence, we found that texture segmentation is not governed by global (statistical) rules, but rather depends on local, nonlinear features (textons), such as color, orientation, flicker, motion, depth, elongated blobs, and collinearity, to name the most conspicuous ones that are both psychophysically and neurophysiologically accepted as being fundamental. Some less clearly defined textons are related to ends of lines or terminators, which occur in the concepts of "corner" and "closure" and which are hard to define for half-tone blobs. Particularly important was the realization that—contrary to common belief—texture segmentation cannot be explained by differences in power spectra. On the other hand, it became obvious that instead of searching for higher-order statistical descriptors, the visual system applies some local spatial filtering followed by some nonlinearity and the results must be again averaged by a next spatial filter stage. This is depicted in figure 9.9b, which illustrates how a Kuffler-type unit [instead of a Mexican-hat-function profile, a simpler spatial filter of 2×2 pixel center excitation (addition) with a two-pixel-wide surround angulus of inhibition (subtraction)] acts on the iso-third-order texture pair of figure 9.8a, followed by a threshold device (Julesz and Bergen 1983). When the output of this nonlinear spatial filter in figure 9.9c is fed to higher

stages in our visual system, a second spatial filtering is performed to separate the two areas of different luminance distributions (which were obtained by means of the threshold device).

One problem with such simple nonlinear filters is their inability to account for the asymmetry problem of human texture segmentation. It is known

Figure 9.9

A demonstration of how a simple local linear filter followed by a nonlinearity (threshold-taking) can segment the iso-third-order texture pair of figure 9.8. From Julesz and Bergen 1983.

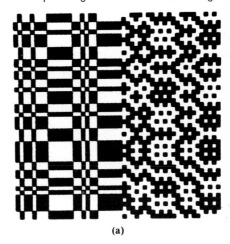

(a)

(b)

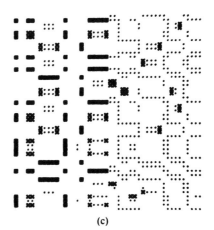

(c)

(Julesz 1981; Gurnsey and Browse 1987; Treisman and Gormican 1988) that very often texture A in B pops out stronger than B in A, as shown in figure 9.10a. For many years I was worried that the asymmetry problem of preattentive texture discrimination might depend on top-down processes and complex figure-ground phenomena. Therefore I was glad to find that the asymmetry effect in figure 9.10a could be explained (Williams and Julesz 1991) by assuming that the nonlinear operation is the subjective contour phenomenon that "closes the gaps." We know from the work of von der

Heydt et al. (1988) that subjective (also called illusory) contours are extracted in V2, and therefore belong to early visual processes. Figure 9.10b yields similar asymmetry of texture discrimination as figure 9.10a, even though the orientation of the gaps is not jittered.

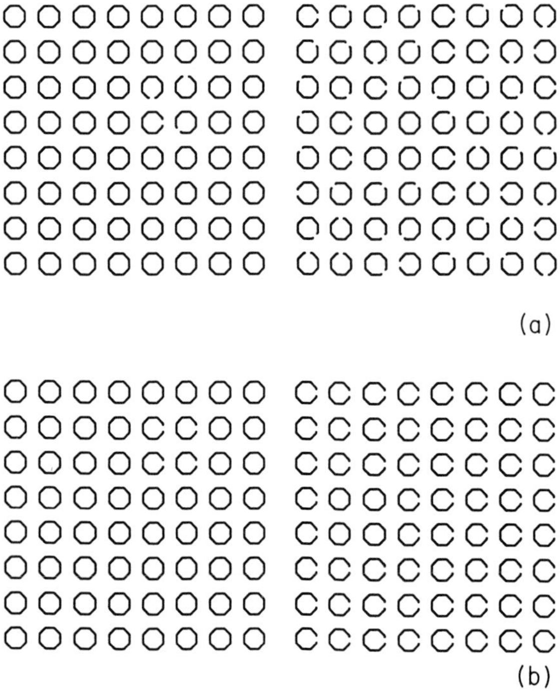

B: I was always amazed how enthusiastic you were when you succeeded in disproving your own conjecture that iso-second-order textures cannot be told apart. When you gave a talk at Caltech reporting the fall of your conjecture, a famous physicist, the co-discoverer of quarks, noted that it must be terrible to have one's life-work seen to be disproved. You gave a glib answer: "It feels like deciphering the grammar of an unknown language, and then finding a few irregular verbs, the textons!"

A: Just as I turned 65, I received an unexpected birthday present: In a seminal paper, John Yellott (1993) revisited my defunct conjecture that iso-second-order textures cannot be told apart. As I found over a decade, texture pairs with the same second-order statistics usually cannot be told apart. Indeed, if one would generate stochastic texture pairs side by side using some ergodic process, say, of a Gaussian or Poisson kind, for eons the textures would not segregate into a discriminable pair. In this statistical sense, my original conjecture is one of the strongest "laws" one could state for psychology. Nevertheless, during two decades I was able with my co-workers to concoct several (non-ergodic) counterexamples, even for iso-third-order textures, that did segregate (Julesz, Gilbert, and Victor 1978).

Yellott defines textures as pictures whose properties stay invariant under translation. My defini-

Figure 9.10

Asymmetry of texture discrimination. (a) The perception of gapped octagons among closed octagons is weaker than vice versa. (b) Similar to a, but the position of the gaps is not jittered. This does not reduce the asymmetry effect. From Williams and Julesz 1991.

(a)

(b)

tion of textures is different from his, yet it is a possible definition of textures since it stresses their stationarity and ergodicity. [Images of objects would vary under positional shifts as they would cover or uncover other objects or textures.] For textures, so defined, Yellott proves that iso-third-order statistics makes them identical. *Thus, all textures with the same third-order statistics are actually identical.* Had I conjectured in the 1960s that textures with identical third-order statistics could not be told apart, I would have made a mathematical—not a psychological—conjecture, since I might have stated a tautology. [For a critique of Yellott's ideas see Victor 1994. Victor stresses that Yellott defines an image, while I always have a stochastic ensemble in mind. And it is the stochastic ensemble that has neurological significance, since organisms evolved to sense an ensemble of textures.]

B: So far you have not mentioned how some of the problematic phenomena in texture segregation, such as the asymmetry problem, affect existing models of texture segmentation.

A: Obviously, the asymmetry problem—that texture A embedded in B can appear very different than vice versa—is a real challenge for any theory, and almost by definition cannot be explained by linear spatial filters. Indeed, in 1988, several texture segmentation algorithms were developed. These were based on linear spatial filters followed by squaring or some other nonlinear operation (Voorhees and Poggio 1988; Bergen and Adelson 1988). [For a definition of spatial filters, e.g. the Laplacian of a Gaussian, or Gabor filters, see below.] For a critique showing that linear spatial filters cannot segment textures, see Julesz and Kröse 1988 and Julesz 1990c. Recently Williams and I demonstrated the nonlinear behavior of human texture discrimination as depicted in figure 9.11 (Williams and Julesz 1991). Here the nondiscriminable iso-

Figure 9.11

A demonstration of the nonlinearity of human texture discrimination. Adding a nondiscriminable texture pair to a highly discriminable texture pair renders the latter nondiscriminable, thus violating the law of superposition. From Williams and Julesz 1992.

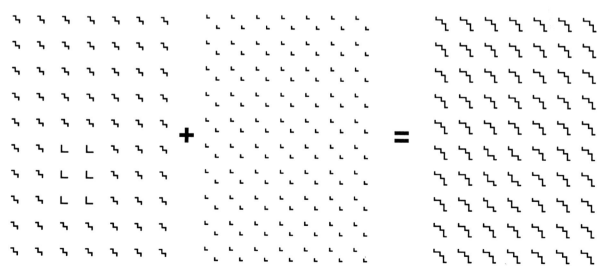

second-order texture pair, invented by Caelli et al. (1978a), is shown on the right side. [This texture pair belongs to the rare cases which have iso-second-order statistics without having random rotation of the texture elements.] We were able to decompose this texture pair into the sum of a highly discriminable texture pair and a nondiscriminable texture pair as shown on the left side. The fact that a discriminable texture pair becomes nondiscriminable when a nondiscriminable texture pair is linearly added shows convincingly the violation of the law of superposition for texture discrimination.

More recently, Fogel and Sagi (1989) and, independently, Malik and Perona (1990) developed texture-segmentation algorithms based on local spatial filters (oriented Gabor filters, or DOG filters, respectively) followed by a quasi-local nonlinear operation (simple squaring by Fogel and Sagi and some inhibition between neighboring elements by Malik and Perona) and a second spatial filter for final segmentation. It was most impressive that it emulated human texture-discrimination performance as measured by Kröse (1987). However, it still could not account for the asymmetry effects. Therefore, it is of great significance that Rubinstein and Sagi (1989) extended their model by determining the variances of the local texture elements' distributions after the nonlinear stage, and found these variances asymmetric, particularly when the orientation of the elements was jittered, mimicking human performance. Their model could account for the textural asymmetries reported by Gurnsey and Browse (1987) and probably will be able to handle some other asymmetries of the kind shown in figure 9.12. In that figure a typical input-output pattern of the Rubenstein-Sagi (1990) algorithm is

presented as it segments a texture pair (A in B) and its dual (B in A). So, it is most heartening that even the textural asymmetry effects that seemed to be based on figure-ground reversals—which in turn depended on enigmatic top-down processes—can be successfully explained by bottom-up processes modeled by relatively simple nonlinear spatial filters.

The Rubenstein-Sagi (1989) model can account for the asymmetry problem by assuming that jitter of line orientation accounts for increase in variance of their filter's output, hence increase in texture-discrimination asymmetry. However, figure 9.11 clearly shows that, in general, the asymmetry problem of texture discrimination does not depend on orientational jitter. Recently, Williams and I extended the texton theory to include illusory contours and "fill-in" phenomena between gaps and nearby elements, which can be regarded as anti-textons (Williams and Julesz 1991). The filling in of the gaps by subjective contours can account for the asymmetry effect, and the fill-in phenomenon between texture elements can explain many other asymmetries.

Anti-textons together with the textons extend the theory of trichromacy, the only real scientific theory in psychology. The theory of trichromacy stated that any color could be matched to a combination of three basic colors, red, green, and blue, such that the boundary between the selected color and the combination colors would become minimal (or disappear without scrutiny). When I introduced textons into psychology, I wished to extend trichromacy to encompass colors as well as textures. I wanted to know whether any texture could be matched to a finite (and not too large) number of textons such that the boundary between any textural array and an array containing a mixture of textons would make their boundary perceptually disappear without scrutiny. It seems now that this can be achieved. The fact that the gamut of colors can be matched by just three colors is in itself amazing. The finding that the infinitely richer variety of 2-D textures could be matched to a mixture of finite number of textons is even more unexpected!

In figure 9.11 it was shown that the law of superposition does not apply for texture discrimination. Whether the mixing of various textural elements that have the same textons as another array with different elements yields always a "metameric match," and whether such matching is a linear or a nonlinear operation, is not yet known. Howard Resnikoff devotes an entire chapter of his interesting monograph *The Illusion of Reality* (1987a) to an early version of my texton theory and argues for the linear superposition of textons. I am skeptical about a linear metameric match, but the possibility

of finding a metameric texton match at all is a most interesting research topic.

As I have spent much of my scientific career in search of the elusive textons, it is almost anticlimactic, yet most satisfying, to find that quasi-local spatial filters can extract texton gradients without having to specify complex concatenation rules between adjacent textons. [I have no doubt that in the near future it will be found that such filters can mimic human preattentive texture discrimination by incorporating several perceptual operations from subjective contours to the "filling in" of gaps.] The reader familiar with speech research will recognize the similarity between "phonemes" and "textons."

Figure 9.12

Output of a nonlinear spatial filter that emulates the asymmetry phenomenon of human texture discrimination as illustrated by dual texture pairs. The first stage of linear Gabor filters is followed by a nonlinear operator (rectifier), which in turn is followed by a second spatial filter. From Rubenstein and Sagi 1990.

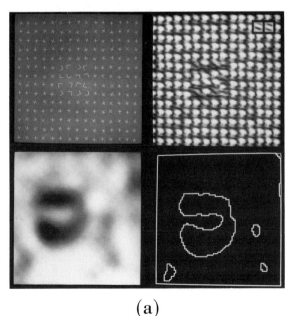

(a)

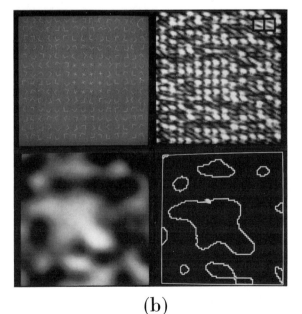

(b)

While phonemes were never well specified, and complex computer algorithms have been used to cope with the many *ad hoc* rules at their various concatenations in order to segment speech, the rudely defined phonemes nevertheless permitted the development of phonetic writing, one of the great discoveries of human civilization. Had the development of phonetic speech coincided with the invention of supercomputers that could automatically segment speech and talk millennia ago, the skill of writing might have never developed. Of course, the fact that our voice organs limit the number of phonemes to a few dozen helped their universal acceptance. Similarly, the main insight from the texton theory was that, of the infinite variety of 2-D textures, only a limited number of textons have perceptual significance and are evaluated quasi-locally in effortless texture discrimination. (I use the term "quasi-local" instead of "local" because line segments, closed loops, corners, etc. have some finite dimensions.) Even though superfast computers will soon perform automatic texture segmentation, practitioners of visual skills—painters, designers of instrument panels, directors of movies, TV shows, and advertisements—can benefit from the texton theory by manipulating the viewer's perception. Indeed, some of the great artists instinctively knew how to create a strong texton gradient to capture attention, or to create a texton equilibrium for which time-consuming scrutiny is needed to discover the hidden images.

Enns (1986) made up arrays of little 2-D perspective cubes with targets (cubes) biased to be perceived in one kind of 3-D depth organization amidst cubes biased in the dual 3-D organization. This depth from 3-D perspective cues yields preattentive texture segmentation ("pop-out"), with the implication that in addition to the textons of brightness, color, orientation and aspect ratio of elongated blobs, flicker, motion, and stereopsis, even perceived depth in 2-D perspective drawings might act as a texton. In my belief, probably, some simple, quasi-local rules of 3-D perspective, occlusion, transparency, etc., are utilized, without the need to invoke top-down processing.

B: You have mentioned only the psychological aspects of texture discrimination. Are there neurophysiological correlates that could explain the psychology?

A: Let me turn then to recent psychological and neurophysiological findings in texture discrimination. Perhaps the most important implication of the texton theory was its division of human vision into a preattentive and an attentive mode of action. Certain texture-gradient-like detections could be performed in parallel without scrutiny, while some other tasks that required identification needed serial search by attention. Recently, Braun and Sagi (1990) made the concept of two visual systems even stronger by showing that while loading attention (by asking the observer to identify a letter) it was possible to carry out simultaneously the detection of texture gradients.

Some recent neurophysiological studies seem to support the texton-gradient notion of our perceptual studies. Van Essen et al. (1989) studied the responses of single units in visual areas V1, V2, and MT (V4) of the macaque monkey to stationary and moving patterns. In V1 and V2 the presence of a static texture surround (e.g. an array of parallel needles) significantly increases the response to a central texture element (single needle) within the classical receptive field if the orientation of the needles in the surround is perpendicular to that in the center. If they are parallel, the neural response is greatly reduced. Another neurophysiological result was obtained by Robert Desimone and his collaborators (Moran and Desimone 1985; Desimone and Ungerleider 1989), who found neurons in V4 whose firing for certain trigger features changes in accordance to the focal attention of the monkey.

B: Could you comment on some of the new learning effects in early vision?

A: Yes. One of the main themes throughout this review was the phenomenological richness of early vision. Without cognitive and semantic cues, rather complex feats of false-target elimination occur in stereopsis and movement perception, asymmetry of texture discrimination takes place, subjective contours are formed, and so on. Even long-term memory effects occur in early vision. We discussed some of the hysteresis effects that accompany the cooperative phenomena of global stereopsis and motion perception. Hysteresis is one of the simplest memory effects, where some action modifies the outcome of a later response. For instance, as was shown by Fender and Julesz (1967), using binocular retinal stabilization (by wearing tight-fitting contact lenses with mirrors attached), an RDS had to be brought within Panum's fusional area (i.e. within 6 min arc alignment) to obtain fusion. But after fusion, the left and the right image could slowly be pulled apart by as much as 120 min arc without breaking fusion. So, the fusional area depends strongly on the prior perceptual states. Another learning effect can be experienced when one

first tries to fuse an RDS with large binocular disparities, as shown in several demonstrations in my monograph (Julesz 1971). We found that it might at first take minutes to achieve fusion, but then even years later one can do it quite easily. This is not a real perceptual (cortical) learning, but rather a procedural (cerebellar) learning. When fusing an RDS with large disparities, the novice tries large convergence movements to bring the corresponding areas of the RDS into Panum's fusional area, and it is this unconscious learning of proper vergence movements that is remembered years later (Julesz 1986a). [See also dialogue 10, item 11, on work in collaboration with Ilona Kovacs.] Here I give only two examples of learning effects in preattentive texture discrimination:

When an observer is presented with some indistinguishable iso-second order texture pairs which, nevertheless, are composed of element pairs with different convex hulls, after several hundred trials they can be effortlessly discriminated (Julesz 1984), as is shown in figure 9.13.

Even more interestingly, Karni and Sagi (1990) report a remarkable long-term learning effect in simple texture- discrimination tasks where learning seems to be local in a retinotopic sense. What has been learned must be relearned for each different area of the visual field. Learning is specific for target orientation as well as for target location, although the effects learned can be erased by changing *background* orientation. These authors briefly presented a few targets of adjacent line segments in an array of horizontal line segments that were tilted from the horizontal orientation. With small tilts, it took several sessions to detect these targets correctly. This improvement was retained for the next sessions in the same retinal quadrant but was not transferable to other retinal quadrants. Changing the orientation of the targets (from left oblique to right oblique) had no effect on the learned performance. However, changing the orientation of the background array (from horizontal to vertical) obliterated learning. These plasticity effects are of great interest, and it seems that perceptual learning in early vision might be a useful tool in understanding the mysteries of human memory.

𝔹: You did not mention that later, in his Ph.D. thesis, Karni also found that consolidation of this

---

Figure 9.13

Long-lasting learning effect of texture discrimination. While the conspicuous triangle/3-prong pops out on the first trial, the iso-second-order target requires several hundred trials to be discriminated from the background. The ordinate represents d', a logarithmic measure of correct responses. From Julesz 1984.

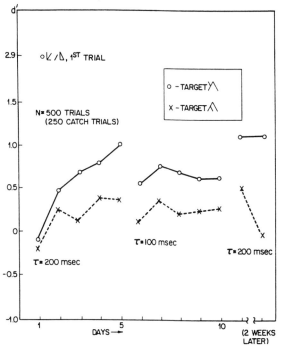

textural learning required sleep. What is your opinion of rapid-eye-movement (REM) sleep in long-term memory (LTM)?

𝔸: I found Karni's work most provocative, but I will refrain from discussing the role of sleep and REM sleep in LTM. I still regard problems of why we sleep and dream as at the edge of metapsychological problems. Of course, it would be delightful if the problem of LTM would be partially clarified during my life, and even more so if the techniques of early vision might pave way to this clarification. Here I only comment on an important aspect of the research by Dov Sagi and his students at Weizmann: the apparent demonstration that in order to learn one has to take part actively at each step of the learning process.

𝔹: Recently you became enthusiastic about another interesting learning phenomenon from Sagi's laboratory. Could you comment on it?

𝔸: Uri Polat and Dov Sagi (1993) found a novel chain-learning phenomenon in early vision. As they tried to increase the effect of two flanking Gabor patches on the visibility of a center Gabor patch, they were able to increase the distance between them with many repeated trials. However, as the distance was increased between the patches, in each session all distances had to be presented; the already learned shorter gaps had to be mixed together with the new (longer) gaps. *If the old and the new conditions were not mixed in each trial, the chain of learned gap distance would break and the learned performance would collapse.* It seems that these new learning phenomena can rewire the early visual cortex in some lasting and novel ways!

DIALOGUE 10
THE ROLE OF EARLY
VISION IN
PSYCHOBIOLOGY
AND VISUAL
COGNITION

Q: Why are you searching for your key here, when I saw you drop it a mile away?

A: There is a street light here!

A: Perhaps the first reason why early vision should be regarded as a model system for psychobiology is told in the epigram: because in this subfield of brain research there is some light! Indeed, the advantages of studying early vision are twofold.

First, it is possible to avoid the enigmatic problems of semantics and of the higher symbolic processes when one concentrates on stereoscopic depth perception (stereopsis), motion perception, and effortless texture segmentation, since they are elicited by computer-generated stochastic displays (dynamic noise) that have well-specified geometrical, topological, and statistical properties but are devoid of meaning.

Second, these psychological phenomena can now be neurophysiologically studied in the input stages of the monkey cortex and, most importantly, the early neural processing stages of the monkey visual system are practically identical to that of *Homo sapiens*. The many dozen higher cortical stages devoted to visual processing in the monkey are not well known, and their relationship to perception and cognition in monkeys and in humans are still a mystery. These enigmatic phenomena of form recognition, gestalt organization, and the many unsolved problems of mental states (which are at present metascientific questions) will be skipped in this dialogue. Although there are interesting speculations—even by Nobel laureates—about the nature of dreams, free will, consciousness, and so on, one can study early vision without knowing what these concepts are, and very

few references will be provided that relate to these subjective ideas.

B: Then is early vision, in the terminology of Jerry Fodor and Zenon Pylyshyn, a "cognitively impenetrable module"? Without cognitive processes the neural machinery of reflexes and preattentive processes is not much more interesting than, say, studying the function of the kidney or the liver. With your random-dot techniques you might have succeeded in stimulating some preattentive psychological systems, however, these systems are not worth studying by self-respecting psychologists.

A: Your point is well taken, but I do not believe that the actions of the simplest nervous systems are at the level of a liver. If a nervous system based solely on hormonal interactions were to exist, your point might be correct. However, to my knowledge, the simplest nervous systems are connected to sensory transducers and their actions become converted into neural spikes, and these neural "codes" are orders of magnitude more intricate than the strictly chemical plants of the liver, the kidneys, or the digestive system. Of course, if some psychologists want to restrict their studies to highly cognitive processes, that is their privilege. About the time I arrived in the United States, just the opposite was the case. Psychologists were still under the spell of behaviorism, and studying mental phenomena that were unaccompanied by motor actions was taboo! It was not gestalt psychology that broke the hold of behaviorism on experimental psychology, but progress in linguistics and the emergence of early vision (and early acoustics). After all, the phenomena of early vision manifest themselves in some observable percepts, even though the underlying subprocesses have to be guessed. While no introspection or pondering could tell apart two different metameric color matches that were perceived as the same color, the finding that three basic colors suffice to carry out such a match (instead of two or four) is a deep insight of early vision. For me, the finding that three primary colors are adequate to span the space of almost infinite hues is a more remarkable insight than the many other achievements of our cognitive arsenal.

B: You are still avoiding my question. I asked whether early vision is intellectually challenging for psychologists. You told me that early vision, with its many unconscious and preattentive processes, is more challenging than studying the functions of the liver, and thus more interesting than the phenomena of physiology. But I do not see how mental phenomena without intimate dependency on consciousness are the proper study of psychologists.

A: Your question reminds me of the intuitionist school of mathematicians, who became worried about the many paradoxes that plagued mathematics when infinite sets were introduced (e.g. "the set of all sets"). To avoid these anomalies they decided to extirpate from mathematics the concept of infinity. Indeed, with the help of this finite mathematics, all the practical problems of the world could still be solved; after all, only finite objects and concepts exist in real-life applications. Yet without infinity mathematics appeared a rather pedestrian undertaking, losing its beauty and many of its intellectual challenges. So, the intuitionists soon disappeared as a movement, since no self-respecting mathematician wished to join such a program.

Similarly, *I think that psychology without consciousness is like mathematics without infinity*. However, there is a great difference between these two domains. In mathematics one has to define precisely what one means by infinity: Is it a *potential* succession, as in an infinite series, or in an algorithmic sequence of ever-continuing steps, or is it an *actual* infinity, as in set theory, where we refer to *all* members of a certain set of numbers or objects? In psychology, on the other hand, one does not have to define what consciousness really is, it is adequate that somehow it is given, and people can agree to a remarkable extent on what states they regard as such.

B: If you could extend your paradigm of early visual perception to include some top-down phenomena that are "cognitive," even though not as complex as genuine cognitive phenomena of logic and symbolic processing, I might become more interested in your field.

A: Until now I adhered to the notion that the majority of problems in vision are bottom-up and belong to early vision. While I believe that this is the case, there are some exciting visual phenomena that appear fundamental yet cannot so far be attributed to bottom-up processing. I am not alluding to important scene-segmentation problems that necessitate form recognition. I already mentioned the problem of knowing from a static two-dimensional retinal projection whether a rabbit's ears belong to the rabbit or to the fence behind it. My point so far has been that, with motion parallax or binocular disparity, one can always determine that the ears are at the same depth as the rabbit, i.e., in front of the fence. Hence, if the ears are also adjacent to the rabbit, then the ears, whiskers, tail, etc., must be parts of the rabbit, and one does not even have to know that the "object" in question is a rabbit or some animal one has already seen. Without motion and binocular disparity information such a segmentation is a genuine cognition problem of great complexity.

The more enigmatic visual phenomena I will now discuss are not based on semantics yet are beyond our grasp. Adopting the terminology of Shimon Ullman (1984), I will call these "problems of visual cognition." One primary example is the problem of how we can perceive in a brief time whether a point is on one or the other side of a complex boundary. I am quite sure that you are able to perceive in a brief flash that the dot P in figure 10.1 belongs to area A and not to area B. As Ullman (1984) explains, the sequential algorithms that have been invented so far can only decide on the position of the dot depending on the size of the area, while in reality the visual system can do it in a jiffy practically independently of the size of areas searched. [I am studying whether indeed the complexity of the boundary interferes with the localization of the dot (by making the boundary a sinusoidally wiggly line or a zigzag line with ever-increasing amplitude and periodicity), but so far I have not been able to get a clear answer.]

B: Ullman's first problem clearly belongs to the more general problem of how serial computation can be replaced by parallel processing, and what is the gain in speed if such a replacement is found. Current debates in the scientific community on replacing serial computer architectures with massively parallel computers, such as hypercubes or "Connection Machines," are being waged by some of the smartest computer hardware and software

experts, and while it seems plausible that parallel computers might be much faster for some specific tasks, it is far from certain whether one could develop a program for a *general-purpose* computer for the most general tasks! I doubt that it will be a psychobiologist who will decide this debate.

A: I agree with you that the psychobiologist might not be the one who will develop the parallel

---

Figure 10.1

Problems of containment. Whether a dot belongs to area A or to area B (separated by a complex boundary) is easy for the visual system to discern; however, as Ullman (1984) stated, no simple parallel algorithm exists.

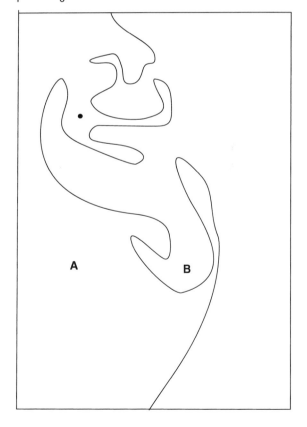

programs needed for visual cognition. But it is the psychobiologist who has to point out that the visual cortex of animals is based on parallel computation—a fact robustly shown by neurophysiologists and easily demonstrated by psychologists. A well-known example is the fact that almost any perceptual task, from form recognition to perceptual constancies, can be performed in about 200–500 msec. Since the synaptic events last about 2–5 msec, the code for a perceptual task must be about 100 instructions. As of now the simplest AI algorithms on the ubiquitous serial computers require tens of thousands of instructions, therefore it is most likely that these perceptual tasks are performed in some parallel way by the nervous systems of animals.

Another well-known example, which can be easily verified, can demonsrate that lexical memory is probably a serial process. If we ask a native speaker of English whether, say, 'cropf' is an existing English word or a nonsense word, the time for decision is about twice as long as if the word we asked was a legitimate English word. Indeed, for English words one would need on average only about half of the time, since 50% of the time the English words would occur in the first half of the memory store, in case of a sequential search, while for nonsense words one had to search the *entire* memory store. In my experiments with texture we found (Bergen and Julesz 1983; Sagi and Julesz 1985) that strong texton gradients would pop out regardless of the number of distractors (a clearly parallel process), while for weak texton gradients search time would increase monotonically (linearly) with the number of distractors (a clearly serial process).

B: Some of your arguments are not as convincing as you state. We know from the work of Saul Sternberg (1966) that some of his memory experiments showed serial search with twice the slope expected. Sternberg concluded that his observers could not terminate the search after an item was found, and called his model a serial non-terminating search, as if observers had a mental inertia and had to conduct an exhaustive search. Townsend (1972), criticizing the Sternberg paradigm, constructed some stochastic processes for which serial and parallel processes gave the same explanation. So, arguing on the basis of search slopes as a function of item numbers is not a simple matter.

A: I grant you that experiments and arguments in cognition are not as convincing as in perception, since the mental phenomena studied are more complex. Nevertheless, in spite of some concocted counter examples, I regard the *definition* of a parallel process as one that does not depend on the number (area) of the items searched as a reasonable definition. As a matter of fact, before the advent of holography and lasers [and coherent Fourier optics in general] I could not conceive of a practical device that could search and find a certain item equally fast, regardless of the item number. However, after the first demonstration of Dennis Gabor's holography using lasers (Leith and Upatnieks 1962) Keith Pennington and I wrote a paper, "Equidistributed information mapping: An analogy to holograms and memory," in which we showed how the central nervous system of organisms could use holographic systems based on Fourier optics to find any item at a great speed regardless of storage size (Julesz and Pennington 1965). It is enough to take the Fourier transform of the item to be searched and multiply it with the Fourier transform of the storage (this mathematical procedure is isomorphic to cross-correlation) and the searched item will pop out with maximum energy relative to the rest. The Fourier transform of the store and the item is obtained if the image of the store and item are placed in the focal planes of an optical lens and then illuminated by coherent light. If image and store are placed in cascade, the item will pop out (at the speed of light). Kabrisky (1966), among others, visualized how the various areas of the cortex were merely sheets of densely packed columns and hyper-columns as first discovered by Mountcastle (1957), and the connections between these cascaded cortical sheets were not light rays but neuron bundles.

The late Harry Blum introduced an entirely parallel geometry based on his brushfire model (Blum 1967). He would start a neuronal brushfire simultaneously at the edges of geometrical objects (triangles, ellipses, etc.,) and would look at those points were the spread would reach the last "grass." These were the "spines" of the objects (called "skeletons" in today's image-processing jargon), and they exhibited remarkable invariant properties. I could easily see how such a model could simulate some phenomena of visual cognition. An attempt along these lines was advanced by Michael Leyton (1992) in his recent monograph *Symmetry, Causality, Mind*. [See also dialogue 14.]

B: Never mind the serial/parallel dichotomy. I would like you to continue with perceptual phenomena that are not merely bottom-up.

A: OK. The first two phenomena that appear to belong to visual cognition belong to my own specialty, stereopsis. One occurs in pseudoscopy, the other is depth from shading. I will quickly discuss these two phenomena, which I regard as purely bottom-up, and then I will turn to phenomena that I cannot explain by bottom-up processes alone.

Pseudoscopy is the viewing of objects with both eyes when the left and right eyes' views are reversed. Except for random-dot stereograms for which no familiarity cues are present, it is a fact that familiar objects do not reverse in depth, particularly convex faces of humans and familiar animals, and familiar objects do not become concave! This perceptual resistance to seeing convex familiar objects as hollow is particularly strong in stereo movies. This emphasis on familiarity that resists stereopsis of reversed disparities is regarded by many as proof that even stereoscopic depth is affected by top-down influences. Therefore it was an important suggestion by van den Enden and Spekreijse (1989) that in pseudoscopy the monocular cues of textural gradients of the objects' surfaces are not exchanged when the two eyes' views are reversed, and this is the reason why familiar objects are perceived as convex. In order to prove their hypothesis, they masked the textures of a human face with a noisy texture, and the face suddenly became hollow. Unfortunately, as pointed out by several critics, the binocular noise mask they used had the inverse disparity of the face (as if the hollowed mask of the face were covered with speckled noise) and therefore it was no wonder that the face reversed in depth. However, I have no doubt that these authors were right, and with correct masking texture (e.g. binocularly uncorrelated noise) one could indeed prove that stereopsis does not depend on familiarity cues, and in the final percept stereopsis dominates all other monocular depth cues.

Depth from shading is another strong monocular depth phenomenon that appears to be top-down. Indeed, shaded objects reverse their depth appearance when viewed upside-down. Astronomers noted this generations ago as they viewed inverted photographs of moon craters surprisingly appeared as convex hills. It is most likely that, since our visual system evolved on Earth, which has only one sun, the "belly" of an object is more in a shadow than the top, and this fact of illumination has been ingrained in our visual system. Ramachandran (1988) and Kleffner and Ramachandran (in press) argue that shape from shading is an early visual process that might serve as an input to motion perception. Jih-Jie Chang and I provided evidence that global stereopsis does dominate depth from motion. We generated anaglyphs that, when viewed monocularly, portrayed convex (concave) spheres due to shading. However, if 10–20% of the pixels that portrayed the shading were also RDSs that yielded stereoscopic depth, then the depth-from-shading effect was either reinforced or juxtaposed by stereopsis. In all cases stereopsis dominated depth from shading. Even if depth from shading is a top-down process, it does not seem to affect stereopsis. If, however, depth from shading is a bottom-up process, then it is even more persuasive that stereopsis operates in the absence of semantics. A demonstration of these stereograms is presented in Julesz 1991. [See also figure 5.4 above.]

Now that we have established that stereopsis is mainly a bottom-up process, let us look for some better candidates for top-down visual processing. An important perceptual process is segmentation of half-tone images with strong shadows. In a provocative paper, Patrick Cavanagh (1991) gives several examples of human faces with strong shadows (depicting a black-and-white image without a gray scale) in which the lightness contours between these black and white shadows yield an unrecognizable face, while the black-and-white image itself is easily recognizable. Cavanagh observes that shadows have two types of borders: attached borders, where the direction of the illumination is perpendicular to the surface normals, and cast borders, where the shadow cast by one surface falls on the second surface. The cast shadow border is not a material border and basically needs to be ignored in order to patch together the pieces of surface that actually belong together. Cavanagh then claims that it is often impossible to ignore these borders without knowing what the original object is. A Dalmatian dog in a black-and-white speckled terrain (figure 2 of Julesz 1974b) belongs to this category, and when viewed upside-down does not fit any memorized image of such a dog and cannot be detected. Only when some memory representation of such an image is available does the dog suddenly appear as a vivid percept.

An even more dramatic demonstration of semantics is provided by the exciting demonstrations of Johansson (1973). At some strategic places of a human (head, torso, arms, and legs), as few as seven luminous dots are attached. In the dark when at standstill, these seven dots appear merely as an aggregate of random dots. Yet when the person starts to walk, dance, throw a ball, climb steps, ride a bicycle, or embrace another person (also portrayed by seven moving dots) the random dots suddenly become alive. We perceive a moving human being, and often we are able to judge the person's sex or age. This phenomenon is vivid and mysterious, as if these few dots had taken out from memory the spatio-temporal essence of a moving human being. Obviously, without a precise memory of human activities these random dots would never have come alive in our mind.

In several other dialogues, learning phenomena in early vision were discussed. This learning is somewhat different from cognitive learning, inasmuch as it is position specific, slow, and often does not need full attention (Karni 1992). The question of finding long-term learning phenomena without semantics is an interesting one. It is known that some patients without long-term memory for lexical items and events can still learn some procedures, like the Tower of Hanoi game. Karni's work raises the question whether such patients (with both temporal lobes damaged) could still learn texton gradients after many repeated trials and also retain this knowledge for many years.

There are many other interesting problems of visual cognition. I will mention the "object-superiority effect," pioneered by Naomi Weinstein and Charlie Harris (1980). Similar to the well-known "word-superiority effect," where a letter embedded in an English text is better detected than amidst nonsense letters, segments of a drawing are better detected when they belong to a real object (e.g. a 2-D drawing of a 3-D object) than when these parts belong to a nonsense drawing. Recent work by Ken Nakayama and Shinsuke Shimojo (1992) on generic views of an object seems to imply that a segment does not pop out when it blends into a real object. I regard this finding as contrary to the object-superiority effect, but it could be that I misunderstand the main implications. By the way, the work by Nakayama and Shimojo (1992) is an important addition to the most persuasive demonstrations by Gunnar Johansson (where a few dots in a

dark background, when in motion, evokes in us the vivid percept of a walking human). They claim that of the many possible views of a 3-D object, the most frequently seen 2-D projections are regarded the canonic representations.

In the spirit of Karl Popper, I hope that the field of perception has an edge over cognition inasmuch as its theories can be falsified and thus qualify to be regarded as scientific. Whether theories in visual cognition can be created that fit the criterion of falsification is a question that I leave for the next generation.

B: You seem to enjoy ending your essays with pathos. Since I regard the basic idea of these dialogues to be expressed by figure 5.1, could you comment on the bottom-up/top-down model of brain function depicted by that figure? After all, your life's work is mainly the study of bottom-up processes of vision. That, in my view, is adequately challenging for neurophysiologists, but it needlessly restricts the scope of psychology.

A: I will devote all of dialogue 11 to defending the bottom-up philosophy underlying early vision. But you are right. Let me make a final comment on the "boxology" expressed in figure 5.1. This also brings me to my four-year association with the Santa Fe Institute, whose participants (particularly Murray Gell-Mann) greatly influenced my recent thinking.

According to Santa Fe Institute philosophy (see the SWARM system of Christopher Langton, whom I quote in the next couple of paragraphs almost verbatim), traditional "reductionist" science is concerned with bottom-up phenomena, and assumes that the dynamics are merely epiphenomena that reflect but do not influence the behavior of the system. However, ignoring the context-setting feedback (the top-down processing), *strict reductionism ignores the possibility for self-organization.*

By contrast, top-down processes alone would correspond to the discarded approach once known as vitalism, in which nonphysical, "vital" organizing principles imposed themselves magically on matter. The vitalists assume that "mere" physical matter cannot, on its own, act in complex ways without being "animated" by some "vital force" (the Greeks called this "quintessence" and supposed it to be a fifth, nonphysical form of existence, beyond the four material forms of Earth, Air, Fire, and Water).

In many real-world systems, top-down and bottom-up processes are coupled in a multi-level feedback loop. Such a system can determine its own boundary conditions, and it is this capacity that provides the basis for the emergence of effectively unlimited complexity. The SWARM project tries to emulate the behavior of a swarm of insects on massively parallel computers. Each individual is coupled both to its environment and to its adjacent neighboring insects (constituting the bottom-up process), and each individual's "state" (as a processor of information) can be globally altered by a feedback command from some statistical evaluator (a top-down process). [For further information see Theraulax and Deneubourg 1992.] Fire ants, termites, and bees are real-life manifestations of such organizations, where the total system exhibits much more complex behavior than its individual members and, what is more, can easily adapt to changes in the environment.

Of course, brains are much more complex in their organization than swarms, because in place of some hormonal coupling from a far distance (perhaps exerted by the queen bee), nerve bundles permit a more specific feedback. The SWARM project, now implemented on the Connection Machine with its many ten thousands of parallel computers, permits a convenient way to fill the gap between models of insect colonies and real brains. It would be most interesting to see how SWARM organization might be approximating the behavior of UTMs, and in what capabilities it falls short of Turing Machines! This is an area of research where model builders, mathematicians, insect physiologists, monkey neurophysiologists, and psychologists of human behavior will collaborate in the future.

[I will return to some of these problems in dialogue 14.]

DIALOGUE 11
A CONDENSED
HISTORY OF MY
FINDINGS

The shah, at age 30, after his coronation, had asked his chief scientist to compile for him the history of mankind. He had long forgotten about it when, on his fortieth birthday, a long caravan arrived carrying several hundred volumes. "How could I read all this stuff with my busy schedule," exclaimed the shah. "Go back and condense it!" On the shah's fiftieth birthday the chief scientist, now very old and feeble, proudly presented his concise history of mankind in twenty volumes. But the shah was not satisfied. "I am not that young anymore, and immensely busy. How could I read these twenty volumes in my lifetime? Go back and shorten it!" Ten years later the son of the late chief scientist arrived with a three-volume set, but the shah was not satisfied. "I am now old, and cannot see well. Condense it even further!" On his seventieth birthday the shah was very ill. The chief scientist's son, now chief scientist himself, rushed to the shah's bedside with a single volume in his hand. The shah looked at the volume and said: "Don't you see that I am dying? Try to condense the history of mankind into a single sentence!" The chief scientist replied: "Well, your highness, men were born, suffered, and then died!" Hearing that, the shah, with a sad smile, nodded and expired.

A: I can sum up the main results of my research—spanning three decades—in a few sentences:

• Contrary to previous beliefs, stereopsis of random-dot stereograms is not a local but a global process.

• Contrary to previous beliefs, effortless texture discrimination was shown to be not a global process based on statistics but a local process based on local conspicuous features (textons).

As a result of recent work on focal attention, I can add the following:

• The fusion of random-dot stereograms suggested at its very inception that stereopsis is an early process. After all, if the disparity is within Panum's fusional limit, then one can fuse an RDS within 60 msec, and in the absence of any familiarity cues. That it takes place at the input of the monkey cortex, as Gian Poggio found, is of great importance. Early vision is bottom-up, and the perceptual phenomena of stereopsis, motion perception, and texture discrimination can be linked to the findings in the early stages of monkey cortex through microelectrode neurophysiology. Thus, the mysterious mind-body problem slowly begins to be solved without much ado.

• If we add focal attention to the bottom-up processes of early vision, then the many other enigmatic top-down processes, from semantic memory to symbolic manipulations of cognition, are not necessary in the great majority of perceptual tasks. It appears that early vision can be subdivided into a preattentive system (resulting in instantaneous pop-out), and an attentive system (based on element-by-element scrutiny). However, in some important cases these are not simply the two extreme points of a continuous psychometric curve; they represent two distinct processing modes—perhaps parallel versus serial mechanisms, or some other qualitatively distinct information processes.

B: What is the point of presenting the essence of your findings in a condensed form? Those who are interested in your work will study it in detail, since in science there is no royal road. Furthermore, some of the outstanding achievements in mathematics, such as the proof of the four-color conjecture and that of the Fermat conjecture, require hundreds of pages of complex explanation.

A: I believe that the essence of any important idea or experiment can be explained in a condensed way, except for a few very sophisticated physical paradigms—say, superstring or relativistic field theories (and I omit mathematics). Furthermore, since there is a limit to how many novel findings one has the good fortune to make, a scientist's real contributions can be summed up in a few pages. Since my work is in vision, and an image is worth 1000 words, I should be able to sum up my contributions with a few demonstrations.

B: To sum up one's life's work in a dozen demonstrations seems quite a challenge. Please go ahead.

A: Let me start with the basic RDS (Julesz 1960), reproduced here as figure 11.1. Nowadays I can generate such an RDS with my HP100LX pocket computer in a minute from scratch, or I can generate a dynamic RDS where the random texture changes 100 frames/sec in real time using some of the fastest computers we own. [Or it can be generated by these faster computers and then displayed in real time on a PC or a Macintosh.] When using the smaller computers, one usually generates a red-green anaglyph and views the display with red-green goggles; however, on several of our larger computers we use a liquid-crystal shutter that alternately presents the left and right stereograms to the appropriate eye. It was with a dynamic RDS that Gian Poggio discovered the first cyclopean units in

Figure 11.1

Basic random-dot stereograms depicting (a) an astroid (diamond), (b) a spiral, and (c) a hyperbolic paraboloid. After Julesz 1971; created by Jih Jie Chang for this book.

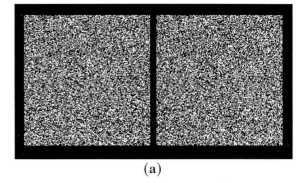

(a)

(b)

(c)

the input stages of the monkey cortex. Nevertheless, for a simple demonstration, I think a static RDS, as portrayed by figure 11.1, gives the essence of my first well-known creation.

In dialogue 5 I discussed the main implications of the RDS. Here I will mention only the main one, which was understood at the very inception of the RDS: that without familiar monocular shapes and contours binocular fusion can be based on disparity alone as a result of some global, correlation-like process.

I also observed (Julesz 1960) that areas presented only to one eye (called the "no-man's-land" in *FCP*) appeared as the continuation of the background, or of the depth plane farthest behind in the scene. I "explained" it by evoking a mechanism that regarded areas seen by only one eye as occluded areas that by definition had to occur behind the other surfaces in front, which are seen by both eyes.

There are a few more demonstrations linked to figure 11.1. First, as figure 11.1 shows, a false target cannot be eliminated by monocular form recognition of each individual target but must be disambiguated by a global process such as cross-correlation. The other demonstration is the "inverse cyclopean" technique illustrated in figure 11.2 (Julesz 1966). Here the monocular symmetry in one eye's view is scrambled in the binocularly fused image, thus showing that most visual processes (e.g. symmetry perception and form recognition) must occur after global stereopsis.

That stereopsis is an early process is based on these kind of demonstrations, and was dramatically confirmed by the neurophysiological findings of Gian Poggio (1984).

Perhaps it is important that (contrary to classical stereograms, which consist of a few line segments), a polarity-reversed RDS cannot be fused as depicted in figure 11.3.

Although I noted on page 73 of *FCP* that when color is added to a polarity-reversed RDS the correlated color can counteract the strong binocular rivalry caused by the polarity reversal, only recently has this observation been proven conclusively and extended to the RDC (Kovacs and

Figure 11.2

The "inverse cyclopean" technique (Julesz 1966). Here the monocular symmetry in one eye's view is scrambled in the binocularly fused image, thus showing that most visual processes (e.g. symmetry perception and form recognition) must occur after global stereopsis. From Julesz 1966.

Figure 11.3

Demonstration that a polarity-reversed random-dot stereogram cannot be fused. After Julesz 1960.

Julesz 1992). This finding will, I hope, finally dispel the notion that the stereo and motion systems are color blind!

Now I will discuss an early (1960) experiment that was published in the Proceedings of the Fourth London Symposium on Information Theory (Julesz 1961) as depicted in figure 4.6 but whose implications have changed in the last 30 years. In this demonstration I took the basic RDS of figure 11.1 and broke up the diagonal connectivities in one of the stereo images. Whenever three adjacent pixels along the ±45 arc deg diagonals had the same color (black or white), the center pixels were complemented. This operation removed the global binocular correlation by only 16%, yet the local similarity between the left and right images disappeared completely. While one image appears as a random aggregate of dots, the other image looks like a maze of horizontal and vertical lines. I also noted that when the two images were blurred they appeared similar and their global correlation became apparent.

Here, then, is a clear demonstration that, instead of some common-sense similarity, similarity in global stereopsis is based on correlation. This is also true for the random-dot cinematogram, as I tried to present in articles in the early 1960s. (Since I could not demonstrate these experiments in print, I only mentioned these findings at lectures. My first article on the RDC was Julesz and Payne 1968.) When the spatial-frequency channels became fashionable, Miller and I showed that fusion is not disrupted as long as a masking noise is added to a stereogram whose SF spectrum is about two octaves below or above the spectral components of the stereogram (Julesz and Miller 1962). Thus, the figure reproduced above as 4.6 was an early dem-

onstration of a stereogram with similar low-SF information but dissimilar high-SF information that did not, however, interfere with fusion, since the spectrum of this masking noise was well above the low-SF spectrum.

While I am discussing stereopsis, let me present an ambiguous RDS (figure 11.4). What might have escaped the attention of many colleagues is that the two surfaces portrayed here, when near each other in depth, can be fused simultaneously. Here is a case that goes beyond transparency. One can easily create a stereogram in which every odd row portrays one surface, and every even row another, and one can perceive a transparent surface hovering in front of another one. What is important, however, is that figure 11.4 is fundamentally different from a transparent stereogram. For a transparent stereogram, *uniqueness* holds. Any corresponding point belongs to only one surface. However, in figure 11.4 we experience *metatransparency*, a condition that does not exist in real life. The uniqueness constraint, which David Marr (1982) and his followers (including Grimson (1981)) regarded as a fundamental constraint, is violated. In my review of Grimson (Julesz 1986c) I pointed out this fallacy of the uniqueness requirement. However, it seems to me that, as long as one does not give it a catchy name, people ignore such a non-common-sense observation. Therefore, I coined the name "metatransparency." [I also coined some other names—"equidistributed information" (Julesz and Pennington 1965), "mental holography," and "psychoanatomy" (Julesz 1971), "textons" (Julesz 1981), and "anti-textons" (Williams and Julesz 1991), to name a few that stuck. As a matter of fact, in the oldest field of psychology, color perception, where the fundamental concept of the three color primaries was known for two centuries, different paradigm groups have renamed the red, green, and blue mechanisms, calling them π mechanisms, or L(long), M(medium), or S(short) mechanisms, and calling adaptation processes by other names, such as "fatigue" and "bleaching," trying to establish their theoretical differences from others, even though the terms refer to the same underlying causes.] However, many observers cannot experience metatransparency and at any instant can perceive only one organiztion in an ambiguous RDS. So, uniqeness in stereopsis is still an open question, but its outcome is merely an experimental problem. For instance, can depth organization in a retinally stabilized ambiguous RDS (when vergence movements are made inoperative) be switched at will?

The last demonstration of my research in stereopsis is the technique of the modified cyclopean illusions, which applies the technique to the Ebbinghaus illusion as illustrated in figure 5.2a. One of the first applications of the RDS was the portrayal of optical illusions by Seymour Papert (1961), who showed that the classical Mueller-Lyer optical illusion can be observed when disparity gradients are used instead of luminance contours.

In *FCP* I went a step further and placed the inducing figures at a different depth from the targets, as shown in figure 5.2c. To my surprise, the illusion seemed to disappear or be greatly reduced. I concluded in 1971 that the lateral inhibition which is responsible for the illusions exists mainly between binocular disparity neurons that are tuned to the same disparities, but not to cyclopean neurons that are tuned to different disparities. *FCP* was mainly devoted to the cyclopean portrayal of optical illusions of aftereffects, etc., by RDSs and RDCs

Figure 11.4

An ambiguous random-dot stereogram demonstrating that two surfaces can be perceived simultaneously. The case of "metatransparency" is shown, since in real life no such case exists. From Julesz 1971.

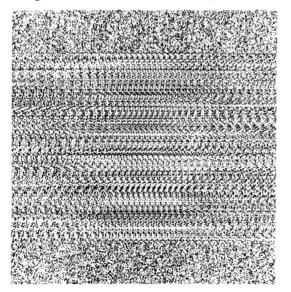
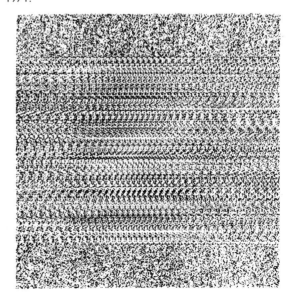

in order to trace their "locus" as being before or after the "cyclopean retina," thus allowing me to make some observations on the lateral interaction between cyclopean neurons—a technique I named "psychoanatomy." Since Gian Poggio (1984) found the anatomical sites of the cyclopean neurons, psychoanatomy has been slowly converted into real neuroanatomy. This ends the list of my contributions in stereopsis that can be demonstrated by a single stereogram.

Unfortunately, the iso-second-order texture paradigm (Julesz 1962), which I regard as a more sophisticated contribution than the RDS paradigm, is too complicated to be demonstrated by a single experiment. But let me try. In Julesz 1962 I demonstrated a texture pair in which one texture was composed of random dots while the adjacent texture was made up of six densely placed triangular patches of equal frequency (figure 11.5). Yet, the repetition of these triangles could not be perceived, except for the all-black one. This demonstration was the precursor of my texton theory, because it clearly showed that preattentive texture discrimination is not a statistical (global) phenomenon, but depends on local conspicuous features (the black triangular blobs), which I later called textons (Julesz 1981).

In Julesz 1971 I showed that texture pairs with the very different power spectra can either be discriminated or not depending on the presence or absence, respectively, of texton gradients (figure 11.6). The opposite is also true: textures with the same second-order statistics, and hence identical power spectra, can or cannot be discriminated, depending again on whether texton gradients are present or absent.

Figure 11.5

An early demonstration that texture discrimination is not statistical. From Julesz 1962. Note the lack of black triangles in the lower right quadrant.

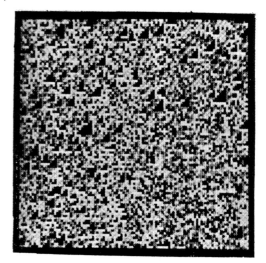

Our most convincing demonstration of how texture discrimination does not depend on global (statistical) parameters (Julesz, Gilbert, and Victor 1976; Julesz 1981) is shown in figure 11.7. Here the three textures agree in their third-order statis-

Figure 11.6

Examples of discriminable and nondiscriminable texture pairs with different power spectra. From Julesz 1980.

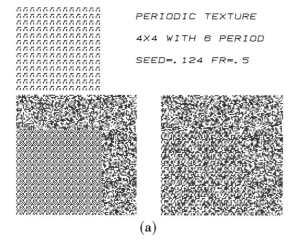

PERIODIC TEXTURE

4X4 WITH 6 PERIOD

SEED=.124 FR=.5

(a)

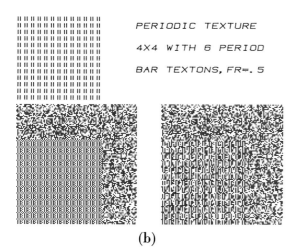

PERIODIC TEXTURE

4X4 WITH 6 PERIOD

BAR TEXTONS, FR=.5

(b)

tics, and differ only in their fourth- and higher-order statistics. The results indicate that the visual system most likely cannot compute subtle differences in fourth-order matrices (which define fourth-order statistics), and discriminate the differences based on elongated blobs with different width, length, and orientation. These are the "textons" underlying texture discrimination. The Gabor patches are also basic textons. They are the generalization of elongated blobs with some periodic flanks, which are useful in SF tuning. I also pointed out that the blank areas between the texture elements also act as textons (Julesz 1984, 1986), an important fact ignored by several critics

Figure 11.7

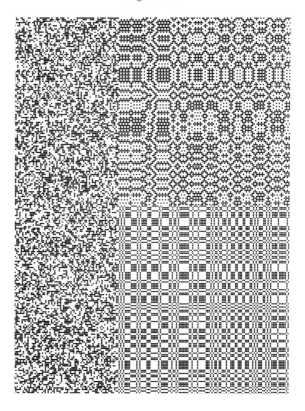

of the texton theory. Doug Williams and I emphasized this fact and named the textons formed by the gaps between elements anti-textons (Williams and Julesz 1991, 1992). In the same publications, we demonstrated that the asymmetry effect of texture discrimination (i.e., texture A embedded in texture B yields stronger discrimination than vice versa, as depicted in figure 9.10) is the result of subjective contours (of the Kanizsa type) perceptually closing the gaps.

I am particularly fond of a demonstration in Williams and Julesz 1991 that shows the nonlinearity of texture discrimination, based on the generalized four-disk method (Caelli et al. 1978). When the aggregate of small Ls are added to the strongly discriminable texture pair in figure 9.11, the resulting texture pair is rendered nondiscriminable. Obviously the law of superposition is violated, which indicates that the preattentive texture-discrimination system is highly nonlinear.

B: As I see it, you were able to guide us through your scientific life, because you skipped many of your other activities that were based on more dynamic experiments, which were inappropriate for the printed page. Is it not unfair to you and your collaborators who worked on these more complex experiments to leave them out in this condensed account?

A: Probably you are right, but for me it was an added pleasure to be able to demonstrate my findings to many people, and share with them the perceptual and intellectual enjoyments of vision. I know of several colleagues who told me that it was through some of these demonstrations that they became hooked on science. In my opinion, no experiment disguised in chi-square statistics and histograms of data can convey the impact on young people of such direct demonstrations. Of course, I have learned much from other experiments (not shown here) we performed as from the insights of my collaborators. I will discuss these in appendix B in detail. In this dialogue I merely present some of the simple "melodies"; the complex pieces with heavy orchestration are discussed elsewhere.

B: While I admit that you gained some unexpected insights in a few select topics of psychology and drummed up an unusually large number of scientists who became interested in these topics, I am quite sure that without you, as computers became prevalent, all these experiments would have been carried out by others in due time. Indeed, I recall how proud you were when one of the reviewers of your monograph *FCP* Ben Barkow (1973) wrote in essence that "if Leo Szilárd were alive and were interested in vision, then he could have written this book." Since Szilárd was one of your heroes, I can see the reason of your satisfaction with this comment. However, it also hinted at the possibility that any clever guy could have come up with your experiments had he had access to a general-purpose computer, which you luckily possessed much earlier than most psychologists. I make these comments not to belittle your contributions, but to clarify matters. My real criticism of your achievements goes much deeper. I regard your paradigm of early vision rather limited, and can hardly wait for the technologies that would go beyond this to permit the scientific study of visual cognition. Returning to your Condensed History, I interpret your epigraph from a slightly different point of view: Is it not sad how little one can accomplish in a lifetime?

A: In a dialogue, I usually like to have the last word. The value of one's achievements is relative. Compared to a Newton or an Einstein very few scientists did accomplish much! I know several scientists whose talents were immense, but their actual scientific achievements fell short with respect to their intellects. I also know some colleagues whose intellect was limited, but accomplished much more than their more gifted fellow scientists. Was this mere luck, or are there some other ingredients beyond IQ that are conducive to creativity? I regard myself a content man, since I accomplished more than my talents entitled me to achieve.

DIALOGUE 12
RECENT FINDINGS
WITH MY CO-WORKERS

My mind works in parallel. A friend, Jerry Lettvin, once told me about an elastic egg-crate model of some membranes through which the eggs (ions) could fall through as long as the crate's partitions were orthogonal to each other, but the eggs got stuck when poisoning deformed the crate and its openings became rhomboid in shape. While this model for membranes is now defunct, it is a good metaphor for my thinking process. For years a few unsolved problems deformed the crate of my mind, and my thoughts got stuck. Only in recent years, with the help of my co-workers, did the scaffolding of my mind's crate became orthogonal again, permitting my thoughts to flow freely. This dialogue is devoted to the surmounting of some of these hurdles.

A: As I become one of the older active researchers in human vision, the problem arises as to whether I should only sum up the highlights of my research, spanning over 30 years, or whether I should prove to you that I am still very active by concentrating on recent findings. Luckily, I do not have to ponder this dichotomy. For several years I was planning to write my second monograph, but I could not do so. A few unanswered questions stood in my way. I am happy to report that the most important of these obstacles have been removed by the adequate solving of some of the difficult problems. As a result, I published a review addressed to physicists: "Early vision and focal attention" (1991). I regard this long article as the backbone of my planned second monograph. Below I will list these scientific hurdles and give some of their solutions. Before doing so, I will give a historic account of my research in what I used to call "cyclopean perception," which nowadays is referred to as early vision.

In the 1960s, the fusion of the random-dot stereogram had already shown conclusively that,

contrary to common belief, stereopsis was not a local but a global process. In the 1970s, the discovery of textons showed that preattentive texture discrimination was not a global process (based on statistics) but essentially a local one. In the decades following these early insights, some others were gained.

Thirty years after the introduction of the RDS technique, its role in vision research has become clearer, although it might take another generation to realize its true significance. After all, stereopsis is a specialized process that yields relative depth from binocular disparity, while recognition of objects (and perspective depth) occur even in monocular vision. How strategic is research in stereopsis if one regards object recognition as the main purpose of vision? Some answers follow.

• The RDS gave conclusive proof that there is no camouflage in three dimensions. Global stereopsis apparently evolved in our primate (lemur) ancestors to overcome the camouflage of insects hiding motionless in the foliage. After this development, stereopsis has helped monocular form perception by performing a very early scene analysis (segmentation) of the environment.

• Psychoanatomy using the RDS is helpful for localizing perceptual processes. [For example, global (short-range) motion must occur after stereopsis.] This can aid neurophysiologists in their tracing of the information flow in the CNS. As early as 1960, the demonstration that stereopsis can occur in the absence of all monocular form (contour as well as depth cues) indicated that it must be an early process. Indeed, Hubel and Wiesel switched from form perception to binocular vision after the first RDS demonstration, in 1960. Gian Poggio's neuro-physiological findings with dynamic RDSs show that cyclopean neurons exist as early as layer IVB of V1 (also called Area 17, or the striate cortex) in the monkey brain (the very input to the visual cortex).

• The global stereopsis of the RDS raised a fundamental problem of brain research: the "false-target elimination problem." This same problem occurs in the monocular motion perception of random-dot cinematograms.

• RDS techniques permit sophisticated analysis of visual processes beyond psychoanatomy. For instance, the role of color in stereopsis and in the magno-cellular pathway can be studied.

• RDS techniques permitted the first nontrivial linking of a perceptual process with neurophysiology.

• RDSs were among the first stimuli to take advantage of the fast, large-storage digital computer, and were introduced at the arrival of such computers in industrial laboratories. Since without a computer it would have been impractical to produce such stimuli in large quantities, here was a genuine example when psychology research gained an invaluable tool. This is now trivial for the younger generation who own their own personal computers, but the arrival of these machines was a most exhilarating experience for my generation!

• Global stereopsis and preattentive texture segmentation are bottom-up processes. By adding focal attention (a top-down process) to these two powerful processes, scene analysis can be explained

without the need for invoking enigmatic semantic information stored in the memory. This in turn paves the way for some of the visual algorithms of scene analysis in machine vision.

• We have evidence that top-down processes (depth from shading, pseudoscopy, etc.) have only a weak influence on global depth perception of the RDS.

B: I was always amazed that Helmholtz, or some early investigator in the last century, did not construct an RDS from sandpaper, using a pair of scissors. However, I thought that one of the main insight that was obtained from the RDS was that it contradicted Kenneth Ogle's claim that monocular contours are necessary for stereopsis. Indeed, such a claim was known to be incorrect a generation earlier, by Helmholtz.

A: I share your amazement. While computers permit ideal camouflage with absolute stimulus control, there must have been dozens of stereo photographs taken from balloons or airplanes of densely textured scenes that emulated random-dot stereograms quite well. In an article by Babington-Smith (1977), one can see the floating ice on the River Rhine in a 1940 aerial reconnaissance photograph of Cologne taken from two nearby vantage points, and the pieces of ice portray interesting surfaces in depth, particularly in the vicinity of the piers of a bridge, where the ice flow is slowed down. For decades I have tried to find some earlier stereo photos; so far, I have failed.

You are also correct that Helmholtz implicitly knew that stereopsis can be obtained without pronounced monocular contours, since he looked at corrugated surfaces with one and then two eyes and noted that binocular viewing enhanced plasticity. Since corrugated paper illuminated from above does not cast luminance contours on our retinae, the observed increase in depth clearly shows that monocular contours are not necessary for fusion. Here is, again, some useful knowledge, already known by Helmholtz, that was forgotten. This lost insight dramatically resurfaced with the introduction of the computer-generated RDS, in which no imperfection—such as cutting some pixel in half—can produce unwanted monocular contours.

B: If you must repeat some of your past work, I would rather hear about your texton theory, which underwent many changes, than about cyclopean perception, which was always a straightforward paradigm!

A: Although I have devoted an entire dialogue to my texton theory and the preattentive/attentive dichotomy in general, let me single out some of our recent findings related to textons.

While RDS research was straightforward, my second paradigm for searching for local features that would yield pop-out in iso-second-order texture pairs had a much more winding path. It took me and my colleagues many years to clarify some of the problems listed here, and much more research is needed to settle these problems in a more conclusive way. I will just list these problems first:

- the asymmetry problem

- anti-textons

- color vs. orientation

- parallel vs. serial scanning and the role of focal attention

- textons vs. nonlinear spatial filters.

Before I go into some details, I will say a few words on scientific style.

Before I arrived in the United States, I was fascinated with thought experiments and mathematics—two activities one can pursue in a poor country. For instance, I was fascinated with Einstein's thought experiments with falling elevators, which led to the theory of general relativity. However, even then I was aware of the limits of thought experiments. After all, the original Einstein equations predicted an ever-expanding universe; Einstein himself regarded this as absurd and modified the equations. Only later, when Edwin Powell Hubble found the Doppler shift of the far galaxies, did Einstein realize that he had been too hasty to have modified his equations. It was obvious to me that thought experiments had their limitations and were only substitutes for real experiments. So, after I arrived at Bell Laboratories, then one of the world's miracles of scientific productivity, I decided to use the most sophisticated experiments I could devise. However, as a devotee of the thought experiment, I decided to modify this tool in a constructive way. I would construct experiments that would require the most complex mathematical and technical tools in order to obtain a dichotomous question whose outcome could not be guessed. For instance, could one perceive depth in an ideally camouflaged stereo pair without monocular contours or form cues? Could one generate texture pairs with identical Nth-order but different (N + 1)th-order statistics and determine the highest N that could still yield perceptual segmentation without scrutiny?

Of course, there remained this: What questions should one pose? It was my mentor and former scientific director at Bell, John Pierce, who taught me that "a good researcher does not attack problems he likes the most, but rather works on problems that became ripe for solution." Of course, these solvable problems should be challenging and fun to work on, and should appear important. Whether a problem is important (perhaps the word "strategic" is better) cannot be assessed at the time of its conception. Only history can tell fashionable problems from strategic ones. Even my two paradigms—the random-dot stereogram and cinematogram (which I introduced in 1960) and the preattentive texture discrimination of texture pairs with iso-second-order statistics (1962)—are still so recent that we cannot be sure of their strategic significance. Nevertheless, from a practical point of view, these two paradigms (and a third: spatial-frequency channels, which was posed by others but which Stromeyer and I helped to pioneer) kept an entire generation of brain researchers busy and earning their living. If they had fun as well, then I am partly assured that I accomplished something.

B: Please stop ruminating over the past and turn to your present work, as you have promised.

A: I am eager to do so. I am particularly pleased to report some interesting recent research, conducted with several new associates and a few old co-workers:

1. Global stereopsis is not color blind (Kovacs and Julesz 1992).
2. Hierarchical processing of random-dot stereograms and cimematograms, and of Glass patterns; difference in spatial integration; Gabor functions, fractals, textons (Kovacs and Julesz 1992).
3. Speed of shifts in focal attention (Saarinen and Julesz 1991; Hung et al., in progress).
4. Anti-textons (Williams and Julesz 1992).
5. The asymmetry problem of texture segmentation can be explained by closing the gap by subjective contours (Williams and Julesz 1992).
6. The preattentive/attentive dichotomy in texture perception (Braun and Julesz, 1992 and in progress).
7. How is the two-diopter chromatic aberration of the human eye lens compensated? Acuity of blue in the presence of red or green. (An abstract (Prasad and Julesz 1991) was published, but since no paper has been published I regard this problem as unsolved.)
8. Except for echo-locating animals, can primates perceive absolute depth? For instance, stereopsis yields only relative depth. Is relative depth adequate to achieve depth and size constancies? (Work in collaboration with Itzhak Hadani. Parts of this study published, other parts in progress.)
9. Depth from shading is dominated by stereopsis. (Work in collaboration with Jih Jie Chang, reported in Julesz 1991.)
10. The mind's eye looks through a telescope. A suggestion of how movement invariance during eye movement can be achieved. (In collaboration with Itzhak Hadani; in preparation. See my comments on Gibson's direct perception.)

11. Extension of Panum's fusional area by extensive learning. The role of sleep. (In collaboration with Ilona Kovacs; still in progress.)

12. Juxtaposing local features (textons) in global perceptual tasks (motion, stereopsis, textural grouping, etc.) to assess their perceptual strength. (In collaboration with Thomas Papathomas and Andrei Gorea. Parts of this study have been published.)

B: I hope you will go into details, since this list of projects is not clear enough.

A: Let me start with a brief discussion.

1. In my first monograph (Julesz 1971, p. 73) I reported briefly that an otherwise-unfuseable polarity-reversed RDS can be made fuseable if the corresponding reversed gray pixels are similarly colored in the left and right images. Thus color can overcome polarity reversal, provided that the reversed contrast is not too large. In spite of this finding that indicated stereopsis cannot be "color blind," a series of papers were published using colored nonfuseable RDSs at isoluminance, with the conclusion that stereopsis does not utilize colors. [After the difficult technical problems of creating isoluminance (at least for the physical stimulus, but not necessarily over the entire visual field) were solved by Lu and Fender (1972), followed by Ramachandran and Gregory (1978), all these authors reported that stereopsis of RDSs portrayed by small pixels did disappear. However, for classical stereograms and for RDSs portrayed by coarse pixels the depth percept lingered on.] Obviously some weird things happen at isoluminance, but the suggestion that stereopsis is color blind is simply not true. Interestingly, only a few researchers have quoted my results as counterevidence to the generally accepted view that stereo is color blind (De Weert and Sadza 1983). In hindsight I understand why this work of mine was generally ignored. Indeed, in 1971 computer-controlled color monitors were in their infancy, and it was difficult to be sure that by adding colors one would not inadvertently interfere with the contrast settings. Thus, Ilona Kovacs and I tried, on a Silicon Graphics IRIS computer, polarity-reversed RDSs under complete color and brightness control. (The stereo separation was achieved by alternately switched liquid-crystal goggles at a rate of 120 frames/sec.) The paper (Kovacs and Julesz 1992, with color stereo plates) provides convincing evidence that without color the polarity-reversed gray RDS cannot be fused, but adding color reestablishes fusion. However, only under strict laboratory conditions is it possible to ensure that polarity remains reversed. We named the polarity-reversed color RDS and RDC *metaisoluminance*. I am glad that my original finding stood the test of time, and I hope that the difficulties of seeing depth in colored RDSs at isoluminance will be understood to be the result of not having luminance contrast alone. It seems that stereopsis utilizes color. That stereopsis is primarily a function of the color-deficient magno system, as Livingston and Hubel (1987) suggested, is provocative but is probably an oversimplification. Nevertheless, while the colored dots of the pattern hover over the colored dots of the background, they are rather formless under metaisoluminance; that is, they do not coalesce into a solid surface.

That stereopsis utilizes color is also evident from the work of Diana Grinberg and David Williams (1985). They bleached the red and green receptors with a bright yellow light, and showed that a dim violet RDS still yielded correct depth percepts. "With the additional assumption that signals from the blue-sensitive mechanism do not contribute to luminance, these results confirm that purely chromatic signals have access to stereoscopic mechanisms" (Grinberg and Williams 1985). The argument for color-sensitive stereoscopic mechanisms is not as direct in the quoted study as we found with our polarity-reversed color stereograms. I just hope that we have finally put to rest the idea that stereopsis is color blind.

2. In a study similar to project 1, Ilona Kovacs and I examined polarity-reversed random-dot cinematograms (RDCs) and random-dot moiré (Glass) patterns (RDGs). Polarity-reversed RDCs are particularly interesting because they yield inverse-phi motion (Anstis 1970). Again, adding corresponding colors to a polarity-reversed RDC resulted in correct motion perception! Thus, the global (short-range) motion mechanism does utilize color as well. Finally, a polarity-reversed RDG, in which the global organization could not be seen, did not yield the global percept when corresponding color was added to the two patterns that we shifted with respect to each other. For details, see Julesz, and Kovacs 1992 and Kovacs and Julesz 1992. [With sparse patterns, however, color can yield global Glass-pattern phenomena under metaisoluminance. This was communicated to me by Thomas Papathomas.] Here I will only mention that we found some interesting unexpected results, such as a strong asymmetry for RDSs depending on eye dominance, and for RDCs depending on precedence. Also, the finding that green-white RDSs and RDCs behaved differently from the red-white ones raises questions about the green visual system, al-

though the culprit might be the TV phosphors used.

3. The problem of the speed of attention shifts, which nowadays I prefer to call *rapid search,* has been particularly worrisome for me, since it plays a pivotal role in my theory of preattentive and attentive texture discrimination. Indeed, small texton differences that do not pop out have to be searched for by time-consuming scrutiny. We developed this texton theory of texture discrimination by using texture pairs with controlled statistical properties and a mask with variable delays (SOA) (Julesz 1981; Bergen and Julesz 1983). Treisman (1982, 1985) and others used RT methodology and found for "conjunction" tasks item-by-item search times as fast as 10–50 msec. Ben Kröse and I were unable to replicate these fast search velocities. We used targets placed on a circle around the fixation point, and presented visual cues (arrows) pointing randomly to various targets in succession. While we were able to find the first cued target rapidly, the attention mechanism became locked onto the cue, as Posner (1978) had reported earlier, and it took more than 150 msec for the attention to get unlocked. Weichselgartner and Sperling (1987) used another paradigm, a sort of "visual RT," by presenting in a window a rapid sequence of alphanumeric strings, which they suddenly cued (e.g., brightened); the observer's task was to report the sequence of the string at and after the cue. The best observers were able to report the cued letter and subsequent ones at a rate of 10 Hz, or a scanning speed of 100 msec/item. These speeds were much faster than eye-movement speeds, and faster than our speeds with moving cues, but were considerably slower than Treisman's (1982, 1985) scanning rates. As was discussed in dialogue 8, Sperling et al.

(1973) could search for a letter in a crowded array of letters at 10 msec/item.

From the classical study by Shiffrin and Gardner (1972), it was clear that that for sparse arrays parallel and serial presentation followed by a mask 50 msec later yielded similar search performance. From this finding they concluded that for these tasks focal attention was not used. So, it was not immaterial to find out whether at higher speeds one could do equally well in a serial presentation when the search for the items was constrained by the order of presentation. Therefore, Jukka Saarinen and I modified the Weichselgartner- Sperling paradigm. Instead of presenting the random numerals on top of one another, we placed them as far apart as possible, on a circle around the fixation point. Whenever a new numeral was portrayed, simultaneously the previous numeral was masked by an effective masking pattern. We found that at a speed of 32 msec/item observers could report four consecutive numerals with good performance; the percentage of correct responses in temporal order was reduced but was still above chance level. For details, see Saarinen and Julesz 1991. Recently, Hung et al. (in progress) extended the Saarinen-Julesz study with 2–4 simultaneously presented numbers followed by a mask 32 and 16.7 msec later and found that simultaneous presentation yielded much better performance than sequential, particularly for faster rates. It seems that in parallel presentation an observer can find the items according to complex search strategies that can improve dramatically with practice. Therefore, it is of considerable interest that, even if the observer has to follow a serial presentation in random sequence, it is possible to catch even the fourth item at 16.7 msec/item. The 32-msec/frame rate is a technical limitation of the usual computer graphic displays with raster scans, and at Rutgers we were able to use new hardware that enabled 16-msec/frame rates. Our preliminary results extend the Saarinen-Julesz findings to items presented at 16 msec/item (Hung, Wilder, Curry, and Julesz, to be published), and it is an interesting question whether the superiority of parallel to serial will expand at ever-increasing presentation rates.

In the light of the work with Saarinen and Hung et al., I now see rapid search and focal-attention shifts in a new light. [See dialogue 8, question 6.] What many authors call "fast shifts of focal attention" should be called "rapid search," and "shifts of focal attention" should refer to an order-of-magnitude-slower process with time constants above 100 msec. The essence of our findings is related to the informational bottleneck—a fundamental problem of psychology that may be more important than attention shifts. As was pointed out by Campbell (1985), among others, there are about 1.5 million alphanumeric characters that can be resolved by the visual system, yet we can only report at most nine characters. This bottleneck, known after the famous paper by Miller (1956) as the "magic number of 7 ± 2," is a robust limit, and nobody who worked with the Sperling (1960) paradigm could extend the number of reported items above nine from the short-term memory. [Very recently, Ilona Kovacs and I repeated the Sperling paradigm, using in place of alphanumeric characters densely packed Gabor patches placed in concentric rings around a fixation point. In these uniform textures observers could read out (and thus see) the orientation of at most nine Gabor patches in any of the rings that were cued about 120 msec after the stimulus presentation (without being masked). However, if, in addition to normal-size Gabor patches, 4-times- larger and 4-times-smaller Gabor patches were placed in these rings, then observers could report (see) $3 \times 9 = 27$ patches correctly. This is a clear demonstration that one can shift attention to different scales. This shift of attention to different scales requires more than 100 msec while the rapid scan to read out the patches in the rings is another kind of process.]

The usual interpretion of this huge bottleneck has been assumed to be at the output of the short-term memory. However, as the result of my findings with Hung et al., it seems that simultaneous presentation of several items is superior to sequential presentation at 33 and 16 msec/item that argues for the bottleneck being at the input stage of the short-term memory. The input device has its preferred protocol for the incoming information that is violated during the sequential presentation in random order.

4,5. Since 1962 I had been interested in another paradigm of mine, the generation of texture pairs side by side with identical second- order (and third-order) statistics and searching for effortless (preattentive) discrimination (Julesz 1962). In most cases stochastic texture pairs with identical second- (and even third-) order statistics could not be discriminated without scrutiny. However, we found counterexamples to this observation. I called those conspicuous local features in discriminable iso-second-order texture pairs textons and suggested a model that would predict their interactions (Julesz 1980, 1986). However, there were two difficulties with my theory. One was the phenomenon of textural asymmetry, the other was the role of anti-textons, a concept that I explained but had not specified in detail. Doug Williams and I suggested explanations both for anti-textons and the asymmetry effect. In dialogue 8 I described this work in detail; see also Williams and Julesz 1991, 1992.

6. Jochen Braun and I are pursuing the preattentive/attentive dichotomy of texture discrimination, using some novel techniques that extend some earlier work by Sagi and Julesz (1985) and Braun and Sagi (1990). We load attention around the fixation point by a demanding task (to tell whether seven Ts contain an L), and simultaneously ask the observer to perform another task (for instance, to judge whether several disks in the parafovea are all of the same color, or to identify the colors of all the disks). We plan to find those primitive tokens that can be identified without scrutiny. We wish to be certain that attention is fixated during the entire presentation time (say, 120 msec) to the center, and be certain that identification of the parafoveal tasks is indeed preattentive. Meanwhile Ben-Av, Sagi, and Braun (1991) have already reported that perceptual grouping, a phenomenon assumed to be rather preattentive, seems to require attention.

Recently, however, we discovered tasks that did not require attention, since the double task was performed as well as the two tasks by themselves, for instance the detection of orientation gradients and color identification. In addition, we found an unexpected result: as the orientation-gradients were reduced, and discrimination performance got reduced, the central and peripheral task remained *independent* (Julesz and Braun 1992). So, there is a nonattentive system that can perceive ever-dimmer texton gradients with reduced accuracy, but without having to borrow attentional resources from a concurrent task!

7. I was always fascinated with the problem of how we can perceive red and blue color patches as equally sharp when there is a difference of more

than two diopters between the sharpnesses of these two colors (due to the chromatic aberration of our eyes). Obviously the speed of accommodation of the eye lens cannot account for this compensation, since middle-aged people lose their accommodation powers yet see red and blue sharply. When K. Venkatesh Prasad defended his Ph.D. thesis on how to reconstruct depth from the amount of blurring in photographs due to the limitations of the depthof fields of optical lenses, and wanted to work with me, it occurred to me that he and I should attack the chromatic-aberration problem outlined above. We presented color Landolt-ring targets for a brief time after a color adapting ring was briefly presented. When the adapting ring was red or green, the blue Landolt-ring target could not be resolved as well as when the adapting ring was blue. When the adapting ring was blue, the blue Landolt ring could be resolved with a gap width about 1 min arc. The finding that blue resolution is reduced when red is present has been reported by John Mollon. However, that blue alone can carry the same acuity as the other colors is rather unexpected and requires careful examination of present TV standards (e.g. NTSC) in which the blue channel has an order of magnitude less channel bandwidth. If this finding were corroborated, it could be of interest to engineers working on new TV standards, particularly for high-definition TV systems. However, because these results exists only as a brief abstract (Prasad and Julesz 1991) and were never published in detail, I regard the problem of chromatic-aberration compensation as unsolved.

Here is an unexpected alternative to the chromatic-aberration paradox: It was commented by Campbell and Robson (1968) that a compound grating of f and 3f SF in phase appeared as a square wave even though the higher odd harmonics were below internal noise. After all, in a highly nonlinear system one could imagine a lookup table that would translate a grating with its third harmonic (of the proper amplitude) to be a square-wave grating. In a similar vein, one could imagine that the highest spatial resolution for blue might be much lower than for green or red, nevertheless, the visual system would treat this finest blue pattern as if it were as sharp as the finest green and red patterns. After all, what is "sharp" is a perceptual phenomenon. It is conceptually not different from the fact that an optic wavelength of 540 nm yields the color "red" and not an auditory pitch.

8. I was always puzzled as to how stereopsis could only yield relative depth and yet one could thread a needle (or hit a nail with an outstretched ruler) better with binocular viewing. That depth perception was not the result of triangulation performed by sensing the convergence angles of the two eyes' axes and knowing one's interocular distance was first shown by Dove in 1841, just three years after Wheatstone constructed the first stereoscope. Dove presented stereograms tachistoscopically (using an electric spark) and found that stereoscopic depth could not be the result of convergence movements of the eyes, since it could not have been initiated during a few microseconds. Since then, it has been amply demonstrated that convergence eye movement is inadequate for binocular depth perception. Instead, a neural machinery performs relative depth processing based on horizontal binocular disparities. Some attempts to introduce vertical disparity into psychology to account for absolute depth are improbable, although vertical disparity might be used in machine vision. So, the question of absolute depth in stereopsis is rather enigmatic. As a matter

of fact, in *FCP* I pointed out that stereopsis did not evolve to enable predators to jump on the prey (since nobody can jump on relative depth) but must have evolved to break camouflage of prey at standstill. It seems that the only role binocular convergence plays in stereopsis is the *scaling* of perceived depth. The smaller the convergence angle, the larger the perceived depth.

Therefore, I was greatly interested in Itzhak Hadani's recent proposals that depth judgments during stereoscopic viewing might be strongly correlated with interocular distance (IOD). Because of my belief that stereopsis cannot yield absolute depth judgments, I believed that IOD would also be a sort of an absolute distance parameter that could not be appreciated by our visual system. Hadani and I aligned in depth a binocularly viewed physical probe (a thin rod) with the perceived depth of a cyclopean center square and its background in a RDS. The difference in depth between the measured square and its background (Z) in millimeters is related to IOD by the following equation:

$$Z = D \cdot \Delta / (IOD + \Delta),$$

where D is the distance to the nearest target (the cyclopean square) and Δ is the binocular disparity (see also Lappin and Love 1992) . We measured a large pool of observers ($N = 45$) ranging from 7 to 63 years, males and females, with and without glasses, with IODs from 4.9 to 7.3 cm, and found the correlation between their measured Z and their IOD was remarkably high. For details see our published graph in the 1992 ARVO Abstracts. It should be stressed that our strong correlation is obtained only if the background falls on the horopter.

I am not sure whether these findings give support to the possibility that absolute depth can be obtained by some added monocular and binocular cues, but I would have never guessed that the exact amount of IOD was known by the visual system. Of course, it might be that the task is performed by proprioception, and we know that moving in the environment and manipulating objects establishes an accurate space sense of our own body and its relationship to the outside world. Just recently there was a neurophysiological article on absolute depth detectors in the monkey cortex that measure the convergence angle of the eyes (Trotter et al. 1992).

9. One of the main implications of the global stereopsis of RDSs has been the realization that stereopsis is basically a bottom-up process in which top-down effects of semantics have a minor role, if any. To my knowledge, there are only two perceptual phenomena that challenge this view. One is pseudoscopy, the finding that familiar objects, particularly faces of humans and animals, refuse to appear concave when the left-right views are inverted. I discussed these two phenomena and their implication to psychology at length in dialogue 7.

B: I did not interrupt you for a while, since unexpectedly you were giving me facts, and *de gustibus non est disputandum*. Yet, the last experiment with Hadani is not as clear to me as the rest. I do not see how this experiment can tell us anything about absolute depth!

A: I wondered about that myself. Before these experiments, I assumed that convergence angles of the eye merely scaled the perceived amount of depth—sort of a 3-D extension of Emmert's Law. Now I am not certain. There must be an effect on depth judgments based on interocular distance, hence convergence angle. Recently Hadani et al. (1994) claim to have solved the passive navigational problem (with the outside world and the observer being still, but the obserever's eye rotating in its socket) and to have determined the absolute depth between the observer and the outside target.

10. The problem of the "mind looking through a telescope" was discussed in detail in dialogue 4. Hadani and I tried to explain the motion invariance of objects at different depths as the eyes and the head move. One explanation is based on our ability to perceive absolute depth (Hadani et al. 1994). However, we wanted to draw attention to another possibility. If the lens of our eye and the cortical magnification factors of our brain form a telescope that collimates the perceived images as they were at physical infinity, then near and far objects move at the same speeds when we move our eyes and head. I discussed this idea in relationship with Gibson's direct perception paradigm in dialogue 4.

11. For decades I used to present to summer students who worked in my department at Bell Labs brief flashes of RDSs with successively increasing disparities. I noticed that after thousands of trials their performance improved dramatically. For a while they had a sharp threshold of binocular disparity, and below their threshold they could tell without mistakes whether the briefly flashed RDS, followed by a mask, portrayed a cyclopean target in front of or behind the surround, or whether the target was uncorrelated (a crucial control). Slightly above threshold, performance rapidly deteriorated

to chance guessing. However, after weeks of trials, observers started to guess correctly the depth in RDSs and then slowly started to actually perceive the cyclopean targets many times above their earlier thresholds, as if Panum's fusional area had been enlarged. It seems as if the arborization of disparity tuned neurons had strengthened with repeated use. These observations of mine were rather anecdotal during those demonstrations, since data was not scientifically collected. After all, at Bell Labs I had no access to many young observers, but at Rutgers I joined forces with Ilona Kovacs and undertook a well-documented study of several observers, young and adult. We found a great plasticity up to an increase of 2 arc deg disparities with training. Indeed, in real life, large disparity detectors are not necessary, because the convergence movements of our eyes can bring the eyes into alignment. However, in our tachistoscopic task, convergence motions cannot take place, and the neural system is forced to cope with unusually large disparities. An account of these experiments will be published soon.

12. One of my earliest interests was the creation of ambiguous RDSs (and RDCs) where the same random-dot array would portray two independent global organizations (Julesz and Johnson 1968). In the case of stereopsis, the same RDS would portray two (sometimes even three) different surfaces in vivid depth. I was interested which one would be seen first, and in whether observers switch to the other global organization at will, or perceive both organizations simultaneously. In FCP I devoted an entire chapter ("Mental Holography") to these problems. Recently, Thomas Papathomas and Andrei Gorea modified the Julesz-Johnson method, juxtaposing the local features in order to see which

of them would dominate the others, thus yielding the corresponding global organization. In collaboration with them, I studied stereopsis, motion perception, and texture segmentation by juxtaposing polarity, color, and orientation of elongated bars. The hierarchy of these features can be found in several of our papers (Papathomas et al. 1988, 1990, 1991). It is interesting that it took a quarter of a century to combine my two paradigms (the ambiguous RDS and the textons) into a new research tool. Gorea and Papathomas's recent concept of generalized contrast will be published soon, and their recent model of texture segregation has great predictive power.

B: I am glad that you and your co-workers are so active. However, I just cannot see much coherence among these many different topics.

A: These topics may seem like a hodgepodge of ideas and results to some, but to me they are all of great importance. Thirty years ago I played with similarly unorthodox stimuli of random textures that I presented to one or two eyes, respectively, and now the implications of these experiments constitute the field of early vision. Whether these newer ideas will coalesce into a more unified whole, or stay jumbled, remains to be seen.

DIALOGUE 13
AUDITORY AND
VISUAL PERCEPTION
COMPARED

A: "Nowhere in auditory theory or in acoustic psychophysiological practice is there anything more ubiquitous than the critical band. . . . And likely, in one way or another, it will be part of our final understanding of how and why we perceive anything that reaches our ears. Students of vision have no such omnipresent entity to worry and console them. The other senses lack the mysteriousness of this unseen—perhaps nonexistent—but pervasive auditory filter." (Tobias 1970, p. 157) I used this as an epigraph to my article "Spatial-frequency channels in one-, two-, and three-dimensional vision: Variations on an auditory theme by Bekesy," in *Visual Coding and Adaptability,* ed. C. S. Harris (Erlbaum, 1980). [This book, masterfully edited though perhaps slightly out of date, contains exceedingly clear articles on visual perception.] I showed that several ideas and findings in auditory perception made by Békésy in 1929 had almost identical analogies in visual perception. By using luminance grating, Blakemore and Campbell (1969) discovered a spatial-frequency adaptation effect, and Blakemore and Sutton (1969) found a spatial- frequency shift phenomenon similarly to Békésy's 1929 findings for auditory spatial frequencies. Of course, Blakemore, Campbell, and Sutton, among others, discovered their visual adaptation phenomena after realizing that the visual analogy of a sinusoidal function was not a sinusoidally wiggling line but a sinusoidally modulated luminance grating. Interestingly, the basic idea of decomposing visual images into sinusoidally modulated luminance gratings was proposed by a television engineer at RCA, Otto H. Schade (1948). It is incredible that it took 40 years from Békésy's auditory aftereffects and 20 years from Schade's work for psychologists to start adapting the visual system with sinusoidal luminance gratings.

After these insights, I was so sure of the visual analogies to Békésy's results that I investigated, with Charles Stromeyer III, the visual analogue of his third auditory result, based on critical-band masking (Stromeyer and Julesz 1972). Thus, the notion of the critical band is as pervasive in vision as it is in audition, and it is interesting that the epigram (quoted from the beautiful book edited by Tobias) was dated a year after the visual critical band was established in 1969 by the Cambridge University group, but the news did not yet reach the ears of the auditory experts.

Years earlier, Ira Hirsh and I had been unable to find deep analogies between the two modalities; we found only complementary functions (Julesz and Hirsh 1972). Audition seemed to serve as the early warning system, while vision's role seemed to be identifying objects and events at closer range. It took me eight years to realize the importance critical bands played in both audition and vision.

My interest in audition, however, dates back much earlier. Just after I joined Bell Labs, I was surrounded by auditory experts, and the much lower auditory information rate permitted me to use computer processing with greater ease than was possible for visual stimuli. Newman Guttman and I started to play with stimuli— somewhat similar to random-dot correlograms—in which a segment of auditory noise was embedded in such a way that this segment repeated periodically at some rate $1/T$ (Guttman and Julesz 1963). So, the repeated auditory noise segment acted as our target. We found that for $T < 30$ msec the percept was a raspy pitch, for 30 msec $< T <$ 100 msec the percept was "motorboating," for 100 msec $< T <$ 1000 msec one heard a "whooshing" sound without effort, and for $1 \text{ sec} < T < 4 \text{ sec}$ one could, with close scrutiny, still perceive the repetition. This experiment of ours was noticed by Ulrich Neisser, who in his book *Cognitive Psychology* regarded us as among the founders of "echoic memory." Since then several investigators have studied this echoic memory and found better auditory analogies for the random-dot stereogram. For instance Michael Kubovy (1981) constructed *cyclotean* stimuli, in analogy to my cyclopean stimuli. When one listened to these stimuli with one ear, only a sequence of some chords could be heard, but when binaurally fused the sequence would portray a melody.

Another early attempt on my part was to compare auditory and visual perception, particularly with regard to whether spatial symmetry—so fundamental in vision—could have an auditory counterpart. Harry Levitt and I constructed "spatial chords" (figure 13.1) such that binaurally we presented, say, pitches $c1(f_1)$, $e1(f_2)$, $g1(f_3)$, $c2(f_4)$, $e2(f_5)$ which were localized between the left and right ears at regular intervals f_1, f_2, f_3, f_4, and f_5 in the head, and called it SCH1 (Julesz and Levitt 1966). Observers with good musical ears could easily discriminate between such spatial chords as we kept the pitches constant while changing their spatial positions. For instance, a large change in space results in a spatial chord $SCH2 = c1(f_5)$, $e1(f_2)$, $g1(f_3)$, $c2(f_4)$, $e2(f_1)$ that is much easier to discriminate from SCH1 than a spatial chord $SCH3 = c1(f_1)$, $e1(f_4)$, $g1(f_3)$, $c2(f_2)$, $e2(f_5)$ in which the spatial changes are less. In general, discrimination between spatial chords depends on the sum of the spatial distance changes alone. So, one reversal of two pitches at a 2-inch interval was identical to two changes of two pitch pairs at 1-inch intervals. However, no patterns of higher complexity, such as symmetrical patterns (which are so crucial in visual perception) could be perceived. That symmetry in melodies cannot be perceived is well known. Musical experts can enjoy symmetry (say, in a fugue) only when looking at the score. However, that even spatial symmetry cannot be perceived by the auditory system was novel to me.

After my friends Newman and Harry left Bell Labs, I stopped my auditory experimentations. Computers had become increasingly powerful, and my interest in vision had became paramount. Furthermore, the epoch-making discoveries of the early 1960s in the visual cortex of the cat and the monkey, by Hubel and Wiesel and others, had no auditory parallel (as is true even now). This lack of neurophysiological correlation with auditory psychophysics is a great handicap, and I would therefore have to stick to vision until this gap was closed. Of course, there is a rich psychological field of phonetics, speech, and language, but since only humans have these abilities it will be necessary to

Figure 13.1

Spatial chords. After Julesz and Levitt 1966.

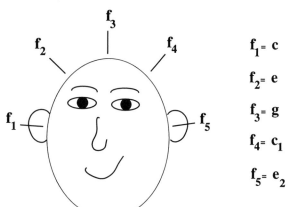

$f_1 = c$

$f_2 = e$

$f_3 = g$

$f_4 = c_1$

$f_5 = e_2$

wait until non-invasive methods, such as PET scans, become feasible.

B: It seems as if you have restricted your comparison between auditory and visual perception merely to the work you and your co-workers did. There must be a large body of similar comparisons by others.

A: You could be right, but to my knowledge there is not much work in audition that would correspond to our concept of visual perception. There are a few excellent books on auditory perception, such as Flanagan 1972, but they are more closely related to the cochlea and its hair cells than to somewhat higher processing stages. Perhaps Bregman and Campbell (1971), Bregman and Rudincky (1975), and Kubovy (1981) have performed experiments that appear analogous to my own in vision.

In my article "Critical bands in vision and audition" (Julesz 1971b) I proposed to experiment in audition with *residue pitches,* discovered by Schouten (1940), which are hidden for the cochlea and which are processed by the auditory nervous system alone. [That a residue pitch, a beat between two nearby frequencies, is not an ordinary pitch was shown by interference experiments in which an ordinary pitch and a residue pitch of the same frequency but with a 180° phase shift did not cancel out.] I proposed—similarly to my cyclopean techniques in vision, where I tried to bypass the earliest processing stages—that all known experiments in audition should use beat frequencies instead of ordinary sinusoidal frequencies, so that even white noise would consist of a spectrum of residue pitches. Could there be cyclotean percep-

tion by the auditory nervous system only without passing through the cochlea? To my knowledge, nobody has launched such a program. This residue-pitch paradigm is not the analogue of the RDS or of Kubovy's binocularly presented cyclotean melodies. Rather, it is analogous to the weakly cyclopean stimulation I discussed in *FCP.* Weekly cyclopean stimulation *d*oes avoid luminance gradients, like random-dot cinematograms or images portrayed by vernier gaps alone. Recently, some colleagues have called the motion elicited by my weakly cyclopean RDC "second-order motion" (in contrast to "first-order motion," which contains moving luminance gradients). Whether such a residue-pitch paradigm will yield sounds that can be heard at all, and if so whether they could yield similar insights to cyclopean vision, remains to be "seen." Here I only argue for a "second-order" auditory perception paradigm that would be able to somehow present the desired information beyond the cochlea, and thus permit the same kind of "psycho-anatomy" I tried with the RDS methodology. [For details see *FCP.*]

B: Perhaps you could end this dialogue with a less speculative theme. I recall you did some work on auditory texture discrimination with statistical constraints.

A: I had almost forgotten about this work, in which I used auditory textures of randomly selected pitch sequences (also called "random melodies") and constrained them with the iso-second-order Markov texture-pair generator, invented by the mathematicians David Slepian and Mark Rosenblatt (1962). Unfortunately, their generalized Markov processes were inherently one-dimensional, while visual textures are inherently two-dimensional. Since at this time we did not yet know how to create two-dimensional texture pairs with identical second-order but different higher-order statistics, I thought to apply the Markov textures for auditory textures that are inherently one-dimensional in time. Again my friend Newman Guttman, a trained auditory expert and musician, came to my aid. We decided to generate random auditory texture pairs using the Slepian-Rosenblatt Markov processes, but the elements of the textures were not loudness values at random but pitches of the diatonic or pentatonic scales. To our surprise, such random melodies could not be discriminated even with effort by trained musicians (Julesz and Guttman 1965). On the other hand, melodies that had identical first-order but different second-order statistics yielded easy discrimination. One could hear, say, that in one melody the pitches of the sounds would increase, while in the other they would decrease. This inability of the auditory system to hear differences in third-order statistics strengthened my belief in my conjecture that such ability is absent in both the auditory system and the visual system. [Although I disproved this conjecture in vision with the discovery of textons, it has not been shown that "auditory textons" exist. Here I refer to auditory textons as counterexamples to the inability of discriminating iso-second-order melodies. In a different paradigm, Ann Treisman (1964) found some primitives I might call "auditory textons." She asked observers to "shadow" a text given in one ear (thus telling aloud with some delay what was heard through this ear), a rather difficult task that draws attention in full to this ear. Simultaneously another text was given in the other ear. What the observers could only hear through the unattended ear were the pitch of the voice (e.g. a male or female speaker), or sudden loudness changes. So pitch and loudness gradients could be regarded as auditory texton gradients.]

Because in 1973 we found the first techniques that could create iso-second-order texture pairs in two dimensions, my motivation to work in audition vanished, and I continued my work in visual texture discrimination with new vigor.

B: Why didn't you mention your early work with Joan Miller on the "electronic sideman," one of the first "expert systems," in the late 1960s?

A: Although Joan Miller and I had great fun with this project, we never published our findings. We felt that it would have taken us too much effort to exhaust this topic, and musical research was outside the charter of my department at Bell Labs. [Joan Miller worked with me on several interesting projects, as is attested by appendix B. She then decided to study for her Ph.D. in mathematics. She is also a good violinist; that explains why she became interested in a musical project.]

A human sideman's ability to accompany a singer without prior access to a score is due to his knowledge of the musical style of the song being performed. It occurred to us that the most valuable information is the last note the singer utters, so that the sideman cannot fully use his limited reaction time. Could a computer that could process this information rapidly beat a human accompanist, since the last notes uttered by the singer are more valuable than the semantic information of large chunks farther in the past stream of notes? We took a melody by Pergolesi and asked a half-dozen colleagues with musical training to write for us a one-finger accompaniment to this brief melody. Most of our colleagues came up with rather similar tunes. It took us several months to find out what these experts did. At our prodding, in the first interviews with them, they could verbalize some of the basic rules of musical harmony. For instance, the right hand's sequence of notes and its left-hand accompaniment should be antiparallel, and parallel melodies should be avoided. These two streams, however, should not separate in their pitches too far. After a limit is reached they should all end in a coda, and so on. We incorporated all this knowledge in our computer program. To our amazement, it composed rather good accompaniments to Pergolesi tunes, sometimes even worked for melodies by Corelli, but failed miserably for Vivaldi or J. S. Bach. That explained to me something I had always felt: that Corelli was not in the same league with Vivaldi. But what about Pergolesi, whose *Stabat Mater* is one of my favorites? Only years later did historians of music discover that—except for a few compositions, including the *Stabat Mater*—an untalented nobleman had forged the pieces attributed to Pergolesi, who had died young. So we created a "musical kitsch detector" that could emulate the style of a period but which failed to grasp the genius of a master. Unfortunately, to this day, the so-called expert systems can handle information better than beginners, compare quite well with some more advanced students of (say) medical diagnosis or income-tax preparation, but fail to reach the competence of the expert!

B: That was rather anecdotal. How can someone who values professionalism expect to entertain me with such a dilettantish project?

A: To me 'dilettantism' does not carry the negative connotation that you ascribe to it. The word comes from the Italian *diletto,* which means "to enjoy." In the 1960s my director at Bell Labs was Max V. Mathews, and my executive director was John R. Pierce. Both were well-known engineers, responsible for many important patents and technical innovations. And yet Max is also known as the father of computer music and as the inventor of several electronic instruments, and John—co-inventor of the traveling-wave tube and the Echo satellite, and recipient of the Marconi Prize and the Japan Prize—is the author of several books on music and the creator of the Pierce musical scale. Famous professional musicians used to converge on Murray Hill in the evenings with their computer disks and without an orchestra; a few hours later they could take home their own compositions in stereo format, as Max's "orchestra program" would convert the prescribed notes into a finished piece, played by many emulated instruments at the tempo, vibrato, and timbre of the composer's desire. I learned from them how science can thrive more in such an enlightened atmosphere that loosened us up than in the usual strictly professional and more regimented traditions of most industrial laboratories. I doubt that in a corporate laboratory, or even in the usual university department of biophysics or communications engineering, the peer pressure would have encouraged such diversions. I regard my 32 years at Bell Labs as the most important period of my scientific life, and this brief story about a little computer-aided variation on a theme by Pergolesi is just a reminder of this period. Of course, such a tradition of tolerance was created over decades. In the 1930s, the beginning of high-fidelity recording and the basic standards for broadcast TV came from a few enlightened industrial laboratories, including Bell, to become a revolutionary trend (and a multi-billion-dollar industry) a generation later. It is also sad how corporate greed can destroy such an atmosphere in a brief period. Of course, there will always be skeptics who insist on professionalism. After all, what is wrong if, say, scientists at Bell Labs continue to invent the best optical communication systems, and professional musicians learn the tricks of music synthesizers independent from each other? Nevertheless, the track record of the relaxed atmosphere of the old Bell Labs is unparalleled. Besides the transistor, it produced the laser, the superconducting magnet, and microwave astronomy (which culminated in the verification of the theory of the Big Bang). Whether such a "Max Planck Institute for the world" will come into existence again remains to be seen. For me, it was a special grace of fate that I could be the beneficiary of the old Bell Labs for 32 years.

B: I found the analogy between auditory pitch perception and visual grating perception quite interesting. Could you elaborate on it?

A: There are many phenomena, such as adaptation to an auditory or a spatial frequency, that are quite similar for both modalities; however, there is a fundamental difference between the two. One can perceive the pitch of an auditory sinusoidal wave regardless of its temporal phase, while a spatial grating must have a well-defined position (phase) to be seen. If one were to jitter the position of a spatial grating, the resulting percept would be a smear. Recently, however, it occurred to me that I have a visual analogue to the phaseless pitch. When I have worked at some arduous task involving textures (such as collecting berries, removing poison ivy, playing chess or *go*, or working on a PC) for hours, before falling asleep I often see these textures in some phaseless form. I see thousands of berries, or see fleeting characters on my monitor, without being able to read the items in detail. This condition is called *palinopsia*. It is my contention that the visual analogue of auditory pitch perception is the floating percept of repeating items in palinopsia.

DIALOGUE 14
FOUNDATIONS OF
CYCLOPEAN
PERCEPTION
REVISITED

. . . I hope that the reader has become familiar with random-dot stereograms and cyclopean techniques in general and can use them for his own research problems. On the other hand, I cannot assure the reader that it constitutes a real paradigm. . . . Only researchers through their results will be able to prove whether or not cyclopean perception is a paradigm.

(last paragraph of *FCP*)

A: *Foundations of Cyclopean Perception* was a youthful work—I started to write it at the age of 40. A quarter-century later, both the field and the author have changed a great deal. In retrospect I still like the book, and I wish I were as young, enthusiastic, and optimistic as I was then. I am also convinced that it was worth writing. Once, when I was visiting Western Australia, friends told me about a captain of a prawn-fishing boat who owned a copy of *FCP* and who looked at the anaglyphs in it while surrounded by the beautiful southern sky. I felt even better when, at meetings, younger colleagues would tell me that *FCP* had hooked them on vision research and had been instrumental in their choice of a profession. Also, whereas more than half of all the scientific papers ever published were never cited (even by their authors), *FCP* became one of the most-cited scientific works in the *Citation Index.*

It took me more than 3 years to write *FCP,* and my friends did not understand why a young man would waste his time on such a futile project instead of doing more research. They did not understand my conviction that, while adding a few more papers on stereopsis would not be much of an achievement, introducing the technique of computer-generated random-dot stereograms would open up a whole new field. The monograph format gave me adequate space to explain the difference between local and global stereopsis, permitted me to describe a new class of ambiguous stereograms, allowed me to draw attention to the false-target-elimination problem of stereopsis and to the spring-coupled magnetic dipole model (one of the first cooperative models of stereopsis), helped me to introduce a paradigm of "psychoanatomy" by tracing the information flow in the brain without a scalpel, and paved the way for the new approach of studying vision through spatial-frequency channels. That many scholarly colleagues refer to *FCP* rather than to my first basic articles, written a decade earlier, shows that a book has more impact than even the best articles.

B: I am also glad that you wrote *FCP.* I am convinced that it was instrumental in your receiving some of the large cash prizes in science, usually not given to psychologists, so that we both could have real turtle soup instead of mock turtle soup—although, since your doctors put us on a diet, and turtles are on the most-endangered list, money seems to have lost much of its value for both of us.

However, I do not like your bragging. Without the work of the late David Marr, who made your book popular among engineers in machine vision and AI, only a few thousand interested psychologists might have read it. After all, it was more than a decade before the book was sold out. Without Marr's insights, particularly his concepts of the "early sketch" and the "2.5-D sketch," the field of "early vision" might not have become so popular during your lifetime.

A: I am indeed indebted to David Marr, who entered the scientific scene around the time of the publication of *FCP* and with whom I had many cordial interactions during his short life. His interest in random-dot stereograms, particularly in the binocular matching problem, was instrumental in linking experimental psychology to machine vision. He shared with me the view that early vision is basically bottom-up, and he created several ingenious models to prove it. [By the way, he liked my spring-coupled magnetic dipole model and treated it separately from other models in his monograph *Vision*.] I am also glad that he posed many metatheories about the function of vision. His insight that the purpose of early vision is to create generalized cylinders that in turn will yield "stick figures" is most persuasive. After all, young children can easily recognize animals made from wires; thus, stick figures might be a promising way to store semantic information of familiar objects. This idea is quite appealing, even though vision existed eons before animals with axial symmetries emerged. By the way, I am glad that Marr took the burden from my shoulder of theorizing. While I worked on *FCP* and lectured on it at MIT during my sabbatical in 1969, some wise colleagues persuaded me to stick to facts and experiments and keep theories to the minimum. For a young scientist this advice was beneficial, and *FCP* is still not obsolete. However, the essence of science is not merely the accumulation of data, but rather the creation of bold theories that organize the data in a unified whole. In these dialogues I have finally started to pose and defend theories, even at the risk that *FCP* will survive long after the dialogues are obsolete.

B: You seem to imply that *FCP* was merely a monograph of novel experiments, without any deep theories. I recall how proud you were of your dual operator theory of perception, which was checked by the famous mathematician Mark Kac. Also, you regarded the spring-coupled magnetic dipole model of stereopsis as a precursor of neural nets.

A: My magnetic dipole model was not ignored. Further, many colleagues understood that I considered it superior to AUTOMAP-1, a computer algorithm of stereopsis that I had developed years earlier (Julesz 1962). Indeed, this dipole model had a great heuristic appeal, while most computer models had their deep structure hidden. On the other hand, my dual-operator theory of perception was completely ignored by all the reviewers of *FCP* and probably by most readers, even though I regard this theory as rather important. What I showed was that there are two kinds of perceptual operators in visual (and auditory) perception (pp. 133–134). One kind expands the stimulus in some eigenfunctions and determines the appropriate eigenvalues. A typical example is color perception, where any color stimulus is decomposed into three eigenfunctions of red, green, and blue, with the appropriate eigenvalues and all three operators act simultaneously. The auditory Ohm's Law and its extension to vision, the spatial-frequency channels, describe similar perceptual operators that also act on the stimulus simultaneously by performing a sort of Fourier decomposition. However, the perceptual act of figure-ground perception constitutes a second kind of operator that tolerates only one state: either the figure or the ground is perceived. I extended this kind of operator to symmetry perception. I showed that every 2-D pattern can be expanded in horizontal, vertical, twofold, and centric symmetrical operators. However, if more than one of these is stimulated by the stimulus, the percept appears to be a random pattern. We combined these two operators by showing, say, a low-spatial-frequency pattern with a symmetry across a horizontal axis and added to it a high-SF pattern with vertical symmetry (Julesz and Chang 1979). These unusual patterns are quite beautiful, as is evident from figure 14.1.

B: There are several reasons why some of your theories were ignored. The most obvious one is that they were not as important as you think. A

Figure 14.1

Two symmetries added such that the one across the horizontal axis has a low spatial frequency while the pattern with vertical symmetry has a high spatial frequency. This permits both symmetries to be perceived. If the two symmetries had the same spectrum, the percept would be a random pattern (Julesz 1971). From Julesz, B., and Chang, J. J., "Symmetry perception and spatial-frequency channels," *Perception* 8: 711–718.

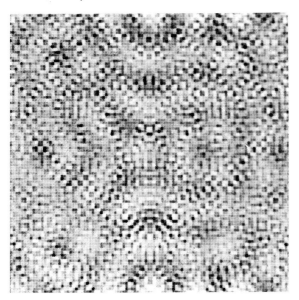

second one might be your mathematical sophistication, which required the appearance of a new generation of mathematically trained psychologists. Also, most people, when confronted with your book, are seduced by the beauty of the demonstrations at the expense of the intellectual content. I can imagine that most of your readers looked through the book instead of reading it. However, this might have a beneficial side. They might have also overlooked your mistakes.

A: There were only three fundamental errors in *FCP*, and I discussed them in detail in *Vision Research* (Julesz 1986).

I wrongly stated that the time needed to fuse an RDS depended on the complexity of the surfaces portrayed. Later I showed (Julesz 1978) that RDS portraying very complex surfaces could be fused in 60 msec (with afterimages erased), provided the correlated areas were within Panum's fusional limit. On the other hand, even the simplest RDS requires a long initial fusion time if the single cyclopean square hovering over the background exceeds Panum's fusional limit. The observer has to learn the proper vergence strategies by first aligning one of the corresponding areas (which is difficult without monocular cues) and then trying to reconverge on the other area slowly (making use of the Fender-Julesz hysteresis effect) without breaking the fusion of the first area. Observers learn this strategy of proper vergence movements unconsciously and can retain it for years. There is some neural learning involved in global stereopsis, as first reported by Ramachandran and Braddick (1973), and some robust perceptual learning [discussed in dialogue 12]. Here I stress that Panum's fusional area increases with the width (area) of the target, as observed for classical bars by Richards and Kay (1974) and for RDSs by Tyler and Julesz (1980). With adequate target dimensions one can achieve fusion in a brief flash (excluding vergence movements) with binocular disparities in excess of 1 deg arc (Schumer and Julesz 1984).

Another erroneous statement (Julesz and Spivack 1967) was based on random-line stereograms with vernier breaks. We assumed that vernier breaks were invisible for retinal mechanisms, and thus superacuity processing by the cortex preceded stereopsis. We did not realize that the breaks in our *dense* line segments, after being convolved with the receptive field profiles, could be seen monocularly. The latter was pointed out by H. K. Nishihara and Tomaso Poggio (1982). With less-dense line segments, they showed, the breaks did not yield monocular luminance changes and hence did not yield stereopsis.

A third finding reported in *FCP* is related to the hysteresis effect (Fender and Julesz 1967). We found under binocular retinal stabilization that an RDS had to be aligned first within 6 min arc for fusion, and then could be slowly pulled by 120 min arc with fusion maintained. Beyond 120 min arc, fusion would break and the RDS had to be brought back within 6 min arc for refusion. The first part of our findings was confirmed by Hyson et al. (1983) and Piantanida (1986); the second part might require some modification. These authors claim that after loss of fusion it is not necessary to bring the RDS within Panum's limit for refusion; it occurs much sooner. Erkelens and Collewijn (1986) retested our findings with an experimental design very different from ours. They stabilized the vergence movements of the eyes but let the observer use conjugate eye movements freely. They

also used 5-inch stereograms in place of our 1-inch ones. Under these conditions, they verified our 120 min arc increased Panum's fusional limit; however, they found a different kind of hysteresis after fusion was lost and the disparity was reduced. We still do not know why their results differ from ours and from Piantanida's. Luckily, the main support for cooperativity of stereopsis comes from other experiments, particularly those reported in Julesz 1964 and in Julesz and Chang 1976.

On the positive side, I reported in *FCP* that stereopsis cannot be color blind. Using polarity-reversed RDSs, which are impossible to fuse, I observed that stereopsis was restored when the corresponding elements of these anticorrelated RDSs were similarly colored in both eyes' views. Had the world paid more attention to this finding, much debate on the color blindness of the stereoscopic system (and the magno-system) could have been avoided.

B: I am glad that you repeatedly correct some of your wrong statements. I think there should be a special journal for this single purpose, enabling authors to correct their own errors. That your brief experiment suggesting that stereopsis is not color blind was overlooked was not a big deal, since you yourself were not sure that the technology available in 1970–71 was foolproof. Only with Ilona Kovacs were you able to make this experiment convincing and to extend it to apparent motion (Kovacs and Julesz 1992).

It is time for me to express my doubt about your best-known teleological comment, your leitmotif in *FCP:* that stereopsis evolved to break camouflage. Only people who think of themselves as "great" scientists make such speculations. It reinforces my belief in the definition of a great scientist: The greater a scientist is, the longer can he impede progress singlehanded!

A: In defense of teleological arguments in psychobiology, I will explain my view of the difference between physics and biology. In the former one concentrates on the *rules* of the "game"; in the latter the *actual history* of the game is perhaps more important. So, teleological arguments are essential in psychobiology, even though they seldom can be accepted as real truth.

B: Your basic assumption in *FCP* is that psychology is merely bottom-up. You treat focal attention as the only top-down process—if such a process really exists—and ignore all the other top-down processes, with their cognitive richness. Isn't that rather naive? I would like to have some convincing answers to this question at last!

A: You are asking two questions here: Is there a point to studying bottom-up processes by themselves? What is the point of concentrating on focal attention alone and ignoring the many other cognitive processes?

The answer to the first question is straightforward. We know from 30 years' psychological and neurophysiological evidence that one can segment visual scenes merely by processing the surfaces of objects and concentrating on differences in their brightness, contrast, color, motion, binocular depth, texture, flicker, etc. It was my role to use monocular and binocular stochastic textures, because these textures were devoid of any higher cognitive cues, and to show that we could still see these surfaces in vivid depth and motion. My access

to the first digital computers that could control these stimuli in space and time was a lucky break for me, as was the advent of low-noise amplifiers and sharp microelectrodes that permitted neurophysiologists to probe the first cortical stages in the cat and the monkey. That some of the random-dot stereograms elicited responses in the input stage of the monkey visual cortex was a recent development that reinforced my belief in the bottom-up processes of early vision.

The second question, on the role of focal attention, is a complex one. Scrutiny of the surfaces and their texture gradients (obtained by early vision) could be most complex. It could be parallel or serial, and it could use cognitive strategies or be restricted to some simpler ones. It would be safe to extend this general scrutiny as the function of consciousness. However, one could restrict the scrutiny to some simpler aspects, such as inspecting some position or scale of detail of the bottom-up phenomena. I regard this restricted scrutiny as related to focal attention. However, if one could inspect in parallel the entire visual field in detail, "focal attention" would be a misnomer. After all, we believe that the entire scene is so complex that all its complexities cannot be perceived at a single glance. Focal attention assumes that there must be a bottleneck in our cognitive processing powers. Since we cannot inspect the entire scene at once, we have to do it piecemeal. Whether this is done element by element in time, or done in parallel but zoomed down to one or more smaller areas, or in some other way is hard to decide. There are hundreds of articles on focal attention, and the findings are not conclusive. We have no direct insight into how we inspect something more thoroughly when eye movements and accommodation are prevented.

(Of course, there are colleagues who are interested in the accompanying eye movements; those are possible to study, but they are not directly yoked to focal attention.) Nevertheless, all of us can inspect an object (say, a face) from a constant distance at different spatial scales. We can concentrate on gross features or on small details of the skin. I regard this shifting to different scales at will as one crucial manifestation of focal attention. Whether one can shift on one or several such scales at once or whether one has to do it in steps is similar to the controversial question of whether one inspects a spot by a single searchlight or in parallel by divided attention. I think it is worthwhile to strip away this simplest aspect of consciousness—which I call attention—because I hope it is ripe for scientific attack, while the study of consciousness in full is still beyond our capabilities.

B: I have always believed more in the genuineness of one's frustrations than in one's assumed successes. Please share your frustrations with the reader.

A: My main frustration—obviously beyond my control—is that during my lifetime I will not learn the secrets of how long-term memory is stored, and probably even my readers will not solve the enigma of qualia. So, let me turn to some more controllable frustrations.

My most unexplainable frustration is my inability to interest ophthalmologists in using dynamic random-dot stereograms with evoked potential recording to diagnose stereo blindness in human infants and to establish the critical period during which rehabilitation might be possible. I just cannot believe that clinicians are not interested in such an important research question with obvious potentially beneficial effects.

My second frustration is the tentative nature of my basic assumption that early vision is processed by the first visual stages of the striate cortex and its neighboring visual areas. Indeed, a recent article by Patricia Goldman-Rakic and co-workers (Wilson et al. 1993) suggests that visual memories for "where" and "what" are stored separately in the monkey's prefrontal cortex. Neurons in a cortical area known as the inferior convexity (IC) retain information about an object's shape and color for a brief time after the object disappears from view. Neurons in an adjacent area called the principal sulcus (PS) encode the object's position. These areas' functions seem to be similar to another dichotomy at an earlier stage, where the inferior temporal cortex (IT) is concerned with object recognition while the posterior parietal cortex (PP) performs spatial perception. Although I am glad that our prediction (Sagi and Julesz 1985) that "*where* and *what* are processed by different mechanisms" has been elaborated further, I am somewhat puzzled that such mechanisms might be duplicated, and some do reside at rather "high" stages that might be called "late vision."

My third frustration—perhaps "regret" is a better word—is that I concentrated mainly on the first segmentation stage of early vision and omitted some important next stages after this early nonlinear filter. Obviously segmentation is not adequate and one has to perform at least two further operations. One is to decide to which of the segmented regions attention should be directed; this is called the *figure-ground problem*. I regarded this crucial process as an important role of focal attention, even though figure-ground segmentation in some cases might occur at a second stage in visual processing. (The enhanced detection inside a closed contour is a clear example, as Kovacs and I have shown.) The second stage has to decide also which of the segmented areas are in front and which are occluded. Regrettably I did not study the role of occlusion in early vision, even though I was among the first to note (Julesz 1960) that in an RDS the half-occluded areas ("no-man's land") were seen at the farthest depth plane. I regarded this phenomenon as the result of some "higher cortical strategy" without embarking on its role in visual perception. He and Nakayama (1994), studying the role of occlusion in stereopsis, suggest that in addition to an early filtering stage there might be a next stage that processes surface appearance, and that it is at this stage that texture segmentation might occur. They also speculate on the interconnection of these two stages: are they simply "feedforward," or does "feedback" exist between them? In the former case the bottom-up philosophy is still valid. For the second case (if this feedback comes from the next stages), the bottom-up concept might be still useful, because I regard top-down influences to come from much higher stages (linked to reasoning and semantic memory).

My fourth frustration is my inability to trace the information flow of stereopsis by non-invasive techniques. Of course, it is very difficult to tell a physicist who dedicated years to inventing and perfecting some positron-emission tomography (PET) device or some high-spatial-temporal resolution magnetic-resonance imaging (MRI) scanner, with the support of some clinical center, what to do with his precious tools! Nevertheless, I am frustrated that so far nobody has been able to trace the neural activity for, say, a dynamic random-dot correlogram

as it would alternate between correlation and uncorrelation (or negative correlation). Obviously, such robust stimuli can be presented as red-green anaglyphs back-projected on a transparent screen, safely away from the enormous magnetic fields generated by these sensitive display devices, and the observer just has to wear red-green goggles. I tried such experiments myself without success, but I only had access to the first-generation PET machines. The second-generation MRI devices seem much more capable. Nevertheless, the literature is filled with reports in which the observer is asked to imagine a color, a word, or a complex event and follow how some auditory, speech, visual, or association area has its metabolic activity change accordingly. I just hope that my younger colleagues will witness soon how single-microelectrode neurophysiology will be taken over by multi-electrode techniques and non-invasive methods, that will permit them to study the human brain in mental action. [In the last moment I came across a paper by Gulyás and Roland (1994), who finally located areas of changes in cerebral blood flow to binocular disparity changes using RDSs, PET scanning, and healthy human observers. Their data indicate that the discrimination of pure stereoscopic information takes place in the polar striate cortex and the neighboring prestriate cortices, as well in the parietal lobe.] Finally, localization attempts by PET scanning in humans are supported by Gian Poggio's neurophysiological findings of the stages of cyclopean stereopsis in the alert monkey. I just hope that soon a finer localization will be achieved with *dynamic* RDS and *MRI* techniques.

My fifth frustration is somewhat similar to my second one, but goes deeper. It relates to my entire philosophy of research based on my belief in the importance of bottom-up phenomena in human perception. In my opinion this strategy helps link psychophysics with the known neurophysiology of the first cortical stages in the monkey. While the psychophysical study of early vision (i.e. devoid of semantics) seems a useful intellectual pursuit by itself, I hoped that trying to impart some neurophysiological insights to the psychological findings might be beneficial. I also stressed the importance of focal attention, the only top-down phenomenon I included in my research. But how shall I interpret the fact the back-projections from V1 to the LGN are far more numerous than the ascending connections? Are these top-down connections at every stage more numerous than the bottom-up ones? Will the advance of neurophysiology and MRI techniques make my belief in the importance of bottom-up pathways obsolete in the next few years? Could it be that this preponderance of descending fibers is related to focal attention, and the main function of the brain is to filter out the incoming information depending on the interest of the organism at the earliest stages? If this is the case, then my research strategy will be vindicated.

B: Could you comment on some thoughts you omitted, or on some recent findings?

A: Unknown to me, at the time I sent my manuscript to the publisher, a new fad started in Japan and is now spreading all over the world—30 years after the creation of the first computer-generated RDS—that might be the nicest 65th birthday gift one could receive. Books and displays of "autostereograms" are now published by the millions. It seems that a new art form has been created through the RDS that has brought delight to mil-

lions of people who otherwise would have missed the aesthetic side of my work. Because these books permitted me to see the enthusiastic acceptance of RDSs by the public, I forgive those who ignore my contributions, misspell my name, misquote my affiliation, or distort the essence of my work with my co-workers. Many of my readers are not familiar with wallpaper-stereograms, also called "autostereograms." To the best of my knowledge, I am also co-inventor with Peter Burt of the computer-generated autostereogram (Burt and Julesz 1980). Autostereograms are based on the wallpaper effect, first described by Sir David Brewster 150 years ago. Brewster noticed that periodic patterns viewed binocularly could jump out in depth. (I even hold a U.S. patent on how to view periodic VLSI chips with stereomicroscopes for purposes of quality control.) I found the stereoscopic fusion of autostereograms still difficult and the monocular periodic stripes disturbing. Therefore, I tried many other techniques to avoid goggles, particularly lenticular lens techniques pioneered by my predecessor at Bell Labs, Herb Ives, in the early 1930s. In order to expand space (as is done in restaurants by placing a mirror on the wall), I wanted to place lenticular RDSs on walls of museums and skyscrapers. Indeed, there are now a dozen museums that have such displays. By the way, lenticular RDSs (whose fusion I explored with Richard Payne in the early 1960s) are "autostereograms" and can be viewed binocularly without the tiny lenticular lenses in front of them, but their fusion is much more difficult than with the lenticular screen. In FCP I have a chapter on "mental holography" where I generalize the concept of wallpaper-stereograms to ambiguous stereograms that can portray more than one three-dimensional shape with the *same* stereogram. Such stereograms were time consuming to generate on the largest computers in 1969, but it was done. Even though I am annoyed by the implication that autostereograms can now exploit my original ideas since computers became more powerful, I am glad that so many people can now enjoy the slow emergence of cyclopean structures in vivid depth. Recently, one of the publishers finally interviewed me, and if the other publishers of these books will give me proper credit and will prompt their readers to drink a glass of sake or wine to my health, so their ocular muscles will relax, they will help the binocular fusion of these wallpaper-stereograms manyfold!

B: We both agree that sharing the beauty of cyclopean perception with millions is a cause for celebration, but why did you spend so much time on a technical detail of how to facilitate binocular fusion? In your first paper in 1960 you supplied flat Fresnel prisms, and in *FCP* you used red-green anaglyphs with inexpensive color filters, and now autostereograms. In autostereograms you do not like the periodic patterns seen monocularly, because you feel that they distract the viewer from the beauty of the cyclopean surfaces. But what if people find it an added challenge to see through these flat wallpaper patterns and perceive the plasticity? So, we should appreciate the efforts of Christopher Tyler (1992) and David Stork (Falk et al. 1986), among others, who used autostereograms in their scientific publications and paved way for the popularity of stereoscopic viewing. I recall some interesting material you used to lecture about but left out of the dialogues.

A: As I told you, in the dialogues I mainly used material that I found too controversial for a textbook. Aristotle (384–322 B.C.) made a useful distinction between the kind of knowledge that is passed from a master to his pupil and the kind of knowledge that is necessary for the pupil to be able to ask questions from his master. Monographs are preoccupied by the first kind of knowledge, while textbooks try to convey the second kind of information. Dialogues present a third kind of knowledge: conversations between masters and/or fools in which the participants can confess their ignorance to each other. Of course, in my undergraduate courses I often tell my students some observations I regard true, and am sure that they are not widely known. I give only one such example that I find useful since most of my readers were born into the digital age. So, I ask my students how small they think a computer could be built that could *compute* the gravitational curvature of the Einstein-Riemann tensor. After some debate we agree that a few thousand gates might suffice where each gate might be the size of a few silicon atoms. Then I mention that a single photon can *obey* the gravitational curvature. A photon is a tiny fraction of such a huge computer and there must be a qualitative difference between the two. Indeed, a computer must be instructed with a program to compute a task. This program has to contain our present knowledge of physical laws. On the other hand, each photon (being an analog device) is coupled to the laws of the universe and obeys them. So, analog machines are quite different from digital computers, and this example might be relevant to workers in AI who want to model brains with digital or with analog neuromimes (artificial neurons), respectively.

B: I hoped for some clearer thoughts, but please continue.

A: I turn now to some important issues that happened recently, or escaped my attention. It occurred to me that throughout the dialogues I rarely mentioned the practical side of my activities as a psychologist in industry. [In appendix B there is mention of some of my patents.] Here, I recall two curious psychological problems that were brought to my attention while I was consulting with the over one million employees of AT&T prior to divestiture:

(a) Our chip designers could trace the complex circuit diagrams of VLSI devices that graced our corridors and could find hidden errors in a jiffy—as if they would just pop out from a labyrinth of wires—but only if the colors were printed in the AT&T convention. The same diagrams when printed, say, in the IBM convention, using different colors, prevented them from detecting these same errors. This enigmatic problem clearly shows the important role color plays in texture vision and memory.

(b) While it is taken for granted that the best way to couple humans to computers is by a "mouse," many people complained that they could not coordinate their eyes with moving the mouse. The reader who cannot imagine the nature of this handicap should try to rotate one hand over his head clockwise while rotating his other hand over his knee clockwise, and then suddenly try to switch to the counter-clockwise direction. I think both of these perceptual problems are of great practical importance, but beyond our grasp.

I return now to a scientific problem that preoccupied me over many years: I did not answer adequately the "paradox" Bart Anderson raised about hysteresis in cooperativity and the Fender-Julesz (1967) hysteresis effect: I always define co-operativity as the simplest system that exhibits order-disorder transitions, multiple ordered states, and hysteresis. There are more complex systems—including self-adapting systems—that exhibit many other behaviors, but, being also cooperative, do exhibit the three properties I assigned to the purely cooperative systems. I never tried to establish how these three properties are interlinked, particularly how hysteresis exhibits order-disorder transitions and transitions between multiple ordered states. For order-disorder transitions, the second law of thermodynamics applies. Thus going from order to disorder is easier than vice versa. Recently Bart and I repeated the Julesz-Tyler (1976) experiment for motion (Julesz and Anderson 1994). Instead of binocular fusion versus binocular rivalry we studied motion of dynamic noise in all directions versus motion restricted within an angle (thus more ordered). It turned out that here again we found neurontropy-like phenomena. It was easier (i.e. took less time) to detect motion when less directed and inserted in more directed motion than vice versa. This hysteresis effect between disorder-order states is somewhat different from hysteresis effects between two or more ordered states. A case in point is the perceptual flipping of the Necker cube in depth or perceiving in the ambiguous old woman/young girl image one of the hidden organization. Here the two images are equally ordered and their order is kept intact by a special long-term memory mechanism whose function is to keep these multiple organizations intact. The hysteresis effects observed as one goes between one of the multiple ordered states to another reflect the structure of the long-term memory more than some subtle difference between the amount of order of the multiple stable states. If these subtle effects were measurable, then we would have a way to define the "complexity" of images. The only puzzle is the Fender-Julesz (1967) hysteresis effect that was discussed in great detail in the book. [Most colleagues are intimidated by the close-fitting contact lenses or expensive eye-tracking devices to study this phenomenon, even though we showed (Burt and Julesz 1979) how one can use the ubiquitous fast computer instead.] This hysteresis, showing the persistence of the fused state, appears opposite to the neurontropy concept of Julesz and Tyler (1976). One way to resolve this paradox is to assume that Bart's interpretation of the hysteresis effect found by Erkelens (1988) is the correct way to assign order and disorder states to dynamic and static states. Unfortunately, Erkelens used very different experimental conditions from that of Fender and Julesz and so the two experiments cannot be compared. More importantly, however, in the Fender-Julesz (1967) study we performed another experiment using temporal occlusion. It turned out that with 50 min arc pulling an occlusion of the stereopair for 5 msec was adequate to break fusion, while at 10 min arc pulling (just outside Panum's limit) could tolerate hundreds of msec without the fused image breaking apart. This robust finding is the main argument for the stability of fusion. So, the paradox between persistence and non-persistence of ordered states under different experimental conditions still remains. Of course, whether this is a real paradox or just the ignorance of our part in understanding the workings of complex systems is an open question.

B: I am surprised that at the end of your book you are still preoccupied with cooperativity. I had hoped to hear from you a few succinct comments worth remembering. Instead, you give long monologues on subtle details. Please turn to a more exciting topic!

A: Before I discuss a really exciting development of recent months, I must answer your criticism. There are, indeed, a few geniuses in physics, such as a Newton or an Einstein, who could look at the ocean at its entirety and postulate some of its rules. However, in psychobiology at present, one can only analyze one drop of the ocean. This has to be done in great detail, so that future scientists can tell apart the significant findings from the chaff. And do not forget that outside of his own field Newton was preoccupied with alchemy in vain, and Einstein could not unite quantum physics with relativity theory. These comments are not made to diminish the monumental ideas of the greatest geniuses of mankind, but instead to draw attention to the fact that even they could not see over the horizon of their zeitgeist. And psychobiology is certainly closer to alchemy than to physics. As an experimentalist I prefer detailed experiments to grandiose theories. Perhaps I can illustrate my point as follows:

A new development in the last few months is related to the work with Ilona Kovacs (Kovacs and Julesz 1994). We found spots of highlighted sensitivity inside closed curves (see figures 8.1–8.3). We showed that local contrast sensitivity is affected within the boundary at far distances from it, and locations of maximal sensitivity enhancement are determined by global shape properties. Our data supports a class of models that describe shapes by the means of a medial axis transformation, implying that the visual system extracts skeletons as an intermediate representation. The first model of that kind was the "grassfire" of Blum (1967, 1973) as I discussed it in dialogue 8. Blum and Nagel (1978) also emphasized the importance of starting the grassfire at different *scales*. We used only one scale so far and compared our psychophysical data by a geometrical procedure that plots the percentage of the boundary points that are equidistant from a given locus within a tolerance of 1%. The agreement between psychophysics and our axis-based representation is excellent. That is why we referred to the Blum model. There are recent psychophysical data, based on observers' ability to bisect distances between contours, supporting the multiscale nature of the representation (Burbeck and Pizer 1994). I am convinced that our sensitivity map, based on contour enhancement, occurs at an earlier stage than the processes underlying the rather sophisticated task of bisecting distances between contours.

So far our assumption of a grassfire model is already quite bold. We need more neurophysiological evidence of cortical propagation times to convert the spatial sensitivity map into a temporal propagation map. To my delight, while correcting the page proofs of the paper, Ilona and I came across a recent paper by Grinewald et al. (1994), who found by direct optical tracing methods some neural locations that are "lit up" by spreading activity in V1 of the cortex of macaque monkey.

Assuming the validity of a grassfire-like model we made a plausible but bold assumption. We generalized our purely spatial results to the temporal domain. Without explicitly stating it, we assumed that perceptual waves emanate from each point of the boundaries of the circles and ellipses we used, and at points where they arrive in close synchrony they enhance each other. At these "synchrony points" the visibility of patches is increased; at other positions the contrast has to be heightened to see the patches. There is one synchrony point for the circle (in its center) while for the ellipse there are two such points that lie on its major axis, similar to the "grassfire model" of Harry Blum (1967, 1973), where his skeletal points are those for which the last grass vanishes as it burns. By the way, the curves do not have to be closed; it is adequate that they are adequately smooth (neighboring Gabor patches have to be quasi-collinear) in order to emit waves that arrive to certain positions in the brain in synchrony.

As I told you, I do not like to drag my coworkers into my metatheories. The next paragraph is merely my own speculation: The grassfire model and our model of perceptual waves that propagate perpendicularly from points on contours have no spatio-temporal periodicity, similarly to Newton's optical theory based on corpuscles. Huygens, a contemporary of Newton, postulated a wave theory, yet it took two centuries to understand that instead of the longitudinal wave propagation of Huygens the electromagnetic oscillation occurs transversely to the light propagation. Whether the brain waves we described with Kovacs exhibit some periodic fine structure, determined by its almost lossless neural medium (not to be confused with the low frequency phenomena at 40–60 Hz, nor with the spiking frequencies of individual neurons) can be only decided after some very critical studies using interference effects. Similarly to Dennis Gabor's idea of holography that had to await the invention of the laser to generate temporally coherent light to make the interference fringes clearly visible, until we find ways to synchronize brain waves in temporally coherent phase, most perceptual interference phenomena will be hidden.

B: I am glad that you toned down your speculations about the spreading grassfire model and the importance of closure you discussed in dialogue 8, and stressed instead a medial axis transformation process. Do you think that your work and speculations on spreading neural activity are related to the brain code?

A: I am stunned by your question. The leitmotif of *Dialogues* was our ignorance of the brain code, and your question implies that you did not listen or—contrary to your claim—you seem to encourage me to fabricate fairy tales. I have already done so in dialogue 3 on solitons. Now, solitons are one-dimensional solutions of very long-lasting waves in nonlinear media. My scientific fairy tale on solitons might be less bizarre if instead one would study coupled (coherent) dipoles of vortices that can last for quite some time in nonlinear media of two and three dimensions, such as brains.

So far I omitted the imaginative and careful work by M. Abeles (1982, 1994) and his co-workers, who use multiple electrodes in cortical hypercolumns of behaving monkey. If there is a candidate for the existence of a brain code in my lifetime it is most likely the *syn-fire* idea of Abeles. To quote him almost verbatim: He and his co-workers studied the spatio-temporal firing patterns of 8–12 neurons in parallel and found thousands of cases when the same pattern repeated many times above chance. In many cases these excessively repeating patterns were associated with behavior in awake monkeys.

A simple neural network that can generate such patterns (and is consistent with the known anatomy of the cerebral cortex) is called the *syn-fire* chain by Abeles. Simulation of activity in such chains revealed that they convert asynchronous excitation into a synchronized volley of spikes that can propagate over many synapses with little jitter in time. A given neuron may take part in more than one link of the syn-fire chain. Cross connections between two syn-fire chains can learn the sequence of firing constellations produced by the chains. By such a process, the two syn-fire chains may bind to create a larger and more stable structure. To me it seems that the study of neural correlations in hypercolumns by nearby electrodes is a promising first strategy. However, in the light of long-range neural activity—discovered by Gilbert and Wiesel (1992)—the concept of syn-firing may need to be extended to remote communication between neurons and verified by neurophysiological techniques.

Obviously the brain code—if it exists—does not have to be based on waves and oscillations, but if it did, similarly to light, electromagnetism, and acoustics, then I could continue with my fairy tale (that started with the solitons) as follows: The 1 mm thin cortex contains trillions of neural pools (looking like a tiny universe) that seem to communicate with each other at far distances. Is it far fetched to assume that the method extraterrestrials use for galacatic communication might be based on the brain code? After all, if our civilization cracks the brain code in the near or very far future, our descendants will realize its sophisticated nature, far more advanced than any communication technology that existed prior to it. Probably the same happened to advanced extraterrestrial civilizations as well. Therefore they adopted the brain code for several reasons: because they felt that Nature brought into being over eons an ultra-efficient communication method in the most complex structures in the universe, the cortices of civilized brains; because they wanted to communicate with intelligent beings, and the least they would expect from them was the knowledge of how their brains worked; and because they realized that they could communicate efficiently only with beings whose brains were similarly organized to theirs.

B: I am sorry that I asked you about the brain code. Your story about extraterrestrial communication is not only quarter-baked and frivolous, but not even original. The Polish science fiction writer Stanislaw Lem has a novel (made also into a movie) entitled *Solaris* describing a planet that acts as a giant computer. It analyzes the brain waves of the circling astronauts and sends them back in modified forms, yielding disturbing thoughts and hallucinations. Of course, I understand that you merely wanted to show how easy it is to go beyond facts by imagination from a respectable model to utter nonsense. I wish that both the brain code and extraterrestrial civilizations were to exist.

For a change, I will make a global comment. As I looked over the transcript of our conversations I noticed a strange thing. Sometimes you defined a contour as the local maxima of a Laplacian operator applied on the luminance distribution of the stimulus. Sometimes you used the difference between two Gaussians instead. From this I guessed that these two operators yield similar results. Then you demonstrated subjective (illusory) contours of the Kanizsa kind (figure 2.3). It was most impressive to see illusory boundaries at places where the

luminance distribution was uniform. Even though these illusory contours appear weaker than luminance defined contours, most people can see them. You also created some illusory contours using sparse RDSs (figure 2.5b) where the illusory contour is clearly visible. But then you review the explanation of the asymmetry phenomenon of texture discrimination (Williams and Julesz 1991, 1992). You explain it by postulating that the asymmetry effect of texture discrimination (i.e., texture A embedded in texture B yields stronger discrimination than vice versa, as depicted in figure 9.10) is the result of subjective contours perceptually closing the gaps. In vain do I search for these illusory contours in figure 9.10; I cannot see them! It appears that there are visible and invisible illusory contours. In your place I would coin another name for invisible illusory contours. You might name them "invisible contours that portray the Cheshire cat's smile." Please continue with your last few comments. You always regarded psychology as the primary source of psychobiological insights into the human psyche, and neuroanatomy and neurophysiology as secondary attempts to understand the workings of the mind. Yet *FCP* is the work of a physiological psychologist who finds the linking of mind and brain the most important activity a psychologist could undertake. Had you insisted on psychological findings alone and ignored the neurophysiology, you might have created a book that would stand the test of time. However, the rapid changes in neurophysiological techniques and insights will soon make your book obsolete.

A: You are probably right. Yet, the quest of a psychologist is not to state some truth that will last forever but is rather vacuous (similar to my iso-second-order texture-discrimination conjecture). Instead, the psychologist should collaborate with the other workers in psychobiology to speed up the understanding of the brain. Even if some problems of the mind—like the essence of sensations and consciousness—might be untractable for several generations to come, I believe that some of the lesser problems of the mind's workings can be understood right now. And we will understand the global manifestations of the mind's working only when we are able to explain them in terms of the underlying neural activity.

B: Since you seem reluctant to publish a second revised edition of *FCP*, do you have any message for readers of that book?

A: On one hand, there has been enormous progress in psychobiology, from psychopharmacological drugs to non-invasive brain scans, since the publication of *FCP*. On the other hand, our ignorance of the brain code keeps *FCP* alive. As a matter of fact, beyond the pleasant task of reading Helmholtz's *Handbook of Physiological Optics* and admiring his genius, the other reason why that book still strikes us as up to date is the surprisingly slow progress of psychobiology. I myself would like to know what fundamental progress has occurred since I wrote *FCP*.

In the history of molecular biology there was a watershed—the discovery that DNA is the hereditary material, followed by the discovery of its structure, the alphabet of the genetic code, and the quick development of a new genetic technology—that made possible the deep understanding and the manipulation of life processes. A book on molecular biology published before this breakthrough usu-

ally has only historic value. Of course, Mendel's guessing of the gene (through some ingenious experiments) paved the way for the breakthrough. So did Darwin's theory of evolution.

Similar precursors of great ideas and findings are at hand in psychobiology. The work of Golgi, Cajal, and Hubel and Wiesel must be fundamental to an understanding of the workings of the brain, whether there turns out to be a fundamental brain code or whether the workings turn out to be performed by a tangle of trillions of special-purpose circuits. Whether my own work with my associates, or the findings of colleagues who shared my paradigms, will have a real impact on the understanding of the human brain is still a question. So let us share the hope that we have contributed something useful to the understanding of the brain. According to the sage, *life is tolerable only because everything changes and nobody knows the future!* This is also my definition of why doing research in such a difficult field is never boring. Therefore, for those not dreaming of making some historic discovery, doing research in visual or auditory perception during the last decades of the twentieth century was—and is—*great fun*.

APPENDIXES

A
INTERACTIONS

Two frogs accidentally fell into a jar of milk, and swam desperately to keep themselves afloat. The pessimist frog realized that it was impossible to climb out of the jar, stopped swimming, and drowned. The optimist frog kept swimming until the milk turned to butter; then he jumped out.

(one of my father's stories)

As I lean back and ruminate over my life, I realize that it has been shaped, directly or indirectly, by the influence of a great many people. My life has been rewarding, and I do not wish to contemplate other scenarios. I am not even sure that only the benevolent "witnesses of my life" deserve my thanks. For instance, a young mathematician of leftist leanings vetoed my appointment to Professor Gombás's physics department because he regarded me as of upper-middle-class origin—a crime in Stalinist Hungary. Had he not prevented my appointment, perhaps I would be now a second-rate physicist. If it is better to excel in a lesser field than to be average in a more prestigious discipline, I might even thank him now.

As I glance through this first paragraph and get irritated with my own chit-chat, my thoughts turn to a more somber topic. Perhaps each day of my adult life I think of family members, teachers, schoolmates, benefactors, and close friends who perished during the tragic years of my youth. Many of them had already achieved, or could have achieved, much more than I, who survived. Let them share the credit for anything valuable I may have achieved.

Concentrating on my benefactors and role models, I want to thank my late parents and my uncle, Miklós (Nicholas) Julesz, a professor of neuro-endocrinology who instilled in me a passion for science and art. Luckily, all three of them survived the Second World War. In particular, I thank my parents for teaching me several languages that proved to be great assets later. I am also very appreciative of my distinguished teachers in Hungary's excellent *gymnasium* system and of the well-balanced university curriculum at the Technical University of Budapest. However, the greatest influence of my youth was my early friendship with Rózsa Péter, who introduced me to the beauty of mathematics. It was an exhilarating experience to learn Gödel's theorem from her at 16. Nevertheless, I am not only thankful to her what she taught me; I am even more thankful that, by introducing me to some really creative mathematicians, she made me realize that mathematics was not for me.

I am also thankful for the pleasant atmosphere of the Academic Institute for Communications Research in Budapest (particularly to its research director, the late Géza Bognár), where in the harsh political climate of 1951–1956 we were permitted to do independent research in communication systems and image encoding. (This institute was the successor of the Research Institute of the Hungarian Post Office, where Georg von Békésy worked for many years.) Indeed, I had the proper climate to finish my thesis on the encoding of visual images, and I earned my degree from the Hungarian Academy of Sciences (a somewhat more advanced degree than the Ph.D. given by Hungarian universities). I probably would have become a system engineer were it not for the Hungarian Revolution of 1956, which led me, my wife, and 200,000 countrymen to escape. I had never believed that the ideas we fought for then would eventually come to fulfillment and result in the liberation of Eastern Europe.

After our arrival at Camp Kilmer, in New Jersey, where most Hungarian refugees were first processed, I was visited by a Bell Laboratories representative, Sergei A. Schelkunoff, Assistant Director of the Mathematical Department. He had never heard of me, but he had been told that a refugee had arrived who had a thesis on information theory and wanted to contact colleagues at Bell Labs. After we introduced ourselves, I asked him whether he was the author of a book on microwave antennas. He was pleasantly surprised that I knew of his book. He was even more surprised when I told him that I had translated his book into Hungarian, and when I quoted parts of the introduction verbatim he took me with him to Murray Hill, where I gave an improvised talk on the encoding of TV signals with optical correlation techniques. On December 31, 1956, I started as a member of the technical staff. (Dr. Schelkunoff died at 95 in May 1992.)

I was offered a choice between working on microwave systems and continuing my work on TV bandwidth reduction schemes, a problem to which an entire department was devoted. I selected the latter—in part because there were still considerable security precautions at Bell Labs, and a refugee from behind the Iron Curtain was still looked at with suspicion. Luckily for me, Sputnik broke this security, and I could start a happy and productive life in a scientific atmosphere unparalleled even at academic institutions. Many of my scientific heroes were there, from Claude Shannon to John Pierce and John Kelly. While probably all my colleagues know about Shannon, the founder of information theory, and about the incredible depth of his insights, and of Pierce, the co-inventor of the traveling-wave tube, inventor of the Telstar communication satellite, and creator of a new musical scale, very

few know about John Kelly, a genius from Texas who died young yet had great influence on all of us who had the good fortune to know him. I refer to his unique idea of information rate (Kelly 1956) in dialogue: 4. If I ever were to write my autobiography, I would devote many pages to his colorful personality and creative mind. Here I will only mention that, with Mohan Sondhi, another engineer friend of mine with an unusually clear mind, Kelly laid the foundations of the echo-suppressor circuits that revolutionized long-distance telephony.

For the reader who is interested in my first years at Bell Labs and in the invention of the random-dot stereogram, I recommend the book *Three Degrees Above Zero* (Bernstein 1984), which contains profiles of me and some other Bell Labs scientists. I also recommend Julesz 1986a, Julesz 1990a, and Julesz 1990b.

Mentors and enemies can promote a scientist's career in strange ways. After joining Bell Labs, I started to read the psychological literature and met some of the first experimental psychologists. I was startled to learn that, according to the notions prevalent among psychologists, stereopsis was an enigmatic problem, based on monocular form recognition, shrouded in the mystery of semantics, and complicated by the many familiarity cues that are needed to recognize, say, a face. As a former radar engineer, I knew that monocular recognition was not necessary, since in aerial reconnaissance one could break monocular camouflage by inspecting aerial images stereoscopically; camouflaged targets would then jump out in vivid depth. Of course, in real life there is no perfect camouflage, so when the first large computers arrived at Bell Labs I used them to create the first ideally camouflaged stereoscopic images with no break or gap between areas of different binocular disparities. As I expected, the correlated areas segregated in vivid depth. This demonstration was greatly opposed by the leading expert on stereopsis, Kenneth Ogle (1964), who was convinced of the need for monocular contours before stereopsis (and who remained so years after my findings were published in spite of his opposition). I quote him verbatim (Ogle and Wakefield 1967, p. 90): "One obtains the impression from some of Julesz's interesting experiments that certain targets yield a stereoscopic depth, but contours cannot be perceived monocularly. However, the stereoscopic depth experienced in the central portion is that of a defined square proximal or distal to the background, determined precisely by the 'lines' he 'cut' in the background pattern of random details in each stereogram pairs. It is difficult to believe that a 'cut' and displacement of random patterns—unless the details of pattern are exceedingly small—result in randomness of the two sides of the cut. Some of the dots could have been split. It may be true that monocularly the contours may be difficult to perceive, but still we wonder if they are not perceivable."

Somehow Ogle incorrectly assumed that computer-generated RDSs were similar to RDSs created by cutting some forms from textured paper and physically shifting them, which indeed present the possibility of faint monocular contour cues. With computer-generated RDSs, the disparity shifts are always integral multiples of the pixel width; therefore, no perceivable monocular contours can exist, since no dot (pixel) is cut! I quote this episode because in hindsight I am convinced that it is more important for a young unknown scientist to have a famous scientific rival than a powerful patron. (Of course, the young scientist has to be

right!) Because I always reproduced the RDSs in my papers, so my colleagues could experience the results directly, the scientific controversy between Ogle and me drew attention to my findings and hastened their acceptance by the scientific community. Of course, this episode does not mean that scientific patrons are not important. I thank, in particular, John Pierce, who was then the executive director of research at Bell Labs. Over the years he became a dear friend, and now that he is in his eighties his creativity, scientific curiosity, and enjoyment of life are still inspirational. When my first paper was rejected by the *Journal of the Optical Society of America* (because of the controversy alluded to above), Pierce helped me to publish it, without any changes, in the *Bell System Technical Journal*. He also permitted me to develop the Fresnel prisms that were provided as stereoscopes (Julesz 1960). I am also indebted to D. B. Judd, who as editor of *JOSA* made sure that my next paper (on the role of contours in stereopsis—Julesz 1963) would be published in his journal by reviewing it himself.

Before writing *Foundations of Cyclopean Perception,* I liked to work by myself (except when I worked on certain topics in acoustics —see dialogue 13) or with a few trusted assistants. I am greatly indebted to my first technician, Richard (Dick) Payne, a mechanical and electronic wizard with whom I pursued many intellectual ventures over 18 years and with whom I wrote the first published paper on cyclopean random-dot cinematograms (Julesz and Payne 1968).

In 1964 I was appointed to head research in vision and neurophysiology in a newly created department called "Sensory and Perceptual Processes." At that time, William Baker was the executive vice-president of research of Bell Labs,

Ed David was executive director of research (soon to be succeeded by Bob Prim), and the director of my department was Max Mathews. My department was a collection of psychologists studying human vision and auditory neurophysiologists studying the auditory tectum of the frog, the lateral line organ of the mud-puppy, and the evolution of the hearing organ in fishes. The first group consisted of George Sperling and Jack Levinson; a few years later I invited John Krauskopf and Walter Kropfl. These illustrious colleagues stayed with me for many years and became famous professors on their own. The neurophysiology group consisted of Willhelm van Bergheijk, Larry Frischkopf, Bob Capranica, and Gerard Harris.

For years I was torn between neurophysiology and psychophysics—the more so since Jerry Lettvin, the famous MIT neurophysiologist (at Rutgers from 1989 till 1993) was for decades an advisor to my group, and so were David Hubel and Torsten Wiesel. It took some frustrated efforts (e.g., deep freezing and electron microscopy on the low- and high- frequency-tuned hearing organs of the green frog and looking for size changes in the synaptic vesicles) to convince myself that "wet" psychobiology required much more patience and luck than psychophysics. Unfortunately, work on frogs and fishes was rather remote from the problems of AT&T, and when I wanted to invite Anthony Robertson to do neurophysiology in the visual cortex of the cat it became apparent that this kind of work might not sit well with the stockholders. Our neurophysiology group was disbanded, but only after each member who wanted to leave Bell Labs found a full professorship. I continued with my psychological group, but whenever I would go on one of my frequent sabbatical leaves I would always go to a university and collaborate with neuroanatomists and neurophysiologists.

At Hans-Luke Teuber's invitation I spent half a year in the psychology department at MIT, where I enjoined interactions with some famous colleagues (e.g., I took a neuroanatomy course from Walle Nauta) and where, in a special seminar, I tried out *Foundations of Cyclopean Perception* on an audience that included Whitman Richards, David Lee, and Charles Stromeyer III.

At Bell Labs I worked with several colleagues outside my department. Harry Frisch, a noted theoretical chemist, became interested in my work on texture discrimination and figure-ground perception, and we applied random geometrical techniques to these problems (Frisch and Julesz 1966).

In 1968, while I was writing *FCP*, Steve Johnson (a well-known computer scientist) joined forces with me, and we were able to create the first nonperiodic ambiguous RDS. (I devoted an entire chapter of *FCP* to ambiguous RDSs.) Several talented programmers who worked on this effort went on to become independent researchers: Joan Miller, Rosanne Hesse, Jerry Spivack, Caroll Boshe, and Ellen Gritz.

During this period I had the good fortune to join forces with Derek Fender at Caltech on some heroic experiments with binocular retinal stabilization. These experiments, in which close-fitting contact lenses were used, established a hysteresis effect for stereopsis and led to the concept of cooperativity (Fender and Julesz 1967). Two decades later our experiments were repeated and extended, with less cumbersome techniques, by Piantanida (1986) and Hyson (1983).

I had also a few guests who visited me for a few months to collaborate with me. John Frisby and I studied a new class of random-line stereograms, and we found some interesting effects of plasticity. Frisby became a professor of psychology and contributed to several AI models of stereopsis. Colin Blakemore visited me for a few days to create the first cyclopean aftereffects to demonstrate the existence of binocular-disparity-tuned neuronal pools. His thesis work on stereopsis in the cat heralded his neurophysiological interests; he now holds the Sherrington Chair at Oxford. The late Fergus Campbell, from Cambridge University, also visited my department, which had the first "visible" lasers, and did the first Young-diffraction experiments to determine the MTF of the nervous sytem by bypassing the aberrations of the eye. I was greatly impressed that the diagonal effect was strictly neural in origin.

Cooperativity was originally observed as the result of a pulling effect (Julesz 1964). However, it was extended in one of the most strategic experiments I conducted in collaboration with Jih Jie Chang (who joined me in 1975) on the pulling effect of stereopsis. That experiment established the cooperative nature of stereopsis even more convincingly than the hysteresis effect did (Julesz and Chang 1976). Ms. Chang and I worked together on several fun projects, particularly on problems of short- and long-term motion perception (Chang and Julesz 1983a,b) and on cooperativity effects in motion perception (Chang and Julesz 1984). She started with me as a sophisticated system programmer, but I soon regarded her as one of my postdocs. Over the years she became an independent researcher in visual perception, and in recent yeras she has published several influential papers. I am indebted to her in the deepest sense, and I am so glad that we were able to start together a new

scientific life at Rutgers. Just before the conference honoring my 65th birthday I learned of her decision to retire, and I am glad that we could honor her as well.

I want to acknowledge my great indebtedness to Walter Kropfl, who came to my department from Walter Reed Hospital, where he had helped Hubel and Wiesel in their epoch-making experiments. He is one of the few experts who can either program a computer or, if the programming language appears inadequate, open the computer and modify the hardware accordingly. For instance, in 1974 he developed a special hardware that sped up commercially available computers by a factor of 16 and permitted us to present complex textures and masking arrays in a few milliseconds using electrostatic monitors.

Before Kropfl succeeded in constructing a computer that made the generation of dynamic RDSs possible, I could only use two uncorrelated stereograms in temporal succession (Julesz and Payne 1968). Seymour Papert (1964) found an ingenious way to generate some special dynamic RDSs that, however, was unable to display general shapes in 3-D. So, the technical problem of how to generate dynamic RDSs in real time became a real stumbling block to lifting cyclopean techniques into the realm of spatio-temporal studies. Therefore, I was mightily surprised when I heard in 1973 that John Ross, at the University of Western Australia, had been generating dynamic RDSs. It turned out that after NASA closed down its tracking stations in Australia many of the largest computers were for grabs. Ross succeeded in getting a few, and he used them to generate dynamic RDSs—a feat that even the rich Bell Labs scientists could not afford. At Ross's kind invitation I spent several very pleasant weeks over two successive years in his psychology department, where we worked on dynamic RDSs and RDCs with gusto (Hogben et al. 1976). Luckily, the following year Kropfl succeeded with his new method, which was even more powerful than any previous attempts, and from then on other colleagues visited us to work with cyclopean techniques.

From 1971 to 1982 I had a most productive time working with the above-mentioned collaborators and with my many postdocs at the "old" Bell Labs.

In this introductory paragraphs of this appendix, where I focused on my youth, I gave the early figures in my scientific life more emotional weight than later ones. However, without the help of the many colleagues, collaborators, students, friends, administrators, and "witnesses of my life" (whom I will list briefly in the next paragraphs) my research could not have unfolded as it did. My special thanks go to the managements of (AT&T) Bell Laboratories, the California Institute of Technology, and Rutgers University. I thank the anonymous "talent scouts" and committees of the MacArthur Foundation, which awarded me its magnificent fellowship prize at a critical time (1983–1989) when the management of Bell Labs and AT&T was changing its views of basic research radically. Here I thank explicitly William O. Baker, former president of At&T Bell Laboratories, and Arno Penzias, vice-president of research, for their continuous support and good will. I also thank Felix Browder, former vice-president of research, and Alexander Pond, former vice-president of Rutgers University, for inviting me and my department to join Rutgers's new "institutes of excellence," and particularly for establishing the Laboratory of Vision Research in January 1989. I thank Rutgers University for continuing support. I received several important prizes, including the Heinecken Prize (1985) of the Royal Netherlands Academy and the Lashley Award of the Philosophical Society in Philadelphia, and I thank the members of their selection boards for singling out my work.

I am most appreciative of the management of Caltech for inviting me twice as a Fairchild Distinguished Scholar and for sponsoring from 1983 until now a visiting professorship in the biology division, where I did much research and gave many seminars and lectures. I am also most appreciative of the enlightened management of the Office of Naval Research for awarding David Van Essen and me a joint grant for many years to study texture perception in monkeys and humans. This grant and the support from the MacArthur Foundation permitted me to have an additional postdoc position. My Caltech stay overlapped with my Bell Labs and Rutgers periods, and interactions with the outstanding colleagues and students at Caltech extended my scientific vista.

My primary thanks go to my collaborators—mathematicians, neurophysiologists, and psychologists. Here I will list in chronological order the colleagues with unusual mathematical talents who took my iso-second-order texture paradigm seriously and helped me to invent such stochastic processes: David Slepian, Mark Rosenblatt, Harry Frisch, Edward Gilbert, Larry Shepp, Terry Caelli, Jonathan Victor, and Persi Diaconis. I am particularly grateful to Terry Caelli, with whom I discovered the first textons, thereby establishing that texture segregation is a local process. In addition, I am indebted to S. Brodie and A. Gagalowicz for their contributions to the iso-second-order paradigm.

After the divestiture of AT&T in 1982, my Sensory and Perceptual Processes Department was briefly reorganized; in the process, I lost Walter Kropfl. Soon after I received the MacArthur Prize, Arno Penzias created the Visual Perception Research Department for me. One of the fortunate events in my life came when Thomas Papathomas, an expert on sparse-matrix eigenvalue problems who had earned his Ph.D. from Columbia in electrical engineering and computer science, asked to join my new department. In only a short time, he planned and installed a very fast high-resolution color graphics system to match large databases (e.g., Cray models for long-term weather forecasting) to human heuristics—one of my old dreams. Soon we ventured into problems of how focal attention can affect spatial-frequency channels. Then we conducted a benchmark test on the Connection Machine by placing in each of the 64,000 computers the Lie germs of the affine transformation group. Afterwards he joined forces with another collaborator of mine, Andrei Gorea, and developed a novel paradigm that makes it possible to juxtapose many attributes, including color, polarity, and orientation, so as to study their role in motion, stereopsis, and texture. Papathomas became a professor of biomedical engineering and my associate director at the LVR at Rutgers.

Finally, I was joined by Itzhak Hadani, from the Technion in Haifa, who is interested in stereopsis and in the mathematical foundation of perceptual constancies. Hadani has interesting ideas and holds an important patent on night goggles. His presence drew my interest to the old problem of whether absolute depth can be perceived and to related questions of autokinetic motion. In the four years he has been with us, his research in passive and active human navigation and autokinetic motion has blossomed. We have also done research together on the role of interocular parallax distance in stereopsis, and on motion constancy (Hadani and Julesz 1992).

After I wrote *FCP*, it became my custom to surround myself with bright postdoctoral fellows. Most of them became distinguished scientists on their own. Here I will mention their contributions and my debts to them in chronological order:

My first postdoc, Charles Stromeyer III (from Harvard), has an unusual knack for successful and surprising experiments, and I am pleased that Harvard has rewarded him with the same appointment that was given to my hero, Georg von Békésy, a generation earlier. Our experiment on critical-band masking in vision (Stromeyer and Julesz 1972) is a highly quoted paradigm. I have had more than a dozen postdocs since, and even an "honorary postdoc": Enrico Chiarucci, who created the cyclopean movie that accompanied *FCP* and who collaborated with me on pioneering work with echoic memory in vision (Julesz and Chiarucci 1973). Chiarucci's main interests were in computer science, and he worked on many interesting problems, from spreading the UNIX operating system to Italy to setting up a data bank in Morocco for translating the Koran into different Arabic dialects. I was devastated when he died suddenly of cancer last year.

My second postdoc was Bruno Breitmeyer, a graduate of Stanford with whom I discovered an up-down asymmetry (instead of a left-right one) for stereopsis (Breitmeyer, Julesz, and Kropfl 1975). From him I learned the importance of metacontrast, which I used in later experiments in texture perception. We also pioneered a paper on the role of temporal transients on low- and high-SF channels (Breitmeyer and Julesz 1975). Like many other former postdocs, he visited me again later, and we tried to find some ingenious ways to separate perceptual processes that rely on retinotopic coordinates from those that are based on egotopic coordinates (Breitmeyer, Julesz, and Kropfl 1982). That some problems with the phosphor time constants may have interfered with the results does not affect the usefulness of the basic idea. Breitmeyer later wrote an influential monograph on metacontrast.

My third postdoc, Christopher W. Tyler, was already an accomplished researcher on his own. Although we worked on many exciting problems of stereopsis, our discoveries of "neurontropy" (an entropy-like process in stereopsis) and of the role binocular rivalry plays in negative correlation (Julesz and Tyler 1976; Tyler and Julesz 1976) were unexpected insights of the sort that come only from cooperative interaction between two minds. Tyler's interest in sinusoidally wiggly lines in stereopsis led him to concepts of disparity gradients.

It was with my fourth postdoc, Peter Burt, that the "forbidden zones in Panum's fusional area" were postulated for the first time and the concept of a "disparity-gradient limit" (Burt and Julesz 1980) was developed. Burt, a most original thinker in computer science and machine vision, was among my few "honorary" graduate students as well—Michael Arbib sent him to work with me on his Ph.D. thesis.

Besides Burt, I had only three more such graduate students. Lloyd Marlowe (sent by Lorrin Riggs), whose random-line stereograms I presented in *FCP*, spent a year with me at Bell Labs; he died tragically soon after moving to Harvard. The other two, whom I acquired during my stay at the ETH in Zürich, were Benno Petrig and Hans-Peter Oswald, were studying with Max Anlicker, but after attending my lecture they decided to do their doctoral work in cyclopean perception. Petrig later became my postdoc.

My year in Zürich (1976) was a rewarding interlude. At the invitation of my dear friend Günther Baumgartner, a noted neurologist and visual researcher, I had the opportunity to develop (with another old friend, Dietrich Lehmann) visually evoked potentials to dynamic random-dot stereograms and correlograms. This technique opened up the field of measuring cyclopean vision in infants and monkeys at the earliest stage.

Before Peter Burt became a postdoc, the fourth postdoc with me was Terry Caelli, a sophisticated mathematician from Australia who wanted to work with me on Lie germs and Lie algebras and on their role in perceptual invariances (a topic to which I devoted an entire chapter of *FCP*). I persuaded him instead to work on preattentive texture discrimination, using the iso-second-order paradigm that led to the discovery of the first textons. I regard this work as of utmost importance to my intellectual development.

Burt helped me to develop (with Walter Kropfl) the GENTEX program, which permitted my later postdocs to generate visual arrays and textures of great sophistication and generality. After turning back to image processing, Burt wrote some really important papers on such original concepts as the Laplacian pyramid.

Benno Petrig, whom I have mentioned already, did his doctoral thesis on VEP measurements on human infants. After he became my postdoc, he, Kropfl, and I improved on techniques of testing human infants by "surrounding" them with dynamic random-dot correlograms projected on a large screen. His findings, together with a follow-up study of a dozen normal infants done with Oliver Braddick, Janet Atkinson, Ivan Bodis-Wollner, and others, established that functional binocularity suddenly manifests itself at 3.5 months after birth. Petrig's findings, together with those from the follow-up study, provide an important first clue to the determination of the "maturational window" for stereopsis and the possible elimination of amblyopia ex anopsia ("lazy eye") due to strabismus.

The next postdoc was Rob Schumer, whose thesis adviser was Leo Ganz of Stanford. Rob worked on aftereffects of sinusoidally corrugated RDS surfaces. Together, we used corrugated RDSs and measured the cyclopean MTF, among other observations (Schumer and Julesz 1984). We also wrote collaborated on the chapter on early vision for the 1981 *Annual Review of Psychology.*

The next postdoc was Jim Bergen, a graduate student of Hugh Wilson with an excellent grasp of mathematics. We linked texture segregation with focal attention. We also showed how iso-third-order texture pairs could be segmented with a linear spatial filter followed by a nonlinearity (Julesz and Bergen 1982). Bergen, like Burt, is now working at the Stanford Research Institute (the successor of the Sarnoff Center), in Princeton.

The next postdoc, Dov Sagi, spent most of his time with me at Bell Labs but also followed me to Caltech. In a series of papers (Sagi and Julesz 1985a,b, 1986, 1987) we suggested a preattentive/attentive dichotomy of vision, following the masking paradigm developed with Burt and Bergen. Sagi, who became a professor at the Weitzmann Institute, visits me often and recently spent a year at the LVR.

Then came Bart Farell, who had worked in cognition. We joined forces and discovered a somewhat global "school of fish" detector that would detect when adjacent oriented elements (e.g. arrows) were quasi-parallel (Farell and Julesz 1989).

Andrei Gorea, a well-established psychophysicist from France, joined me next at Bell Labs. While our collaboration was interrupted by my car accident, we managed to obtain the unexpected finding that stick figures resembling human faces were more easily detected than random aggregates of sticks even when the observer did not consciously recognize the face (Gorea and Julesz 1990).

At the same time, Ben Kröse, from the Netherlands, whose thesis work was on the psychological quantification of texton-gradient strength, was working as a postdoc in my laboratory at Caltech. Studying search strategies of focal attention, we found no evidence for a scan path or for zooming, but we found a parallel and a serial process operating simultaneously (Kröse and Julesz 1989).

The last postdoc at Bell Labs, and my first at Rutgers, was Doug Williams (also a graduate student of Hugh Wilson), whose work on cooperative phenomena in motion perception had impressed me. We worked on the asymmetry problem of texture discrimination and on anti-textons. We found that subjective contours would fill in gaps and that some other fill-in phenomena could account for many asymmetries in perception (Williams and Julesz 1991, 1992).

I invited Jukka Saarinen to Rutgers because his interest in seeing texton gradients in the periphery matched my own. We succeeded in measuring the speed of rapid search, a problem that preoccupied me for years (Saarinen and Julesz 1991).

My present postdoc is Jochen (Achim) Braun, who started as a postdoc with Dov Sagi and who therefore is my "scientific grandson." In light of the aforementioned findings, we load attention to the center by a difficult method that requires time-consuming scrutiny. Simultaneously we ask how some other detection or identification tasks in the periphery (e.g., orientation, color, size) can be done preattentively (i.e., independent of target number). A brief report of this work, which is still in progress, is available (Braun and Julesz 1992).

Ilona Kovacs, a cognitive psychologist from Budapest, came to me on a Soros Foundation scholarship. After some impressive joint research on the role of color under metaisoluminance (Kovacs and Julesz 1992) and on the extension of Panum's area under intensive learning, I extended her scholarship and asked her to become a research fellow till 1995. Her research with me led to the concept of metaisoluminance (Kovacs and Julesz 1992). At present we are working on an outstanding idea of hers leading to a genuine visual topology.

Recently I offered a postdoctoral position to Bart Anderson, who last worked at Harvard and who is interested in stereopsis and cooperativity— problems matching my own. I am looking forward to an exciting collaboration.

My 14 winters at Caltech had a great influence on me. Teaching the smartest undergraduates I ever encountered, together with excellent graduates and postdocs, was a most delightful experience, and interacting with the faculty extended my vista. I am most appreciative of interactions with John Allman, Derek Fender, John Hopfield, Christof Koch, Carver Mead, and particularly David Van Essen (with whom I worked for a decade). My walks and discussions with Max Delbrück and Murray Gell-Mann are most memorable. Also, during my stay I frequented the Helmholtz Club at Irvine University, run by Francis Crick and attended by psychobiologists and their guests.

I am most grateful to the following people, who took kind interest in me and in my work: Phil Anderson, Günther Baumgartner, Georg von Békésy, Francis Crick, Salvador Dali, Gerald Edelman, Paul Erdös, Richard Gregory, Leon Harmon, David Hubel, John Krauskopf, Jerry Lettvin, Murray Gell-Mann, Don Glazer, Mark Katz, Ben Logan, David Marr, Alexander Melzak, Vernon Mountcastle, Tommy Poggio, Manfred Schroeder, Anne Treisman, Henk van der Tweel, Roger Shepard, George Sperling, Saul Sternberg, János Szentágothai, Gerald Westheimer, Torsten Wiesel, and Semir Zeki.

I also have some scientific heroes among the younger generation, but I might harm them if I were to reveal their identities. However, I will give tribute to two of my favorite young scientists who, before their untimely deaths, extended early vision beyond my dreams: David Marr and Svatoslav Prasdny. I am deeply indebted to them.

I am most proud of my dear friends Werner Reichardt and Gian Poggio, whose work affected my own. In 1985 Werner and I shared the Dr. H. P. Heinecken Prize; unfortunately, he died before he could read this acknowledgment. In 1989, Gian and I shared the Karl Spencer Lashley Award. Gian's finding that global stereopsis occurs even earlier than anyone had guessed—at the very input to the cortex—was the greatest scientific satisfaction I experienced.

Recently, Ákos Fehér, an expert in computers and visual displays, joined my laboratory and helped us in many sophisticated projects.

There are many scientists, mathematicians, philosophers, and artists—not explicitly quoted here—whose work consciously or unconsciously affected my thinking and my outlook on life. For example, the epigraph by Leibniz was brought to my attention by Daniel C. Dennett [whose 1992 book I really enjoyed even though I side with John Searle (and his Chinese-room argument) and do not believe that algorithms of AI will eventually become conscious and could have sensations]. The idea that one can share with the layman some of the deepest concepts of mathematics I learned from the beautiful book by Rademacher and Toeplitz (*Von Zahlen und Figuren*, translated as *The Enjoyment of Mathematics*) when I was 16. These authors concentrated on simple but deep theorems (which they called beautiful simple melodies), instead of difficult theorems (heavily orchestrated symphonies) that could be understood and solved by professionals only. By concentrating on early vision and ignoring the heavy pieces of cognitive psychology I tried to emulate their example.

It occurred to me to look up the author index of *FCP* and my book chapters. In these longer reviews of mine there are dozens of colleagues named, whose work lives in my thoughts though not mentioned explicitly in *Dialogues*. Just to name a few: J. C. R. Licklider, whose binaural localization of auditory noise caught my fancy; N. S. Sutherland, who pioneered neurophysiological linking with psychological adaptation phenomena; Jacob Beck, who defined perceptual grouping in a novel way; and Tony Movshon, who pioneered the linking of neurophysiological findings with microstimulation to the behavior of monkeys. I thank them all.

I cannot thank all my friends by name—outside and within my specialty—whose kindness and wisdom sustained and influenced me in countless ways. Here I thank only four of my oldest friends: Peter Lengyel, a pioneer of deciphering the genetic code, who kept me up to date on the miraculous developments of molecular biology; Victor Roth, who shared with me his knowledge and philosophy of life, including the quotation in the last paragraph of *Dialogues;* Andrew Gabor, inventor of the daisy wheel and the silent typewriter, with whom I started my career as an engineer and who reminds me of nostalgic intellectual achievements and quests had I remained an engineer; and Peter Földes, an expert on satellite antennas and an accomplished painter, who proved to me that it is possible to excel in both the sciences and the arts.

I started this appendix by thanking my parents; I will finish it by thanking my wife, Margit, for her love, wisdom, and care over 40 years—for providing me an oasis beyond my scientific pursuits.

B
PUBLICATIONS, WITH COMMENTS

The Years in Hungary

1. Julesz, B. Network theory. Lecture notes (1950), Technical University, Budapest. In Hungarian.

2. Julesz, B., Analysis of TV signals by correlation methods. Ph.D. thesis, Hungarian Academy of Science, 1955. This is my first scientific paper. I measured the power spectra of various TV images, from faces to soccer crowds. This I did indirectly (since Hungary did not broadcast TV yet) by measuring the autocorrelation functions optically (illuminating two cascaded identical transparencies with a spatial shift between them and integrating the flux with a selenium photodetector). From the obtained autocorrelation functions I took their Fourier transforms, which—according to the Wiener-Khintchine theorem—resulted in their power spectra. It turned out that the power spectra of natural scenes had a $1/f$ or $1/f^2$ shape, such that mass scenes were almost flat, while faces in close-up had sharply decaying spectra with diminishing high spatial frequencies. So, I proposed a transmitter-receiver system such that the transmitter signal was delayed by one frame and was transmitted with a flat power spectrum (yielding a maximum signal-to-noise ratio), and also transmitted the amount of preemphasis the receiver had to use for the next frame. This increased the fringe area of reception considerably, and was the precursor of other variable preemphasis schemes later used in reducing hiss in tape recordings (one of the best-known such technique is the Dolby system). My thesis was not published, since after its defense I escaped from Hungary. It was this thesis and my interest in correlation methods of image encoding that helped me join Bell Labs.

3. Julesz, B. Report on comparison of PCM and FM systems, Budapest, 1955. In Hungarian.

The Years at Bell Laboratories

4. Julesz, B. Method of coding television signals based on edge detection. *Bell System Technical Journal* 38: 1001–1020 (1959). This, my first published English paper, presaged my interest in visual perception. I tried to save TV bandwidth by transmitting only the extrema of TV signals and letting the receiver interpolate a linear transient between adjacent extrema. While the information saving was modest, I emphasized the psychological implications of my results. It turned out that the visual system was not sensitive to the exact shape of short luminance gradients. Whether it was convex, concave, or linear could not be perceived. I was limited by the one-dimensional scanning of the images, and proposed that a two-dimensional scheme might have been more successful. I even proposed a two-dimensional interpolation technique using soap-bubble-like schemes. My interest in finding two-dimensional extrema, and thus the edges (boundaries) of objects, led to my most important paper, which is listed next.

5. Julesz, B. Binocular depth perception of computer-generated patterns. *Bell System Technical Journal* 39: 1125–1162 (1960). This is my first and most cited psychological paper. I think this article contains several insights which I did not emphasize in *FCP* and which are often missed even by experts. For instance, I pointed out that the no-man's-land, seen by one eye only, is perceived as the continuation of the depth plane farthest behind. Also, I showed, using perturbations, the various effects

that addition, subtraction, multiplication, and division had on stereopsis and binocular rivalry. The effects of such operations on motion perception and stereopsis are now being studied by Werkhoven et al. (1991), among others.

6. Julesz, B. Binocular depth perception and pattern recognition. In *Proceedings of the Fourth London Symposium on Information Theory,* ed. C. Cherry (Butterworth, 1961). This article was the summary of the talk at London in 1960 in which I first introduced my computer-generated random-dot stereograms to an international audience. It is a condensed version of [5], but it contains RDSs of somewhat better quality. During the few months between the two articles, a very good computer-driven optical display device was built in my department at Bell Labs.

7. Julesz, B. Conditions for stereopsis on binocular rivalry of contours. *Journal of the Optical Society of America* 52: 1327 (1962). Abstract of a brief talk; an introduction to [14].

8. Julesz, B. Towards the automation of binocular depth perception (AUTOMAP). In Proceedings of IFIPS Congress, Munich, 1962. To my knowledge, this is the first computer simulation of global stereopsis, and because its stages of successive approximations, it emulates cooperative computation. It clearly showed the robust nature of cooperative models once the strategic nature of the false-target elimination problem was realized.

9. Julesz, B. Visual pattern discrimination. *IRE Transactions on Information Theory* 8: 84–92 (1962). This is my second-most- important paper. In it I introduce the study of scrutiny-free (preattentive) texture discrimination, using texture pairs with identical second-order statistics. This paper is completely unknown to cognitive psychologists interested in the Treisman paradigm, and the journal is defunct.

10. Julesz, B., and Miller, J. E. Automatic stereoscopic presentation of functions of two variables. *Bell System Technical Journal* 41: 663–676 (1962). Some nice and complex mathematical surfaces are depicted by computer-generated RDSs. Nowadays I can generate better quality stereograms (even at movie speeds), yet these were the best one could obtain in 1962 on the IBM 704.

11. Julesz, B., and Guttman, N. Auditory memory. *Journal of the Acoustical Society of America* 35 (11): 1895 (1963). This, my first auditory paper, establishes the limits of echoic memory.

12. Julesz, B. Effects of contour flicker of apparent motion on retinally stabilized images. *Journal of the Optical Society of America* 53 (11): 1336 (1963). I used close-fitting lenses on my own eyes to obtain retinally stabilized images, and I showed an important difference between physically real and stroboscopic (apparent) motion.

13. Guttman, N., and Julesz, B. Lower limits of auditory periodicity analysis. *Journal of the Acoustical Society of America* 35: 610 (1963). A sequel to [11].

14. Julesz, B. Stereopsis and binocular rivalry of contours. *Journal of the Optical Society of America* 53 (8): 994–999 (1963). I tried several subtle perturbations of contours in RDSs, such that the contours were either on the inside or the outside of the pixels, yielding dramatic perceptual differences. I systematically tried many relations, and hoped that

mathematicians would come up with a theory of stereopsis. I regard this as among my best papers and am astonished that so far no one has improved on it.

15. Julesz, B. Binocular depth perception without familiarity cues. *Science* 145: 356–362 (1964). This, my first review article in *Science,* established that global stereopsis is a parallel and cooperative process by measuring perception time with masking.

16. Julesz, B., and Pennington, K. S. Equidistributed information mapping: An analogy to holograms and memory. *Journal of the Optical Society of America* 55 (5): 604 (1965). This is one of the first attempts, if not the very first one, to draw attention to a deep analogy between Fourier-transform holograms and memory properties of brains. We pointed out that equidistributed information storage goes beyond holograms and optical interference patterns. Even complex organisms that contain the same chromosomes in each of their cells obey this principle.

17. Julesz, B., and Guttman, N. Higher-order statistics and short-term auditory memory. In Proceedings of the Fifth International Congress on Acoustics, Liege, 1965. A study of auditory texture discrimination using Markov melodies having identical second-order statistics. Such melodies cannot be told apart. Before 2-D non-Markov iso-second-order textures were invented, the 1-D musical textures (melodies) were the only useful applications, since visual textures are inherently 2-D.

18. Julesz, B. Some neurophysiological problems of stereopsis. In *Proceedings of the Symposiumon Information Processing in the Sight Sensory System,* ed. P. Nye (Caltech,1965). In this article I made the prediction that if binocular disparity tuned cortical neurons were to be discovered they would most likely not be orientationally sensitive. Many years later, Gian Poggio (1984) found such nonorientatinal cyclopean neurons in the monkey cortex.

19. Julesz, B. Texture and visual perception. *Scientific American* 212 (2): 38–48 (1965). My first popular article on my work in texture and depth perception.

20. Julesz, B. Visual perception and Roentgenography. In Proceedings of the Conference of Teachers of Radiology, Philadelphia, 1965. Invited talk and paper on the application of RDSs to x-ray fluoroscopy.

21. Julesz, B. Binocular disappearance of monocular symmetry. *Science* 153: 657–658 (1966). The first publication of the inverse cyclopean technique that shows that monocularly perceived symmetrical patterns and text can be scrambled in the stereoscopic view, rendering them invisible. In my psychoanatomical investigations, this technique strengthens the insight that stereopsis is a very early process, prior to many perceptual phenomena—including symmetry perception.

22. Frisch, H.L., and Julesz, B. Figure-ground perception and random geometry. *Perception and Psychophysics* 1: 389–398 (1966). A sequel to my studies using random geometries. We show that figure ground perception does not depend on the tessellation (triangular, square, or hexagonal) of the array. This indicates that it depends only on the first-order moment, the area fraction of black and white, but not on higher-order moments, such as the perimeter/area fraction, that would depend on the tessellation used.

23. Julesz, B. Perception time of binocular depth and information measure. In Proceedings of the Fourth Canadian Symposium on Communications, Montreal, 1966. A sequel to [15] with emphasis on perception time of stereopsis.

24. Julesz, B. Random patterns and visual perception. In Proceedings of the Symposium on Human Use of Computing Machines, Bell Laboratories, 1966. A paper given at a prestigious symposium for university presidents intended to advance the use of computers.

25. Julesz, B., and Levitt, H. Spatial chords. *Journal of the Acoustical Society of America* 40 (5): 1253 (1966). A brief abstract of research on musical chords presented binaurally.

26. Julesz, B. Computers, patterns and depth perception. *Bell Labs Record* (September 1966): 261–266. A popular article on my work with RDSs and texture discrimination, with a front-surface mylar mirror used to help stereoscopic fusion.

27. Fender, D., and Julesz, B. Extension of Panum's fusional area in binocularly stabilized vision. *Journal of the Optical Society of America* 5 7(6): 819–830 (1967). This report of a sophisticated experiment using binocular close-fitting lenses with attached mirrors showed for the first time that Panum's fusional area can be extended over 2 deg arc when the stereograms are fused first and then slowly pulled.

28. Julesz, B. Some recent studies in vision relevant to form perception. In *Proceedings of the Symposium on Models for the Perception of Speech and Visual Form,* ed. W. Whaten-Dunn (MIT Press, 1967). This article (submitted in 1964) shows that pre-senting the sides of polygons in serial order yields a unified percept at longer presentation rates than when shown at random order. It is also the first multi-dimensional scaling study (using the non-parametric method of Roger Shepard) of preattentive texture discrimination. It shows that luminance and orientation are the two main axes.

29. Julesz, B., and Spivack, G. J. Stereopsis based on vernier acuity cues alone. *Science* 157: 563–565 (1967). This paper has a basic flaw. We thought that the vernier breaks in our stereograms could not be processed by the retinae; however, at great densities this is not the case, as was pointed out by H. K. Nishihara and T. Poggio (1982). So, our claim that vernier acuity is utilized by stereopsis (i.e., that stereopsis occurs after vernier acuity processing) is not substantiated, although it is not disproved either. Nevertheless, in this paper the idea of false-target elimination is illustrated for the first time.

30. Julesz, B. Suppression of monocular symmetry during binocular fusion without rivalry, *Bell System Technical Journal* 46: 1203–1221 (1967). A more elaborate article on the inverse cyclopean technique.

31. Julesz, B. Cluster formation at various perceptual levels. In *Proceedings of the International Conference on Methodologies of Pattern Recognition,* ed. S. Watanabe (Academic Press, 1968). My views on stereoscopic and texture perception using models that search for clusters of nearby feature extractors tuned to similar trigger features.

32. Julesz, B., and Payne, R. A. Differences between monocular and binocular stroboscopic movement perception. *Vision Research* 8: 433–444

(1968). While in 1960 I worked both with random-dot stereograms and cinematograms, I concentrated on the first. I could not demonstrate the latter on the printed page, and I felt that these perceptual phenomena were so beautiful that they deserved to be shared. This is the first detailed report on RDCs, both without and with monocular cues. We also show that cyclopean motion detectors have longer time constants than ordinary motion detectors tuned to luminance.

33. Julesz, B., and Johnson, S. C. Mental holography: Stereograms portraying ambiguously perceivable surfaces. *Bell System Technical Journal* 47: 2075–2093 (1968). Here we extend the wallpaper effect from parallel planes at various depths to surfaces of any shape that can be portrayed simultaneously with a single RDS. The creation of such ambiguous RDSs required many days on the fastest mainframe computers of the day.

34. Julesz, B. Perception during the eclipse of monocular cues. *Psychology Today* 2: 16–23 (1968). A popular article on cyclopean perception, using red-green anaglyphs and goggles for the first time.

35. Julesz, B. Problems of pattern recognition and perceptual psychology. In *Pattern Recognition,* ed. L. Kanal (Thompson, 1968). A review of my work for experts in machine vision.

36. Julesz, B., and Johnson, S. C. Stereograms portraying ambiguously perceivable surfaces. *Proceedings of the National Academy of Sciences* 61 (2): 437–441 (1968). A condensed account of [33] intended for a more diverse readership.

37. Julesz, B. Stereopsis as an aspect of perception. In *Encyclopaedia of Linguistics, Information and Control* (Pergamon, 1968). My first encyclopedia article on global stereopsis.

38. Julesz, B. Binocular depth perception. In *Processing of Optical Data by Organisms and by Machines,* ed. W. Reichardt (Academic Press, 1969). A review article on global stereopsis, and a precursor to *FCP.*

39. Julesz, B. Foundations of cyclopean perception. *Journal of the Optical Society of America* 59: 1544 (1969). This introduction to my ideas, prepared for a seminar I gave at MIT in 1969, is another precursor to *FCP.*

40. Julesz, B. Optical constancy phenomena. In *Processing of Optical Data by Organisms and by Machines,* ed. W. Reichardt (Academic Press, 1969). A sequel to [38] and another precursor to *FCP.*

41. Julesz, B. Pattern discrimination. In *Processing of Optical Data by Organisms and by Machines,* ed. W. Reichardt (Academic Press, 1969). A sequel to [38] and [40] and another precursor to *FCP.*

42. Julesz, B., and White, B. Short-term visual memory and the Pulfrich phenomenon. *Nature* 222: 639–641 (1969). Using dynamic RDSs having corresponding stereo frames delayed in time, we show the short-term memory required for the Pulfrich effect. This work paved the way for future studies to measure delays in myelin diseases.

42a. Julesz, B., Slepian, D., and Sondhi, M. M. Correction for astigmatism by lens rotation and image processing. *Journal of the Optical Society of America* 59: 485 (1969). An elaboration of my conjecture that a rotating slit is equivalent to the optics of a pinhole (or a rotating cylindrical lens is equivalent to a spherical lens), using Bessel functions. The conjecture is only true for white line drawings on a black background and not vice versa, since the Fourier transform of the stimulus has to be divided by the absolute value of the spatial frequency (generalized integration), so low spatial frequencies cannot be present. Later we learned that similar ideas were incorporated in the Radon transform and are the basic equations in computer tomography.

43. Julesz, B., and Hesse, R. I. Inability to perceive the direction of rotational movement of line segments. *Nature* 225: 243–244 (1970). Here we show that a small array of clockwise-rotating needles embedded in a large array of counterclockwise-rotating needles (with random phases) will perceptually segregate unless the needles in the two arrays rotate with the same velocity. This shows that movement detectors can analyze the speed of orientation changes, but not their direction.

44. Julesz, B. The separation of retinal and central processes in vision. In *Psychotomimetic Drugs*, ed. D. Efron (Raven, 1970). This article warns of the dangers of poisoning one's brain with hallucinogenic drugs. Anyone who takes them for curiosity's sake should at least view an RDS to see whether central or retinal stages are affected.

45. Julesz, B. Binocular depth perception in man: A cooperative model of stereopsis. In Proceedings of the Fourth Congress of the Deutsche Gesellschaft für Kybernetik, 1970. This contains my first explicit proposal of a cooperative model for global stereopsis.

46. Julesz, B. Critical bands in vision and audition. In Proceedings of the Seventh International Congress on Acoustics, Budapest, 1971. An attempt to introduce cyclopean methodology into audition by using residue pitch in place of regular pitch to operationally skip the cochlea, with its hair cells, and portray the auditory information on the neural network.

47. Julesz, B. *Foundations of Cyclopean Perception* (University of Chicago Press, 1971). My first monograph is an extension of my research with random-dot stereograms and cinematograms and texture discrimination. It also discusses most of the perceptual phenomena from optical illusions to aftereffects in the absence of luminance gradients. It is still relevant, mainly because it is more experimentally than theoretically oriented.

48. Blakemore, C., and Julesz, B. Stereopsis depth aftereffect produced without monocular cues. *Science* 171: 386–388 (1971). A report on the first cyclopeanly produced aftereffects showing the existence of binocular-disparity-tuned neurons in the human cortex.

49. Julesz, B. Cyclopean perception and neurophysiology. In Proceedings of Seminar on Neurophysiology of the Visual Mechanism Using Single Unit Recording at Various Levels in the Visual Pathway, Canberra, 1972; also in *Investigative Ophthalmology* 11 (6): 541–548 (1972). A review article based on a talk presented at an important seminar of invited speakers from the United States and Australia.

50. Stromeyer, C. F. III, and Julesz, B. Spatial frequency masking in vision: Critical bands and spread of masking. *Journal of the Optical Society of America* 62 (10): 1221–1132 (1972). A report of

the first attempt to establish a deep analogy between critical-band masking in audition and vision.

51. Julesz, B., and Hirsh, I. J. Visual and auditory perception: An essay of comparison. In *Human Communication: A Unified View,* ed. E. David, Jr., and P. Denes (McGraw-Hill, 1972). Working with the auditory expert Ira Hirsh, I attempted to compare low-level and high- level perceptual phenomena in audition and vision.

52. Julesz, B. Binocular depth perception. In *From Theoretical Physics to Biology* (Karger,1973). A review of global stereopsis prepared for the distinguished scientists at the Institute de la Vie in Versailles at the invitation of Mark Kac.

53. Julesz, B., Gilbert, E. N., Shepp, L. A., and Frisch, H. L.. Inability of humans to discriminate between visual textures that agree in second-order statistics—revisited. *Perception* 2: 391–405 (1973). A novel paper for integral geometry, co-authored by two professional mathematicians (Gilbert and Shepp) and a physical chemist (Frisch). Several new methods for creating non-Markov two-dimensional texture pairs are discussed, and the conjecture that humans are unable to perceive texture difference beyond second-order statistics is further corroborated. A particularly useful method was the use of a four-disk technique to generate texture pairs with identical second-order but different third-order statistics.

54. Harmon, L. D., and Julesz, B. Masking in visual recognition: Effects of two-dimensional filtered noise. *Science* 180: 1194–1197 (1973). Using high-spatial-frequency-filtered and block-sampled picture of Abraham Lincoln, we showed that quantization noise masked the original low-SF information and that critical-band filtering restored the face.

55. Julesz, B., and Chiarucci, E. Short-term memory for stroboscopic movement perception. *Perception* 2: 249–260 (1973). Attempting to establish echoic memory for vision, we found a 520-msec limit, below which our observers were able to detect repetition of dynamic noise segments without scrutiny. This was the first use of robust statistical analysis in psychology. Joan Miller was of great assistance.

56. Julesz, B. Synergetics, cooperative phenomena in multi-component systems. In *Proceedings of the Symposium on Synergetics, 1972, Schloss Elmau,* ed. H. Haken (Teubner, 1973). A review article for physicists, stressing the cooperative phenomena of global stereopsis.

57. Julesz, B. Hierarchical systems in visual perception. In *Cooperative Effects,* ed. H. Haken (North-Holland, 1974). A sequel to [56], also intended mainly for physicists.

58. Julesz, B. Two-dimensional spatial-frequency-tuned channels in visual perception. In *Proceedings of the International Symposium on Signal Analysis and Pattern Recognition,* ed. G. F. Inbar (Wiley, 1974). A review of my work with spatial-frequency channels in vision, intended for colleagues working in AI and machine vision.

59. Julesz, B. Cooperative phenomena in binocular depth perception. *American Scientist* 1: 32–43 (1974). In this popular article reporting on my recent work on global stereopsis I characterize my spring-coupled dipole model of global stereopsis as a two-dimensional extension of the zipper.

60. Frisby, J.P., and Julesz, B. Depth reduction effects in random-line stereograms. Perception 4: 151–158 (1975). We show that random-line stereograms that have orthogonal line segments in the corresponding views can be still fused, but with reduced depth. This plasticity effect of depth gives support to Whitman Richard's view that stereopsis can be the mixture of two types of disparity-tuned neurons for near and far depths, respectively. Gian Poggio found such cyclopean neural units in the monkey cortex, but the majority of the cyclopean neurons respond to sharply tuned binocular disparities.

61. Breitmeyer, B., Julesz, B., and Kropfl, W. Dynamic random-dot stereograms reveal an up-down anisotropy and left-right isotropy between cortical hemifields. *Science* 187: 269–270 (1975). This paper reports on the great advantage of perceiving farther objects above the mid-line and closer objects below the mid-line—a result already guessed by Helmholtz (1896). This up-down asymmetry is in contrast with the expected left-right asymmetry, which proved to be absent. Also, we found some large cyclopean scotomas in several observers for specific disparities. They were unaware of these, since convergence movements can shift the 3-D stimuli to other disparities that are more sensitive.

62. Julesz, B., and Miller, J. E. Independent spatial frequency tuned channels in binocular fusion and rivalry. Perception 4: 125–143 (1975). Here we showed for the first time that global stereopsis uses apatial-frequency channels, and that if the binocular masking noise is an octave away from the spectrum of the RDS then fusion is possible even if the masking noise yields strong binocular rivalry.

63. Julesz, B., and Frisby, J. P., Some new subjective contours in random-line stereograms. *Perception* 4: 145–150 (1975). This sequel to [60] offered a 3-D analogue to subjective (illusionary) contours.

64. Frisby, J. P., and Julesz, B. The effect of orientation difference on stereopsis as a function of line length. *Perception* 4: 179–186 (1975). In this follow-up to [60] the lengths of individual line segments were varied.

65. Breitmeyer, B., and Julesz, B. The role of on and off transients in determining the psychophysical spatial frequency response. *Vision Research* 15: 411–415 (1975). An article following up Bruno Breitmeyer's idea that the role of on-and off-transients is different on the SF response.

66. Julesz, B. Experiments in the visual perception of texture. *Scientific American* 232 (4): 34–43 (1975). My second *Scientific American* article emphasizes texture discrimination with iso-second-order texture pairs. This was the last report on texture perception before the texton theory was formulated.

67. Julesz, B. Anisotropies and scotomas of binocular disparity detectors in humans. In *Orthoptics, Past, Present, Future: Transactions of the Third International Orthoptic Congress, 1975* (1976). An article bringing the work described in [61] to the attention of ophthalmologists and optometrists.

68. Julesz, B., Breitmeyer, B., and Kropfl, W. Binocular-disparity-dependent upper-lower hemifield anisotropy and left-right hemifield isotropy as revealed by dynamic random-dot stereograms. *Perception* 5: 129–141 (1976). A longer report on the

research reported in [61], with more plates on cyclopean field tracing.

69. Julesz, B., Petrig, B., and Buttner, U. Fast determination of stereopsis in rhesus monkey using dynamic random-dot stereograms. *Journal of the Optical Society of America* 66 (10): 1909 (1976). An abstract of work based on a novel technique of measuring visually evoked potentials to dynamic RDSs, as reported in [81].

70. Julesz, B., and Chang, J. J. Interaction between pools of binocular disparity detectors tuned to different disparities. *Biological Cybernetics* 22: 107–119 (1976). My first joint paper with Jih Jie Chang is an extension of [15] showing that a small area of an unambiguous RDS can perceptually pull the entire organization of an ambiguous RDS if the disparity of the unambiguous target is close to the disparity of one of the competing surfaces of the ambiguous RDS. The time constant of this pulling was found to be 60 msec. This pulling effect is the most direct evidence that global stereopsis is a co-operative process.

71. Julesz, B., and Tyler, C. W. Neurontropy, an entropy-like measure of neural correlation in binocular fusion and rivalry. *Biological Cybernetics* 23: 25–32 (1976). In this paper we show that perceiving order to disorder (i.e., fusion to loss of fusion) is much easier than vice versa. Some observers with a strong binocular rivalry mechanism can even perceive differences between negatively correlated and uncorrelated dynamic RDSs.

72. Hogben, J. H., Julesz, B., and Ross, J. Short-term memory for symmetry. *Vision Research* 16 (8): 861–866 (1976). An article noting that symmetry perception in dense random-dot textures is similar to the perception of dynamic RDS with delay, but that the time constants are different.

73. Frisby, J.P., and Julesz, B. The effect of length differences between corresponding lines on stereopsis from single and multi-line stimuli. *Vision Research* 16: 83–87 (1976). This study of the plasticity effect of depth in RDS summarizes my collaboration with Frisby.

74. Tyler, C. W., and Julesz, B. The neural transfer characteristics (neurontropy) for binocular stochastic stimulation. *Biological Cybernetics* 23: 33–37 (1976). A sequel of [71] showing that order to disorder can be perceived in a few msec, whereas the reverse takes an order of magnitude longer.

75. Julesz, B. Perceptual limits of texture discrimination and their implications to figure ground separation. In *Proceedings of the Conference on Formal Theories of Visual Perception, Nijmegen, Holland, July 1976,* ed. E. Leeuwenberg and H. Buffart (Wiley, 1977). A summary of my work in depth and texture perception, presented at an important meeting. Among other figure-ground phenomena, I stress the fact that when an area becomes figure the higher spatial frequencies are better perceived.

76. Julesz, B. Recent results with dynamic random-dot stereograms. *Proceedings of the Society of Photo-Optical Instrument Engineering* 120: 30–35 (1977). This review of my work with RDSs, prepared for imaging scientists and photo-optical engineers, contains the first reports of two patents for the quality inspection of chips. One patent involves the use of a miniature RDS to help align stereo microscopes for use in inspection tasks where seeing VLSI chips in depth is crucial. The other patent involves the use of an RDS with a disparity equal

to the distance between periodic circuits on a wafer to force the inspector to align chips in one eye with the neighboring chips seen in the other eye, resulting in binocular rivalry for the few defective chips. (Previously, the microscope platform had to be moved laterally in rapid succession to obtain stroboscopic motion.)

77. Burt, P., and Julesz, B. Expanded Panum's area for dynamic random-dot stereograms. *Investigative Ophthalmology and Visual Science* 26 (3): 287 (1978). The Fender-Julesz (1967) hysteresis effect revisited with a new methodology that does not need image stabilization. The hysteresis effect has been generalized to *dynamic* RDS. Observers fixated a central band of a 3 degree square RDS while the upper and lower halves moved rapidly into depth with equal but opposite disparities. When these surfaces reached a test depth at 180 msec, one or both were briefly decorrelated. Observer's task was to detect the decorrelated surface(s); this was possible only when he fused both surfaces prior to the test. He performed best when he fixated midway between the surfaces without eye movements. When surfaces moved from zero to large disparities the "breakpoint" for fusion was 42 min.arc, but when surfaces moved from large to small disparities refusion occurred at 18 min.arc.

78. Tyler, C.W., and Julesz, B. Binocular cross-correlation in time and space. *Vision Research* 18: 101–105 (1978). A summary article expanding on [73] and [74], addressed to psychologists (who generally do not read *Biological Cybernetics*).

79. Julesz, B., and Oswald, H. Binocular utilization of monocular cues that are undetectable monocularly. *Perception* 7 (3):. 315–322 (1978). Hanspeter

Oswald (a graduate student who worked with me during my one-year sabbatical at the ETH in Zürich) and I used EOG techniques to measure eye movements to cyclopeanly portrayed moving bars. Without monocular luminance cues (real cyclopean condition) the latency of eye movements was considerably larger than with monocular contrast cues. We also determined the latency time for monocularly presented moving bars with small contrast. We found conditions for which neither a monocularly presented bar with weak contrast nor did a cyclopean bar elicited pursuit eye movements, yet when a cyclopean bar was shaded with the same luminance contrast as the former stimulus the two together elicited follow-up motion. This experiment indicated that luminance and stereopsis information were combined at a later stage, and we suggested that this was achieved by probability summation.

80. Julesz, B. Global stereopsis: Cooperative phenomena in stereopsis depth perception. In *Handbook of Sensory Physiology, VIII: Perception*, ed. R. Held, H. W. Leibowitz, and H. Teuber (Springer-Verlag, 1978). This chapter in an important handbook is a continuation of *FCP*.

81. Lehmann, D., and Julesz, B. Lateralized cortical potentials evoked in humans by dynamic random-dot stereograms. *Vision Research* 18: 1265–1271 (1978). A joint effort with Dietrich Lehmann (an expert on evoked potentials in the Neurology Department of Kantonspital in Zürich) demonstrating that VEPs to dynamic RDSs will originate on the contralateral side of the cyclopean target. Using multi-channel electrodes, we found such lateralization, thus showing for the first time that cortically evoked potentials are indeed gener-

ated in the cortex, since an RDS cannot be processed by the retina. A modified form of this technique was used in [69], [91], [98], [99] and [101], for a quick determination of stereopsis in human infants and adults and in monkeys.

82. Caelli, T., and Julesz, B. On perceptual analyzers underlying visual texture discrimination: Part I. *Biological Cybernetics* 28 (3): 167–175 (1978). Using the four-disk method to generate iso-second-order texture pairs, we found that textons (which we then called "quasi-collinearity") popped out from these texture pairs and yielded preattentive texture discrimination.

83. Caelli, T., Julesz, B., and Gilbert, E. On perceptual analyzers underlying visual texture discrimination: Part II. *Biological Cybernetics* 29 (4): 201–214 (1978). The second part of [82], containing a discussion of the generalized four-disk method. This generalization increased manyfold our repertoire of methods for generating iso-second-order textures in two dimensions. With these added methods we discovered additional textons, which we named "corner" and "connectivity." These names were only crude descriptors, and many other stimulus parameters now used for the texton gradients had not yet been identified.

84. Julesz, B., Gilbert, E. N., and Victor, J. D. Visual discrimination of textures with identical third-order statistics. *Biological Cybernetics* 31 (3): 137–140 (1978). We were able to generate (and give existence proof of) texture pairs with identical third-order but different fourth-order statistics, using 2-D cellular automata (invented by John von Neumann). Preattentive texture discrimination of iso-third-order texture pairs seemed to be the result

of local conspicuous features of elongated blobs with different sizes, aspect ratios, and orientations, and obviously the visual system cannot analyze fourth-order global (statistical) parameters.

85. Julesz, B. Visual texture discrimination using random-dot patterns: Comment. *Journal of the Optical Society of America* 68 (2): 268–270 (1978). This is a comment on a paper that had confused our second-order statistics (also called dipole statistics) of randomly thrown dipoles of all lengths and orientations with diagram statistics (usually for Markov processes), where the dipoles are adjacent samples.

86. Julesz, B., and Caelli, T. On the limits of Fourier decompositions in visual texture perception. *Perception* 8: 69–73 (1979). We took the Fourier transforms of discriminable iso-second-order texture pairs and showed that, in agreement with theory, their power spectra agreed, while their phase spectra appeared random. This supported our view that discrimination was based not on global features (i.e. the Fourier spectra) but on conspicuous local feature differences, which we named *texton gradients*.

87. Caelli, T., and Julesz, B. Psychophysical evidence for global feature processing in visual texture discrimination. *Journal of the Optical Society of America* 69 (5): 675–678 (1979). In this paper we demonstrated psychophysically, and analyzed mathematically, the dependence of discrimination between texture pairs of dipoles on the distribution of their scattered orientations and on their densities. We showed for the first time that the first-order statistic of dipoles (i.e., blob textons) deter-

mines texture discrimination, and that therefore a global process underlies it.

88. Julesz, B. Random-dot correlogram test for eidetic imagery, Open Peer Commentary: Twenty years of haunting eidetic imagery: Where's the ghost? *Behavioral and Brain Sciences* 2: 583–629 (1979). In *FCP* I devoted a section to an eidetiker studied by Stromeyer and Psotka (1970) without having tested the validity of their claims; I included that material because it showed the usefulness of cyclopean techniques by providing an RDS test that could not be faked. In this peer review, I turned to the question of testing super-eidetikers

89. Julesz, B., and Chang, J. J. Symmetry perception and spatial-frequency channels. *Perception* 8: 711–718 (1979). One of the most important mathematical insights in *FCP* was my conjecture that all 2-D functions can be decomposed into four components (with horizontal, vertical, twofold, and centric symmetries), and that only one eigenvalue can exist (that is, only one of these organizations is permitted; otherwise the percept is a random array). In this article we show that all these organizations can be perceived simultaneously if their spatial-frequency spectra fall into separate critical bands.

90. Braddick, O., Atkinson, J., Julesz, B., Kropfl, W., Bodis-Wollner, I., and Raab, E. Cortical binocularity in infants. *Nature* 288: 363–365 (1980). I asked Oliver Braddick and Janet Atkinson, two psychologists from Cambridge University, to come to Mount Sinai Hospital in New York to study the onset of functional binocularity in infants, using the techniques developed in [91]. We found that in normal human infants VEPs to dynamic random-dot correlograms appear at 3.5 months. In spite of much effort on my part, this is the only occasion when I was able to collaborate with ophthalmologists, even though the determination of the critical window for stereopsis may be the key to preventing amblyopia ex anopsia (lazy eye) in cases where strabismus causes stereo blindness and not vice versa.

91. Julesz, B. Kropfl, W., and Petrig, B. Large evoked potentials to dynamic random-dot correlograms and stereograms permit quick determination of stereopsis. *Proceedings of the National Academy of Sciences* 77 (4): 2348–2351 (1980). An improvement on measuring VEPs to dynamic random-dot correlograms by using projection TV monitors, which enabled us to surround the observer with the cyclopeanly pulsating stimulus (between correlation and uncorrelation). The generation of these correlograms and the averaging of the VEPs was performed by a small computer.

92. Burt, P., and Julesz, B. Modifications of the classical notion of Panum's fusional area. *Perception* 9: 671–682 (1980). In this paper we showed that nearby objects warp the fusional space, and that even within Panum's fusional area only those objects (dots) whose disparity gradients are below a critical constant can be fused. Christopher Tyler, working with wiggly lines, proposed similar notions but did not postulate a disparity gradient limit.

93. Tyler, C. W., and Julesz, B. On the depth of the cyclopean retina. *Experimental Brain Research* 40: 196–202 (1980). In this article we summarize several findings of [74] and [78], add a few more, and propose a novel way to handle global stereopsis.

94. Julesz, B. Spatial nonlinearities in the instantaneous perception of textures with identical power spectra. *Philosophical Transactions of the Royal Society* B290: 83–94 (1980). In this summary and elaboration of the texton theory, presented at a prestigious symposium. I tried to rename the corner and closure textons "crossing" and "zero terminator number," respectively, in order to avoid the topological concept of closure, which had led to much confusion.

95. Julesz, B. Spatial-frequency channels in one-, two-, and three- dimensional vision: Variations on an auditory theme by Békésy. In *Visual Coding and Adaptability,* ed. C. S. Harris (Erlbaum, 1980). In this didactic paper I tried to establish a deep analogy between auditory experiments performed by Békésy in 1929 and visual experiments based on spatial-frequency channels performed 40 years later.

96. Burt, P., and Julesz, B. A disparity gradient limit for binocular fusion. *Science* 208: 615–617 (May 1980). A succinct version of [92] for the wide readership of *Science*. Both papers (submitted in 1979) portray computer-generated autostereograms—to my knowledge the first in print.

97. Julesz, B. A theory of preattentive texture discrimination based on first-order statistics of textons. *Biological Cybernetics* 41: 131–138 (1981). A precursor of [105] including several demonstrations that textures with different power spectra cannot be discriminated in the absence of texton gradients.

98. Bodis-Wollner, I., Barris, M. C., Mylin, L. H., Julesz, B., and Kropfl, W. Binocular stimulation reveals cortical components of the human visual evoked potential. *Electroencephalography and Clinical Neurophysiology* 52: 298–305 (1981). This article presents some clinical applications of dynamic RDSs—particularly the measurement of optical pathway delays in myelin-related diseases, such as retrobulbar neuritis.

99. Petrig, B., Julesz, B., Kropfl, W., Baumgartner, G., and Anliker, M. Development of stereopsis and cortical binocularity in human infants: Electrophysiological evidence. *Science* 213: 1402–1405 (1981). A maturational study of the onset of the development of functional binocularity and stereopsis in human infants. In addition to finding a sudden onset of VEP to random-dot correlograms at age 3.5 months, there is a doubling of VEP response of the stimulus frequency of alternation, similar to the response at 6 months of age. It could be that functional binocularity emerges at 3.5 months whereas stereopsis requires 6 months.

100. Julesz, B., and Schumer, R. A. Early visual perception. *Annual Reviews of Psychology* 32: 575–627 (1981). An extensive review of work on early vision.

101. Miezin, F. W., Myerson, J., Julesz, B., and Allman, J. M. Evoked potentials to dynamic random-dot correlograms in monkey and man: A test for cyclopean perception. *Vision Research* 21: 177–179 (1981). Using techniques described in [91], we measured VEPs to dynamic random-dot correlograms in adult humans and monkeys, and found similar responses.

102. Julesz, B. Figure and ground perception in briefly presented iso-dipole textures. In *Perceptual Organization,* ed. M. Kubovy and J. R. Pomerantz (Erlbaum, 1981). A review of the texton theory

and of its implications for figure-ground phenomena, presented at a workshop of distinguished psychologists—many of them with gestaltist leanings.

103. Julesz, B. Perception of order reveals two visual systems. *Leonardo* 14 (4): 311–322 (1981). A review of the texton theory and the preattentive-attentive dichotomy of human perception written for visual artists.

104. Julesz, B. Psychologically determined receptive fields in monocular and binocular texture perception. In *Neural Communication and Control,* ed. G. Székely, E. Labos, and S. Danjanovich (Pergamon, 1981). A review of perceptual receptive fields prepared for a satellite meeting of the International Congress of Physiology in Debrecen, Hungary.

105. Julesz, B. Textons, the elements of texture perception and their interactions. *Nature* 290: 91–97 (1981). An invited article on the state of the texton theory for a general readership.

106. Julesz, B. Theoretical and clinical advances in global stereopsis. In *Advances in Physiological Sciences,* ed. E. Grastyan and P. Molnar (Pergamon, 1981). A second review paper prepared for the 28th International Congress of Physiology, held in Budapest.

107. Julesz, B., and Kropfl, W. Binocular neurons and cyclopean visually evoked potentials in monkey and man. *Annals of the New York Academy of Sciences* (1982): 37–44. A review article discussing previous findings with cyclopeanly evoked VP.

108. Breitmeyer, B. G., Kropfl, W., and Julesz, B. The existence and role of retinotopic and spatiotopic forms of visual persistence. *Acta Psychologica* 52:. 175–196 (1982). The ideas used to distinguish between retinotopic and spatiotopic (ego-centered) visual phenomena based on iconic memory were novel, yet the results were marred by the afterglow of the phosphors used in the TV tube.

109. Julesz, B. The role of terminators in preattentive perception of line textures. In *Proceedings of the Conference on Recognition of Pattern and Form, 1979* (University of Texas at Austin, 1982). A report of experiments with texture pairs composed of line segments of different number of terminators.

110. Julesz, B. From images to surfaces: A computational study of the human early visual system. *Journal of the Optical Society of America* 72: 1292 (1982). A book review.

111. Julesz, B. Binocular depth perception in normal adults and its early development. *Fortschritte der Ophthalmologie* 80: 378–383 (1983). A review of developmental work on the onset of stereopsis, written for ophthalmologists.

112. Chang, J. J., and Julesz, B. Displacement limits for spatial frequency filtered random-dot cinematograms in apparent motion. *Vision Research* 23: 1379–1385 (1983). A critical study, performed with random-dot cinematograms, showing that the maximum displacement limit increases with the size of the cyclopean target.

113. Chang, J. J., and Julesz, B. Displacement limits, directional anisotropy and direction versus form discrimination in random-dot cinematograms. *Vision Research* 23 (6): 639–646 (1983). An exxtension of [112] showing that elliptically filtered RDCs that produce elongated blobs have

the maximum disparity limit according to the size of the blob orthogonal to the motion.

114. Bergen, J. R., and Julesz, B. Parallel versus serial processing in rapid pattern discrimination. *Nature* 303: 696–698 (1983). A tachistoscopic study showing that texture (texton) gradients (Xs in Ls) yield immediate (preattentive) discrimination, whereas Ts in Ls require time-consuming scrutiny (depending on the number of elements).

115. Julesz, B. Textons, rapid focal attention shifts, and iconic memory. Open peer commentary: The impending demise of the icon: A critique of the concept of iconic storage in visual information processing. *Behavioral and Brain Sciences* 6 (1): 25–27 (1983). In this peer review I dispute Haber's feeling that his lifelong research on iconic imagery was wasted.

116. Burt, P., and Julesz, B. The disparity gradient limit for binocular fusion: An answer to J.D. Krol and W.A. van de Grind, *Perception* 11: 621–624 (1983). Our original idea of a binocular disparity limit, presented in [92] and [96], was developed in our earlier critique of a paper by Krol and van de Grind. This is an answer to their reply to our critique.

117. Julesz, B., and Bergen, J. R. Textons, the fundamental elements in preattentive vision and perception of textures, *Bell System Technical Journal* 62 (6): 1619–1645 (1983). A didactic article combining my texton theory with my spatio-temporal masking studies with Jim Bergen [114]. We show, among other things, that discrimination of iso-third-order texture pairs can be accomplished by a linear (size-tuned) spatial filter, followed by a

nonlinearity (i.e. threshold). Here we argue for a preattentive/attentive duality of vision.

118. Bergen, J. R., and Julesz, B. Rapid discrimination of visual patterns. *IEEE Transactions on Systems, Man, and Cybernetics* 13 (5): 857–863 (1983). This article argues for a continuous theory of visual texture discrimination in which the preattentive/attentive dichotomy proposed in [114] and [117] merely represents the two ends of the psychometric curve.

The Years at Bell Laboratories and Caltech

119. Hyson, M., Julesz, B., and Fender, D. H. Eye movements and neural remapping during fusion of misaligned random-dot stereograms. *Journal of the Optical Society of America* 73 (12): 1665–1673. The Fender-Julesz hysteresis effect revisited, with binocular close-fitting contact lenses under suction and with light sources attached. Instead of retinal stabilization, the position of the eyes was measured. Mike Hyson conducted the experiment; Derek Fender and I participated in its evaluation. The results were in agreement with [27], and the possibility of neural remapping was hypothesized.

120. Julesz, B. The role of analog models in our digital age. Open peer commentary: The quantized geometry of visual space: The coherent computation of depth, form, and lightness. *Behavioral and Brain Sciences* 6 (4): 668–669 (1983). Commenting on Steve Grossberg's neural models, I bring attention to my old spring-coupled-magnetic-dipole model of stereopsis, which I think can give excellent heuristic to some of the complex filling-in phenomena Grossberg is treating with nonlinear partial differential equations. This peer commen-

tary contains several interesting comments by specialists and gives an excellent insight into Grossberg's influential work.

121. Julesz, B. A brief outline of the texton theory of human vision. *Trends in Neurosciences* 7: 41–45 (1984). This brief summary of the texton theory reached many workers in psychobiology who had not been familiar with it.

122. Julesz, B. Adaptation in a peephole: A texton theory of preattentive vision. In *Sensory Experience, Adaptation and Perception,* ed. L. Spillman and B. Wooten (Erlbaum, 1984). In this review paper honoring the 65th birthday of Ivo Kohler, I tried to connect some of the predictions of the texton theory with Kohler's sensory-adaptation experiment.

123. Schumer, R. A., and Julesz, B. Binocular disparity modulation sensitivity to disparities offset from the plane of fixation. *Vision Research* 24 (6): 533–542 (1984). A report of experiments in which Rob Schumer and I, using sinusoidally corrugated surfaces portrayed by dynamic RDSs, obtained a cyclopean modulation transfer function.

124. Chang, J. J., and Julesz, B. Cooperative phenomena in apparent movement perception of random-dot cinematograms. *Vision Research* 24: 1781–1788 (1984). An attempt to extend cooperativity to motion perception using random-dot cinematograms.

125. Julesz, B., and Papathomas, T. V. On spatial-frequency channels and attention. *Perception and Psychophysics* 36 (4): 398–399 (1984). My first paper with Thomas Papathomas discusses the relation between focal attention and spatial-frequency channels.

126. Julesz, B., and Moffatt, G. T. The texton theory of vision sheds light on how we see. *AT&T Bell Labs Record* (May 1984): 4–7. In preparing this article for an audience of AT&T employees and their associates, I had the assistance of a professional writer. That it won a "best technical paper" award shows how much more I could have achieved if my English style had been more polished.

127. Julesz, B. Toward an axiomatic theory of preattentive vision. In *Dynamic Aspects of Neocortical Function,* ed. G. Edelman, W. Gall, and W. Cowan (Wiley, 1984). The first axiomatic formulation of the texton theory.

128. Julesz, B., and Harmon, L. D. Noise and recognizability of coarse quantized images. *Nature* 308 (8): 211–212 (1984). An answer to a critique of our [54].

129. Chang, J. J., and Julesz, B. Cooperative and non-cooperative processes of apparent movement of random-dot cinematograms. *Spatial Vision* 1 (1): 39–45 (1985). An article on our work with RDSs and RDCs, with particular emphasis on cooperativity.

130. Sagi, D., and Julesz, B. Detection versus discrimination of visual orientation. *Perception* 14: 619–628 (1985). In this paper we demonstrate that, although orientation differences (yielding texture gradients) in textures can be preattentively detected, identifying the orientations requires scrutiny and depends on the number of these gradients. This paper stirred considerable controversy among cognitive psychologists, and our unorthodox claim is still under debate.

131. Sagi, D., and Julesz, B. Fast noninertial shifts of attention. *Spatial Vision* 1: 141–149 (1985). Here we show that, contrary to some reports in the cognition literature, focal shifting from one target to another is practically noninertial and therefore does not depend on the distance between the targets to be scrutinized.

132. Julesz, B., and Papathomas, T. V. Independent channels in stereopsis. *Investigative Ophthalmology and Visual Science* 26 (3): 242 (1985). An abstract on spatial-frequency channels in global stereopsis.

133. Julesz, B. Preconscious and conscious processes in vision. In *Pattern Recognition Mechanisms,* ed. C. Chagas, R. Gattas, and C. Gross (Pontifical Academy of Sciences, 1985). A review paper given at a prestigious workshop on consciousness, held at the Pontifical Academy in the Vatican and organized by Sir John Eccles. Here I regarded preattentive processes as unconscious and attentive ones as conscious—an oversimplification, but one that was of interest to some eminent scientists who participated.

134. Sagi, D., and Julesz, B. Where and what in vision, *Science* 228: 1217–1219 (1985). This review paper brought the unorthodox findings in [130] to a wider readership. Our conjecture that detection of 'where' is preattentive whereas identification of 'what' is attentive requires further research, since there are coarse where and fine where (and coarse what and fine what). Jochen Braun and I have been investigating these problems in recent years.

135. Julesz, B. Computational vision, a link between psychology and robotics *Contemporary Psychology* 31 (11): 872–874 (1986). In this review and critique of Grimson's 1981 monograph on AI models of stereopsis, I elaborate on the noncooperative model of Marr and Poggio.

136. Sagi, D., and Julesz, B. Enhanced detection in the aperture of focal attention during simple discrimination tasks. *Nature* 321: 693–695 (1986). A suggestive paper that measures the aperture of focal attention by showing that attending to a target is not passive but lights up its neighborhood. The only problem with our paradigm is that by its very nature the observer cannot keep his criterion constant. I would like to see someone improve on our technique and find ways to measure the enhancement of detecting a test spot in the attentional aperture by ensuring that observer's detection criteria remain constant.

137. Julesz, B. Preattentive human vision: Link between neurophysiology and psychophysics. In *Handbook of Physiology, Neurophysiology Section 5, Higher Functions of the Nervous System,* ed. F. Plum (American Physiological Society, 1986). A discussion of my views on linking monkey neurophysiology with human psychophysics of early vision.

138. Sagi, D., and Julesz, B. Short-range limitation on detection of feature differences. *Spatial Vision* 2: 39–49 (1987). In what may be my most significant paper with Dov Sagi, we show that textures are formed only when the distance between elements is less than a critical value, about twice the average element size. Thus, with increased target number, as long the elements are less dense than this critical distance, search time increases monotonically; however, above a critical density texton gradients are formed and search becomes effortless.

139. Julesz, B. Stereoscopic vision, *Vision Research* 26 (9): 1601–1612 (1986). A sequel to *FCP* in which I give a historical account of the discovery of the RDS, review research on global stereopsis since 1971, correct three inaccuracies, and pay tribute to my friend Gian Poggio, who found the first cyclopean neurons that are triggerred by a dynamic RDS in such early stages as layer IVB of V1 (the striate cortex) in the behaving monkey.

140. Julesz, B. Texton gradients: The texton theory revisited, *Biological Cybernetics* 54: 245–251 (1986). This is one of the last papers on the state of the texton theory before I revised it with the help of Doug Williams. However, I emphasize here the importance of both the textons in the texture elements and the textons that are created between the spaces of texture elements. (Later, for didactic reasons, we named the latter *anti-textons*.)

141. Schiavone, J. A., Papathomas, T. V., Julesz, B., Kreitzberg, C. W., and Perkey, D. J. Anaglyphic stereo animation of meteorological fields. In Proceedings of the International Conference on Interactive Information Processing Systems for Meteorology, Oceanography, and Hydrology, 1986. In this extension of cyclopean techniques from three to four dimensions, we portray large databases as 2-D planes stacked above one another. An observer can shift the positions of these planes so that correlated events at different times can coincide, thus making this correlation effortlessly apparent.

142. Papathomas, T. V., and Julesz, B. A spatiotemporal stereo paradox. *Supplement to Investigative Ophthalmology and Visual Science* 28 (3): 294 (1987). This ARVO abstract reports a successful attempt to extend Roger Shepard's ever-increasing auditory staircase to stereoscopic vision.

143. Papathomas, T. V., and Julesz, B. Animation with fractals from variations on the Mandelbrot set. *Visual Computer* 3: 23–26 (1987). We conjectured from computer-generated animation that when the Mandelbrot set is raised to the Nth power and $N \to \infty$ the result converges to an open circle. This conjecture was later proved mathematically (Devancy, Goldberg, and Hubbard 1986).

144. Papathomas, T. V., Schiavone, J. A., and Julesz, B. Stereo animation for very large data bases: Case study—meteorology. *IEEE Computer Graphics and Applications* 7 (9): 18–27 (1987). A sequel to [141].

145. Papathomas, T. V., Schiavone, J. A., and Julesz, B. Applications of computer graphics to the visualization of meterological phenomena, *Computer Graphics* 22 (4): 327–334 (1988). A further sequel to [141].

145A. Julesz, B. (1987) Vision: The early warning system. In *The Oxford Companion to the Mind*, ed. R. Gregory (Oxford University Press, 1987). A brief encyclopedia chapter on the texton theory of preattentive vision.

146. Julesz, B., and Kröse, B. Features and spatial filters. *Nature* 333: 302–303 (1988). A "News and Views" article that accompanied—and convincing countered— two papers in which it was claimed that a properly selected stage in a linear Laplacean pyramid followed by a nonlinearity could segment textures.

147. Papathomas, T. V., and Julesz, B. Stereoscopic illusion based on the proximity principle. *Perception*

18 (5): 589–594 (1989). A detailed description of [142].

148. Papathomas, T. V., and Julesz, B. The application of depth separation to the display of multivariable phenomena. In *Dynamic Graphics for Statistics,* ed. W. Cleveland and M. McGill (Wadsworth, 1988). Here ideas discussed in [141] are applied to multivariate functions.

149. Papathomas, T. V., Julesz, B., and Chodrow, S. E. True 3D animation for displaying VLSI modeling data. *IEEE Computer Graphics and Applications* 8 (1): 6–9 (1988). An application of the methods described in [141] and [148] to the display of voltage and current flow in VLSI models.

150. Farell, B., and Julesz, B. Perception of static directional flow fields. *Perception* 18 (2): 155–172 (1989). A report of the discovery of static "school of fish" detectors sensitive to arrow-like targets pointing in a similar direction.

151. Papathomas, T. V., Gorea, A., Julesz, B., and Chang, J. J. The relative strength of depth and orientation in motion perception. *Investigative Ophthalmology and Visual Science* 29 (3): 401 (1988). The first participation in this interesting paradigm by Andrei Gorea and Thomas Papathomas.

152. Papathomas, T. V., and Julesz, B. Lie differential operators in animal and machine vision. In *From the Pixels to the Features: Proceedings of the COST 13 Conference,* ed. J. Simon (North-Holland, 1988). Invited chapter. The research reported here was the outcome of a benchmark test of the Connection Machine. We placed in each of the 64,000 parallel computers the Lie germs of the

affine transformation group, and we obtained a mathematical description of a device that would detect only targets that moved, say, ballistically. While I do not believe W. Hoffman's claim that human perception can be modeled by Lie groups, I do agree with him that it can be a powerful tool in machine vision.

153. Julesz, B. Global stereopsis. In *Strabismus and Amplyopia,* ed. G. Lennerstrand, G. von Noorden, and E. Campos (Macmillan, 1988). A summary of my efforts with my co-workers to diagnose stereo blindness in early infancy, and an attempt to draw the attention of ophthalmologists to our ideas.

154. Julesz, B., and Papathomas, T. V. Asymmetries in binocular motion perception from disparity and rivalry differences. *Investigative Ophthalmology and Visual Sciences* 29 (3): 266 (1988). An abstract on experiments with stereoscopic motion and how binocular disparity and rivalry affect it.

155. Julesz, B. Texture perception. In *Encyclopedia of Neuroscience,* ed. G. Adelman (Birkhauser, 1987).

The Years at the Rutgers Laboratory of Vision Research and Caltech

156. Julesz, B. AI and Early Vision—Part I. In *AI and the Eye,* ed. A. Blake and T. Troscianko (Wiley, 1990). A review of my research in stereopsis, motion, and texture perception.

157. Julesz, B. AI and Early Vision—Part II. In *Proceedings of the SPIE/SPSE Symposium on Electronic Imaging, Conference on Human Vision, Visual Processing and Digital Display,* ed. B. Rogowitz (SPIE, 1989). A sequel to [156] for an audience

composed mainly of engineers and experts on machine vision and visual displays.

158. Kröse, B. J. A., and Julesz, B. The control and speed of shifts of attention. *Vision Research* 29 (11): 1607–1619 (1989). An article disproving the zoom-light theory of focal attention and arguing for a mixed parallel and serial search strategy.

159. Schiavone, J. A., Papathomas, T. V. and Julesz, B. Visualization of meteorological data: a review of computer graphics applications. Presented at Fifth International Conference on Interactive Information and Processing Systems for Meteorology, Oceanography and Hydrology, Anaheim, 1989. A sequel to [141].

160. Papathomas, T. V., Gorea, A., and Julesz, B. The strength of color and luminance in eliciting motion perception. *Investigative Ophthalmology and Visual Science* 30 (3): 388 (1989). An ARVO abstract on the use of the Gorea-Papathomas paradigm.

161. Gorea, A., Papathomas, T. V., and Julesz, B. Color against luminance in motion perception. Presented at European Conference on Visual Perception, 1989; also in *Perception* 18: 536 (1989). An ECVP abstract on research similar to [160].

162. Papathomas, T. V., Gorea, A., and Julesz, B. Color does resolve ambiguities in apparent motion perception. AT&T Bell Laboratories Technical Memorandum 11223–890306-01TM (1989). A report on work mentioned in [160] and [161].

163. Van Essen, D. C., DeYoe, E. A., Olavarria, J. F., Knierim, J. J., Fox, J. M., Sagi, D., and Julesz, B. Neural responses to static and moving texture patterns in visual cortex of the macaque monkey. In *Neural Mechanisms of Visual Perception*, ed. D. Lam and C. Gilbert (Portfolio, 1990). An article linking the texton theory of human texture discrimination to corresponding neural analyzers in V1 and V2 in the monkey cortex. We found units that had classical elongated receptive fields to a single line segment, but when surrounded by an array of parallel line segments their responses were inhibited, while an orthogonal family of lines inhibited them much less.

164. Julesz, B. Concepts in early vision. In *International Symposium on Synergetics of Cognition*, ed. H. Haken and M. Stadler (Springer, 1990). A summary of my work aimed at physicists interested in lasers and complex synergistic systems.

165. Gorea, A., and Julesz, B. Context superiority in a detection task with line-element stimuli: a low-level effect. *Perception* 19: 5–16, (1990). We showed subjects simple faces, composed of line segments, embedded in random line segments, and found that texture (orientation) gradients were better detected in faces than elsewhere, even though observers were not aware of the faces. The effect was weak but statistically significant, and it raises questions about the roles of some top-down processes in early vision.

166. Papathomas, T. V., Gorea, A., and Julesz, B. Juxtaposition of orientation, luminance and polarity in perceptual grouping. *Investigative Ophthalmology and Visual Science* 31: 105 (1990). An extension of [162] in which we juxtapose luminance, color, and orientation in order to establish a hierarchy of strengths for perceptual grouping.

167. Chang, J. J., and Julesz, B. Low-level processing of disparity-tuned binocular neurons takes

precedence of shape from shading. *Investigative Ophthalmology and Visual Science* 31 (4): 525 (1990). An ARVO abstract in which we report that monocular shape-from-shading effects (e.g. convex or concave spheres) can be dominated by stereopsis if about 20% of the sphere's texture is an RDS.

168. Julesz, B. Early vision is bottom-up, except for focal attention. *Cold Spring Harbor Symposia on Quantitative Biology—The Brain* 55: 973–978 (1990). A brief outline of my work on stereopsis, motion, and texture perception with random noise stimuli, which I named *early vision*. For didactic reasons I include one top-down process in my studies: focal attention.

169. Julesz, B. Consciousness and focal attention: Answer to John Searle. *Behavioral and Brain Sciences*. 16 (1): 191–193. (1993).

170. Julesz, B. Early vision and focal attention, *Reviews of Modern Physics* 63 (3): 735–772, (1991). A major invited article directed at physicists, and the backbone of my coming monograph *The Enjoyment of Vision by Eye and Intellect* .

171. Julesz, B. Some strategic questions in visual perception. In *Representations of Vision: Trends and Tacit Assumptions in Vision Research,* ed. A. Gorea (Cambridge University Press, 1991). An article presenting my views on solved, unsolved, and metascientific problems of vision.

172. Williams, D., and Julesz, B. Filters vs. textons in human and machine texture discrimination. In *Neural Networks for Perception, Vol. 1—Human and Machine Perception,* ed. H. Wechsler (Academic Press, 1991). A work discounting some earlier attempts to explain the asymmetry effect on the basis of increased noise. Instead, we solve the asymmetry problem of texture discrimination by experimentally demonstrating that physical gaps are perceptually closed by subjective contours. We also extend the texton theory by formally introducing the concept of antitextons.

173. Saarinen, J., and Julesz, B. The speed of attentional shifts in the visual field. *Proceedings of the National Academy of Sciences* 88: 1812–1814, (1991). A paper in which we succeeded for the first time in showing shifts of attention speeds of over 30 msec/item. The items were presented in random positions at 30-msec steps and at a distance from each other (to avoid lateral inhibition) and masked immediately. Observers were able to report up to four items with orders of magnitude better than chance; however, the sequential order of the items was often incorrect. These focal attention shifts measured with our masking techniques are in agreement with search speeds reported in the cognitive literature (usually based on RT techniques). See [202].

174. Julesz, B. Early vision, focal attention, and neural nets. In *Neural Networks: Theory and Applications* (Academic Press, 1991). A summary of my work for AI experts and engineers. I stress that, because focal attention is crucial in search tasks, attempts to exploit the scanning behavior of eye movements during inspection tasks are doomed to failure.

175. Papathomas, T. V., Gorea, A., and Julesz, B. Two carriers for motion perception: color and luminance. *Vision Research* 31 (11): 1883–1892 (1991). A review article that establishes the roles of color and luminance in motion perception.

176. Williams, D. W., and Julesz, B. Perceptual asymmetry in texture perception. *Proceedings of the National Academy of Sciences* 89: 6531–6534 (1992). A succinct review of our efforts to solve the asymmetry problem. In addition to elucidating the role of subjective contours in closing gaps, we disprove earlier attributions of the asymmetry effect to Weber's Law.

177. Hadani, I., Ishai, G., and Julesz, B. The autokinetic movement and visual stability. *Investigative Ophthalmology and Visual Science* 32 (4): 900, Proceedings of ARVO Meeting, April 1991. An ARVO abstract applying theoretical work by Hadani and Ishai to autokinetic phenomena.

178. Williams, D., and Julesz, B. Fill-in between texture elements is critical for texture segregation. *Investigative Ophthalmology and Visual Science* 32 (4): 1038, Proceedings of ARVO Meeting, April 1991. An ARVO abstract summarizing the work published in [176].

179. Papathomas, T., Gorea, A., and Julesz, B. Link between textural grouping and visual search for the conjunction of color and orientation. *Investigative Ophthalmology and Visual Science* 32 (4): 1039. An ARVO abstract summarizing some of the work published in [175].

180. Prasad, K. V., and Julesz, B. Neural time-constants involved in compensating for the chromatic aberration of the human eye. *Investigative Ophthalmology and Visual Science* 32 (4): 1273. An ARVO abstract of some work in which we attacked the still-unsolved problem of why the 2-diopter accommodation error between red and blue (due to the chromatic aberration of the eye lens) results in equally sharp perception of both colors.

181. Hadani, I., and Julesz, B. Interpupillary distance and stereoscopic depth perception. *Investigative Ophthalmology and Visual Science* 33 (4): 707. Proceedings of ARVO Meeting, May 1992. Discussed in dialogue 12.

182. Julesz, B., and Kovacs, I. Stereopsis is not colorblind (except for green). *Investigative Ophthalmology and Visual Science* 33 (4): 1332. Proceedings of ARVO Meeting, May 1992. See [184].

183. Julesz, B. Some recent findings in early vision and focal attention. In *Spatial Vision in Humans and Robots,* ed. L. Harris and M. Jenkin (Cambridge University Press, 1993). A precursor of dialogue 12.

184. Kovacs, I., and Julesz, B. Depth, motion and static flow perception at metaisoluminant color contrast. *Proceedings of the National Academy of Sciences* 89: 10390–10394 (1992). Polarity-reversed RDSs and RDCs cannot be fused or yield reversed-phi motion. However, if corresponding dots have the same color, then stereopsis is restored and reversed-phi becomes real-phi motion. Thus, the stereopsis and motion systems are not color blind, although the perceived dots in depth or motion do not form a solid surface.

185. Hadani, I., and Julesz, B. Perceptual constancy and the mind's eye looking through a telescope. (in progress)

186. Braun, J., and Julesz, B. Early Vision: Dichotomous or Continuous? Psychonomic Soc. Meeting, St. Louis, November 11, 1992 . Preliminary talk and abstract.

187. Julesz, B. (1993) Illusory contours in early vision and beyond. *Giornale Italiano di Psicologia*

20 (5): 869–877. A historical survey of subjective contours.

188. Kovacs, I., and Julesz, B. (1993) A closed curve is much more than an incomplete one: Effect of closure in figure-ground segmentation. *Proceedings of the National Academy of Sciences* 90: 7495–7497. Though it is too early to judge, results seem to imply a field theory of visual perception. Closed segments of a curve are better seen among a clutter of line segments than an open curve. The inside of the closed curve has patches of varying visibility according to a field theory.

189. Kovacs, I., and Julesz, B. A closed curve is much more than an incomplete one: Effect of closure in completion of segmented contours. *Investigative Ophthalmology and Visual Science* 34 (4): 1084. Proceedings of ARVO Meeting, May 1993. A precursor to [187].

190. Ramanujan, K. S., Papathomas, T. V., Gorea, A., and Julesz, B. Similarities between motion perception and texture grouping. *Investigative Ophthalmology and Visual Science* 34 (4): 1237. Proceedings of ARVO meeting, May 1993.

191. Chang, J. J., Anderson, B. L., and Julesz, B. Panum's limiting case exhibits greatest stability and clearest depth when consistent with the geometry of occlusion. *Investigative Ophthalmology and Visual Science* 34 (4): 1438. Proceedings of ARVO Meeting, May 1993.

192. Julesz, B. *Dialogues on Perception* (MIT Press, 1995).

193. Kovacs, I., and Julesz, B. Closed contours facilitate the detection of interior targets. *Perception* 22 suppl.: 4. Summary of [189].

194. Hadani, I., and Julesz, B. (1994) Computational aspects of motion perception during self-motion. *Behavioral and Brain Sciences* 17: 293–355. Peer commentary on Alexander H. Wertheim's "Motion perception during self-motion."

195. Julesz, B. Subjective contours in early vision and beyond. Presented at Partitioning Data Sets: With Applications to Psychology, Vision and Target Tracking, DIMACS Workshop April 1993, Rutgers University, Piscataway, N.J. Similar to [187], but with some added comments for engineers.

196. Julesz, B., and Anderson, B. L. Motion hysteresis, cooperativity, and neurontrophy. *Investigative Ophthalmology and Visual Science* 35 (4): 1389. Proceedings of ARVO meeting, May 1994. A paper by Williams et al. is revisited, and we show that their findings do not support the persistency of ordered motion, but belong to the neurontropy kind. Thus more ordered motion when briefly inserted in a stream of less ordered motion takes more time to perceive than vice versa.

197. Anderson, B. L., and Julesz, B. Motion parallax and subjective occluding contours. *Investigative Ophthalmology and Visual Science* 35 (4): 2162. Proceedings of ARVO meeting, May 1994. An interesting demonstration of how a moving pattern can yield a subjective contour, based on occlusion.

198. Kovacs, I., and Julesz, B. Maps of global sensitivity change inside closed boundaries. *Investigative Ophthalmology and Visual Science* 35 (4): 1627. Proceedings of ARVO meeting, May 1994. A brief precursor to [199], but containing the sensitivity maps for circular and elliptical curves.

199. Kovacs, I., and Julesz, B. (1994) Perceptual sensitivity maps within globally defined visual shapes. *Nature* 370: 644–646. Discussed throughout *Dialogues*, particularly in dialogue 14.

200. Papathomas, T. V., Kovacs, I., Gorea, A., and Julesz, B. A unified approach to the perception of motion, stereo, and static flow patterns. A didactic paper on establishing perceptual hierarchy between many visual attributes.

201. Julesz, B. Some afterthoughts. In *Early Vision and Beyond*, ed. T. V. Papathomas, C. Chubb, A. Gorea, and E. Kowler (MIT Press, 1995). Here I summarize my recent work and thank the participants and contributors who came to the conference to celebrate my 65th birthday.

202. Hung, G. K., Wilder, J., Curry, R., and Julesz, B. Simultaneous better than sequential for brief presentations. Here we repeat the Saarinen-Julesz (1991) experiment, but with two important differences: the speed is increased from 32 to 16 msec per frame and the display is both sequentially and simultaneously shown. Simultaneous presentation is superior to sequential, particularly with increasing rates. We interpret these findings as suggesting that the bottleneck for information transmission is not the short-term memory but occurs at the input stage of the memory buffer. These implications are discussed in detail in several dialogues.

Patents and Technical Memoranda

1A. Interpolation Between Extremals of Television Signals. I am particularly fond of this paper, since it established my reputation at Bell Labs. I gave the first version to my department head, Bob Graham, an exquisite speaker of the English language, who glanced at it and promised to read it but never mentioned it afterwards. Then a capital idea struck me. I asked a dear friend, the late Leon Harmon, to correct the manuscript and translate it into correct English, but to ignore its scientific content. When I gave the revised manuscript to Bob Graham, he glanced at it, then sat down and read it on the spot. Then he turned to me and asked whether it was the same manuscript I had given him before, and who had written it. I told him that it was the same paper with the English corrected by Leon. He looked me in the eyes, perhaps for the first time, and later that day he assigned me my first technical assistant. So, it was this brief paper that established me as a genuine member of the technical staff, a year before I began working with random-dot stereograms. See also [4].

2A. Supplement to the Technical Memorandum: Interpolation Between Extremals of Television Signals, MM-57–134–50, December 1, 1957. An extension of [1A] with detailed circuit designs for patent consideration and with with some comments on how one-dimensional interpolation schemes between extrema could be implemented by a soap-bubble-type analog device to process the information in real time, years before computers could achieve similar feats.

3A. IDENTRACKING—A Detection Procedure in Which the Identity of Outlined Moving Objects is Continuously Preserved. Bell Labs memo MM-58–134–18, July 1, 1958. This is my first important paper. The basic idea of establishing the identity of a wire object is the insight that this can be accomplished without semantics (silhouettes are already too complex). This paper heralds my later interest in problems of vision in which the enigmatic processes of semantics and long-term memory are not necessary.

4A. Automatic Reconstruction of 3-Dimensional Images From 2-Dimensional Projections. Bell Labs memo MM-58–134–32, October 15, 1958. A precursor of my AUTOMAP-1 model, prior to the invention of the RDS. It worked only for polyhedra.

5A. Automatic Depth Evaluation From Stereo Plane Projections, MM-59–123–7, January 30, 1959. A sequel to [3A] written around the time the idea of the RDS was first implemented.

6A. Some Recent Studies in Vision Relevant to Form Perception. Invited paper delivered at Symposium on Models for the Perception of Speech and Visual Form, Boston, November 1964. Bell Labs memo MM-65–1223–1, January 12, 1965. See [28] above.

7A. The PARCEPTRON: An Optical Voice Recognition Device. Bell Labs memo MM-64–135–1, 1222–12, 2813–30, December 8, 1964. A joint patent with Chape Cuttler and Keith Pennington on combining acoustic and coherent optics ideas to achieve speaker-dependent voice recognition. Optical fibers of random lengths were made to mechanically resonate to the speaker's voice, and a hologram was made of the light emitting from the end of these fibers. The holograms could store thousands of utterances.

8A. Equidistributed Information Mapping, An Analogy to Holograms and Memory (co-author: K. Pennington). A first draft of our ideas on coherent holograms, animal memories, and equidistributed information storage, published later as [16]. This is regarded by many as the first realization that holograms might be related to memories in animals.

Patents

B. Julesz. 2,974,195. Economy in TV Transmission. Dated March 7, 1961. See [1A].

C. C. Cutler, B. Julesz, and K. S. Pennington. 3,543,237. Pattern Recognition Apparatus and Method. Dated November 24, 1970. See [7A].

B. Julesz, B. T. Kerns, and M. E. Terry. 4,023,911. Stereopsis Test Patterns for Adjustment of Stereomicroscopes in the Inspection of 3-D Objects. Dated May 17, 1977. See [76].

B. Julesz. 4,032,237. Stereoscopic Technique for Detecting Defects in Periodic Structures. Dated June 28, 1977. See [76].

GLOSSARY

Note: Starred items are adapted, with permission, from the glossary of P. S. Churchland and T. J. Sejnowski's book *The Computational Brain* (1992). The reader might also consult R. Gregory's *Oxford Companion to the Mind* (1987).

*accuracy** The minimum distance that can be perceived between the centers of two stimuli presented in nonoverlapping regions of a sensory space. Also termed *acuity* or *hyperacuity*. Not to be confused with resolution.

*acetylcholine** A chemical in the nervous system that acts as a neurotransmitter when binding to nicotinic receptors and as a neuromodulator when binding to muscarinic receptors.

adaptation paradigm** Habituation. It is assumed that if a sustained stimulation by a certain atribute (feature) causes the threshold for this atribute to increase, then some neurophysiological analyzer (detector) may exist that was fatigued by that feature.

*agnosia** An inability to recognize visual objects that is due to an inability to combine components of a visual image into a complete percept. Associated with damage to inferotemporal cortex. Agnosia can be very specific, as in the case of prosopagnosia.

amacrine cell** A retinal interneuron receiving input from bipolar cells and projecting to retinal ganglion cells, other amacrine cells, and bipolar cell axons. Amacrine cells do not have a conventional axon and do not fire action potentials.

*amnesia** Loss of all declarative memory for times before (retrograde) or after (anterograde) the amnesic episode. Associated with damage to temporal lobe or diencephalic structures such as the mammillary bodies and medial dorsal nucleus of the thalamus.

*amygdala** A collection of nuclei deep in the temporal lobe, reciprocally connected to the hypothalamus, the hippocampus, and the thalamus. A part of limbic system, it controls emotional behavior and associated autonomic responses.

anaglyph** A way of presenting stereo pairs so as to aid fusion. The left and rught images are printed in red and green, respectively, so that red-green goggles help to separate the information to the corresponding eyes.

*antagonist** A chemical that binds to the receptor of a particular neurotransmitterr and prevents the neurotransmitter from activating the receptor.

*apparent motion** The percept of motion from a stimulus of two discrete images that are spatially separated and alternately turned on and off. Wertheimer's original demonstration of apparent motion was created by alternately shining lights behind two slits, one vertical and the other slightly rotated about 30° from vertical. When the interval between the two slits was of the right duration (aproximately 60 msec), observers reported experiencing the flashing bars as a single bar moving between the two positions.

architecture** The structure of a neural network, generally referring to the numbers and types of processing units and their internal organization (such as layers and connections between layers).

*association cortex** Areas of neocortex not involved in the processing of primary sensory and motor information. These areas combine sensory information from several modalities and produce motor plans. Once thought to form most of the neocortex in primates, it is now believed to be a relatively small fraction.

autocorrelation** A mathematical operation in which a function is multiplied by itself but at a shifted input and then summed (integrated) over all values. In case of a stochastic function it is defined as $\Sigma xy\, p(x,y)$, where $p(x,y)$ is the second-order (dipole) statistics. For black-and-white images the dipole statistics is the autocorrelation function. The Wiener-Khinshin Theorem states that the Fourier transform of the autocorrealtion is the power spectrum.

*autonomic nervous system** The division of the nervous system innervating (efferent only) the viscera, skin, smooth muscle, and glands. Divided into the sympathetic and parasympathetic systems.

axon The principal output process of a neuron. Often branched, sometimes myelinated, it conducts action potentials from the soma to the presynaptic terminal, where the action potential is transformed into a chemical signal. Can carry information a long distance.

axon hillock Initial segment. Beginning of axon process coming from the soma. Contains a high density of sodium channels, and thus is the site for action potential initiation.

backpropagation A learning algorithm for adjusting weights in neural networks. The error for each unit (desired minus actual output) is calculated at the output of the network and recursively propagated backward into the network. This makes it possible to decide how to change the weights inside the network to improve its overall performance (the credit-assignment problem).

basal forebrain The structures (including the septum, the nucleus basalis, and the diagonal band of Broca) that send cholinergic and GABAergic fibers to the forebrain. Probably important in memory and arousal systems.

basal ganglia Forebrain nuclei, including the caudate nucleus and putamen (these two make up the neostriatum), the globus pallidus, the substantia nigra, and the subthalamic nuclei. Lesion data indicate that this system is involved in the generation of voluntary movement.

binocular rivalry Periods of dominance and suppression of one eye's view relative to the other eye's view when discordant images (such as vertical and horizontal stripes) are presented one to each eye and are perceived as alternating with a period of about l sec.

bipolar cell A retinal interneuron connecting a photoreceptor to a retinal ganglion cell. Bipolar cells are divided into on-center and off-center cells (depolarized and hyperpolarized, respectively) by light activation of photoreceptors.

blind spot The region in which the retinal axons and blood vessels exit the eye. No photoreceptors are present.

brain stem The base of the brain, made up of the medulla, the pons, and the midbrain. It contains many motor and sensory nuclei (including taste and hearing) and many fiber tracts going both rostrally to the rest of the brain and caudally to the spinal cord.

calcium A divalent cation maintained at a low concentration inside neurons and most cells. Used for intracellular signaling, such as release of transmitter from presynaptic terminals and induction of long-term potentiation. May be the most important ion in the universe.

catastrophe theory A theory in differential topology, founded mainly by René Thom, according to which in four dimensions (three spatial and one temporal) only seven kinds of discontinuities can exist. These discontinuities, called *elementary catastrophes,* are known as fold, cusp, swallowtail, butterfly, hyperbolic umbilic, elliptic umbilic (hair), and parabolic umbilic.

caudal Toward the tail end of an organism.

cell death A process, occurring naturally during development, whereby up to 75% of initial cells in a structure die. The cells that survive tend to be those that were most active, or were well connected, during their critical period. In some creatures, such as the nematode, neurons are genetically programmed to die.

cellular automata A parallel computer (invented by John von Neumann) composed of a two-dimensional lattice of cells, each of which performs a computation based on its own input and the output of its neighboring cells.

center surround A contrast-sensitive receptive field displayed by retinal ganglion cells and lateral geniculate nucleus cells and consisting of a circular center that generates an excitatory (on- center) or an inhibitory (off-center) response to a light stimulus, surrounded by an annulus of the opposite polarity.

cerebellum A structure posterior to the pons on the brain stem consisting of cortex and deep nuclei. Has a role in the high-level control of motor activity. Lesions lead to characteristic motor deficits.

chaos A term now applied to dynamical systems exhibiting highly intricate behavior (typically generating fractal state spaces) which may be understood as the operation of a deterministic system of equations.

*chaotic behavior A pattern of activity that appears random (i.e, .cannot be predicted) and is very sensitive to the initial conditions of the system generating the activity. Occurs in some nonlinear networks that feed back activity to their own input units.

*closed loop A neural circuit operating with negative feedback. Important in homeostatic systems and motor systems, such as eye tracking. Feedback circuits are able to maintain a stable operating point.

*coarse coding A term describing the selectivity to stimuli of units mediating a distributed representation. Coarse coding means that the response selectivities of units overlap, because the units have broad tuning curves. This allows phenomenon such as hyperacuity.

*color constancy A phenomenon by which objects appear to be the same color despite wide changes in the spectral composition of the ambient lighting.

*commissure Fibers joining functionally similar areas from each half of the brain across the midline. The corpus callosum, a central commissure, is the largest fiber tract in the brain.

*complex cell A neuron of visual cortex displaying nonlinear response properties. Receptive fields are large and oriented, but the position of the stimulus within the receptive field is not critical. Many complex cells are sensitive to motion.

*computer A physical system computing some function where the inputs and outputs are taken to represent the states of some other system by an external observer. This definition includes the digital electronic computer but also covers slide rules and tic-tac-toe machines.

*cone A photoreceptor in the retina made up of three classes with peak wavelength sensitivities at about 430, 530, and 560 nm, termed blue (short-wavelength), green (middle-wavelength), and red (long-wavelength) systems, respectively. Found at high density in the fovea. Responsible for color vision at high light levels (scotopic vision).

congruency A geometric concept: coinciding exactly when superimposed.

conjugacy An equivalence relation between a difficult or unexplored task (operation) and a familiar one whose solution is already known.

*connectionism The term (introduced by Jerome Feldman) for a style of computation that emphasizes the pattern of the connections in a network of neuronlike elements. Usually uses semi-linear activation functions connected by variable strength weights, but includes more complex units such as higher-order units and radial-basis function units.

*content-addressable memory Representations that are accessed not by presenting some filing system reference number but by presenting a partial or distorted form of the representation itself. The output is then the completed representation (pattern/vector completion). This task can be performed by a type of associative network with as many output units as input units.

cooperativity In physics, cooperativity refers to states in which some set of elements (e.g., atoms or molecules) interact so as to form coherent, macroscopic structures. The term originated in the chemistry of ligands. The interaction is between neighboring elements (excluding far interactions) and is assumed to be nonlinear (excitation or inhibition).

*corpus callosum The largest fiber bundle in the brain. Consists of cortico-cortical axons crossing the midline and integrating the functions of the two cerebral hemispheres. Also allows neurons in the two hemispheres to synchronize their activity.

correspondence problem The problem, in stereopsis, of knowing which features in one eye's image to match with which features in the other eye's image. Can be solved by the human visual system even for stimuli made up of identical, randomly positioned dots. Also know as the *false-target elimination* problem.

cortical column A description of the organization of the visual cortex into columns of cells that prefer oriented stimuli (first described by Mountcastle in 1975 in the motor cortex, and in visual cortex by Hubel and Wiesel in 1960). For instance, a single column represents a given visual direction. As one moves upward or downward in the column, the preferred orientation of the cell shifts to a slightly rotated variant of the neighboring orientations, and the column as a whole spans the entire range of orientations. See also *ocular dominance columns.*

*critical period The phase of development during which the components of a brain area are organized, often under the influence of sensory experience (e.g., into ocular dominance columns). If this organization is prevented (e.g., by sensory deprivation) during the critical period, it will occur with difficulty or not at all later in life. Also called the maturational window.

*declarative memory Memory for explicit experiences and facts, directly accessible to conscious recollection. This type of memory is lost in amnesia.

*dendrite The input process of a neuron, upon which synapses are made. Consists of a number of branching, tapering cables extending from the soma. Conduction of current from the synapse to the soma is often assumed to be passive, though voltage-dependent conductances are known to exist on dendrites in some neurons.

2-deoxyglucose (2-DG) An analogue of glucose that is taken up by active cells but not metabolized.

*depolarize To make the internal surface of a neuronal membrane more positive with respect to the external surface, usually by the entry into the cell of positively charged ions (sodium and calcium).

*dichromat A person missing one of the three cone systems, usually red or green. Dichromats lack a whole dimension of color vision.

Dirac function A mathematical function of infinetisimal width whose integral yields a finite (energy) value.

disorder-order transition The transformation of a system from a state characterized by a relatively high degree of disorder (or entropy) to a state that is more structured (i.e., has a lower entropy).

*disparity A mismatch in the relative spatial location of images of the same object on the retinae of the two eyes, due to the spatial separation of the eyes. Cells in visual cortex tuned to specific retinal disparities relative to the plane of fixation are thought to mediate stereopsis.

*distributed representation Representation of information as activity across a large number of units. This allows generalization to occur because of overlapping patterns of activity for related items and makes the information resistant to damage. Also known as *vector coding.*

*dopamine Catecholamine neuromodulator. Dopaminergic neurons are found in the midbrain. Loss and malfunction of dopaminergic neurons are implicated in Parkinson's disease and schizophrenia, respectively.

*dorsal Toward the back of an organism.

*efference copy A signal from a motor axon collateral to an earlier point in the circuit controlling motor behavior. Allows a network direct access to its own output.

eidetic memory Photographic memory.

élan vital A mysterious "life force" often referred to by the philosopher Henri-Louis Bergson in the era before the code of life was broken by molecular biologists.

*end stopping A property of hypercomplex cells and special simple cells in visual cortex whereby the response to an appropriately oriented bar decreases if the bar extends out of the excitatory part of the receptive field into an inhibitory zone. This property makes hypercomplex cells good candidates for representing curvature.

*energy landscape Activation space or weight space of a network with an extra dimension ("height") representing the energy of the whole network. For a network relaxing to the solution of an optimization problem, the minimum energy level (global energy minimum) represents the optimal solution to the problem. For other networks, the energy landscape can be thought of as an error surface, with the global minimum representing least error.

*energy minimum The state a system is in if changing the activity of any unit results in an increase in energy of the system. A local energy minimum is an attractor because all the states around the minimum in the energy landscape will converge to the minimum upon relaxation. A global energy minimum is the lowest possible energy state of the system. For optimization networks, such as Hopfield networks or Boltzmann machines, the global energy minimum is the optimal solution to the constraint-satisfaction problem the network is configured to solve.

*episodic memory The division of declarative memory concerned with past events in a person's life. This system has a temporal structure—each event is stored in association with some particular time, as in an autobiography.

esotropia Cross-eyedness (strabismus) in which the eyes deviate nasalward.

*exclusive or (XOR) A binary function taking two inputs, each of which can be 1 or 0, and producing an output of 0 if neither or both of the inputs are 1, and 1 if only one of the inputs is 1.

exotropia Cross-eyedness (strabismus) in which the eyes deviate temporalward.

*extrastriate visual cortex A large region of visual cortex outside of the primary visual cortex, area V1. Has more than 24 subdivisions, including V2, a belt of cortex around V1 that receives input from V1; V3, an area that receives input from V2 and projects in separate pathways to V4 and MT; V4, a visual area at the junction of temporal, occipital, and parietal cortices where neurons are responsive to the wavelengths and orientations of stimuli; MT, in the medial temporal region (also called area V5), which has neurons with receptive fields that are large and characterized by motion selectivity; and MST, a visual area in the medial superior temporal lobe where cells respond preferentially to rotation and expansion or contraction of images.

fatigue Adaptation; habituation.

*feature detector A unit in a network that responds to a particular systemacity in its input, such as an edge (continuous boundary). Unsupervised nets can structure themselves via weight changes to represent these features without an external teacher.

*finite-state automata Devices taking sequences of input vectors and producing sequences of output vectors. Their state transitions may depend on an internal, finite memory. They can be modeled by recurrent networks.

four-color problem The classical problem, solved only recently with the help of computers, of how any map in the two-dimensional Euclidean plane can be colored by four colors without any neighboring state having the same color. (A simplified version of this problem, using five colors on the surface of a torus, can be solved with high school mathematics.)

*fovea The small central area of the retina containing the highest density of cone photoreceptors and thus providing high spatial resolution. Intervening neural layers are spread to the side to allow light maximum access to the photoreceptor.

*frontal lobe An area of neocortex involved in planning, movement, and speech.

Fourier transform A computational method for representing almost any function as a linear combination of sine and cosine functions. May be considered to be a method of decomposing a complex pattern into some set of elementary or base functions that allow various properties of the pattern to be quantified (such as the amount of energy present at a given frequency). The inverse transform can be used to reconstruct the orignal pattern by linearly combining (i.e., adding) the weighted basis functions.

fractals Geometric structures that may not be characterized with integer-dimensional representations. Intuitively, fractal forms are "rough," in contrast to the smooth (or differentiable) surfaces studied in the calculus. The underlying premise of the calculus is differentiation, which requires that, as you look more and more closely at a smooth function, it eventually becomes a straight line (the tangent to the curve). Fractal patterns do not become straight lines under magnification. Rather, more and more structure is revealed as a fractal is magnified. Self-similar fractals are those in which the magnified sections of a curve are strict copies of the larger scales; stochastic self-similarity requires only that the magnified sections of the curve be statistically similar to the coarser levels.

fusion The state of seeing a single world despite the fact that the two eyes views receive slightly disparate images.

*GABA A common inhibitory amino acid neurotransmitter in the brain, g-aminobutyric acid, that binds to GABA-A receptors, directly opening chloride-permeable ion channels, and to GABA-B receptors, opening potassium-permeable ion channels via a second-messenger system.

ganglion A discrete collection of nerve cells, often a nodular mass defined by connective tissue.

Garden of Eden configuration A term introduced by E. Moore, who showed that in a self-reproducing machines (automaton) there must exist a state that cannot reside in the machine.

gestalt Global organization that emerges from multiple interactions among features in an image.

*glial cells A variety of small cells thought not to generate active electrical signals as neurons do. They support neurons by buffering the extracellular fluid, scavenging debris, and providing physical structure and myelin.

*glutamate An excitatory amino acid neurotransmitter that causes the opening of ion channels permeable to sodium, potassium, and sometimes calcium. Principal excitatory transmitter in cortex.

Gödel-like problems Statements whose truth cannot be proven. Also called *undecidable propositions.*

*Golgi staining Impregnating a small, random sample of neurons in a piece of tissue with silver deposit. The stain spreads through the entire dendritic tree and fills some of the axon. The staining of axons is more complete in neonatal tissue, which is less myelinated.

*habituation Decrease in the behavioral response to a repeatedly presented stimulus. Shown to be due to a decrease in the synaptic efficacy between sensory and motor neurons in aplysia.

*hair cells Sensory cells located in the vestibular organ and the cochlea. When stereocilia (hairs) projecting from the cell are displaced by the movement of surrounding endolymph, the cell is depolarized or hyperpolarized, depending on the direction of displacement.

*hardwired A term describing neural connectivity, meaning that all connections are specified by the genes and thus are essentially fixed and unmodifiable.

*Hebbian synapse A synapse that changes its efficacy according to Hebb's rule: the strength increases when both presynaptic and postsynaptic elements are active. The synapse may decrease in strength if there is presynaptic activity without concurrent postsynaptic activation.

*hidden units Units in a neural network equivalent to biological interneurons, i.e., not input or output units.

*Hopfield network An associative network that relaxes to the solution of an optimization problem. Such a network can implement content-addressable memory.

horizontal cells Retinal interneurons receiving input from and providing feedback to photoreceptors. These cells do not fire action potentials; indeed, their axons may be electrically isolated from their somata. Some horizontal cells have electrical synaptic couplings between them.

horopter A curved surface wrapping around the visual field and defined as the set of points from which light falls on the same retinal location in the two eyes. Near the fovea these points are in the plane of fixation of the subject.

*hyperacuity Perceptual detection of intervals smaller than the resolving power of any single transducer. In visual perception, hyperacuity can be spatial, stereoscopic, or chromatic.

*hyperpolarize To make the internal surface of a neuronal membrane more negative with respect to the outside, usually by the exit from the cell of positively charged ions (potassium).

*hypothalamus A structure below the thalamus that regulates autonomic, endocrine, and visceral integration.

hysteresis A lag between the cause and the effect of a process (such as magnetization of a ferromagnetic substance).

*iconic memory Very brief (< 1 sec) memory of the preceding visual image, susceptible to masking by subsequent stimuli. May be due to a transient physical change in the sensory transduction system. Its auditory analogue is echoic memory.

*inferotemporal cortex Aa area in the anterior temporal lobe concerned with the visual recognition of objects. Neurons from this area are reported to respond specifically to complex objects, such as hands.

information theory Theory describing information as the negative entropy of a system. A powerful version created by Claude Shannon defines the channel capacity of a communication system. As long as the information rate is below this capacity, there exist codes that permit the error-free transmission of this information.

*invariance A phenomenon displayed by the visual system whereby the image of an object is recognized as the same object regardless of changes in size, rotation, and velocity. Also called size, rotation, or velocity constancy. Invariant recognition of objects reduces the amount of memory required to store the representations of the objects.

*just-noticeable difference The minimum difference between two stimuli that can be detected. It increases in proportion to the magnitude of the reference stimulus.

Kuffler units Simple receptive fields in the optic nerve of the cat, with a circular center area of excitation (inhibition) surrounded by an antagonistic annulus of inhibition(excitation).

Laplacian pyramid A multi-resolution representation of visual data. A Laplacian operation reduces the data to the locations where the second derivatives of the luminance distributions cross zero, giving a rough but imperfect representation of "edges" in a scene. The pyramid structure is generated by performing this operation on a number of blurred copies of the highest resolution image and retaining all such ouputs in an ordered pyramid that spans from coarse to fine.

*lateral Away from the midline, relative to a particular landmark. Each nucleus has a lateral portion, such as the lateral geniculate nucleus.

*lateral geniculate nucleus A nucleus of the thalamus that receives input from the retina and projects primarily to layer 4 of primary visual cortex. Often referred to as a relay nucleus, its function is largely unknown. It may have some role in visual attention, or more generally in regulating the flow of information into primary visual cortex.

*lateral inhibition A phenomenon, exhibited by many perceptual systems, that increases the signal strength (activity) of a unit at a point, relative to the background, by inhibiting surrounding units. This reduces the salience of constant fields and enhances the salience of borders and point sources.

law of superposition A test of the linearity of a system. If for inputs A and B the outputs are $f(A)$, and $f(B)$, respectively, then for a linear system the output for $A + B$ has to be $f(A + B)$.

Lie algebras and germs Infinetisimal transforms that can describe invariances, particularly under affine transformations such as translations, expansions, and rotations.

*ligand A substrate bound by a receptor, such as a neurotransmitter or a neuromodulator.

*limbic system A term designating C-shaped structures bordering the corpus callosum (including the cingulate gyrus, the orbitofrontal cortex, the hippocampus, and the amygdala) that are devoted to motivation, emotion, and memory. Strongly connected with the hypothalamus, these structures control the interaction between emotion and visceral function via the autonomic system.

*limit cycle The state that a system giving a periodic output (e.g. an oscillator) is in if it returns to producing the baseline output pattern after perturbation.

*linear function A function where the relationship between the elements of one domain and the elements of another (the range) can be described by a straight line. Thus, the output of a linear function to a combination of inputs is just the sum of the outputs to each input presented separately.

*linearly separable function A function in which the input space can be segregated with a straight line. A networks must have hidden units to solve nonlinearly separable functions. In high-dimensional spaces, the separating surface of a semi-linear unit is a hyperplane.

*locus coeruleus A nucleus in the brain stem filled with norepinephrine-containing cells projecting widely to almost the whole central nervous system. Has a vital role in controlling the stages of sleep and wakefulness.

*long-term depression A decrease in the efficacy of a synapse. Found in the cerebellum when the presynaptic parallel fiber input and a Purkinje cell are simultaneously stimulated. Found in the hippocampus when the presynaptic input is stimulated and the postsynaptic cell is hyperpolarized or the postsynaptic cell is depolarized without presynaptic activation. Also found in neocortex.

*long-term memory Long-lasting, potentially permanent store of information about past experiences. Thought to be due to physical, plastic changes in the structure of the brain.

*long-term potentiation Persistent increase in synaptic strength, lasting hours to days after a brief high-frequency stimulation of synaptic inputs. First described in the hippocampus, but found in many brain areas. May be a mechanism for storing long-term memories. Can be homosynaptic (change restricted to stimulated synapse) or heterosynaptic (other synapses on postsynaptic cell changed).

*lookup table A simple computational principle based on precalculating the answers to a problem and storing them in an organized way allowing speedy access.

*Mach bands A brightness illusion, occurring at a high-contrast edge, whereby a thin, very dark band appears on the dark side of the edge and a thin, very light band appears on the light side of the edge. Can be explained by the phenomenon of lateral inhibition.

*magnetic-resonance imaging (MRI) A method of mapping the spatial distribution of atomic nuclei, such as hydrogen and phosphorus, based on the precession of nuclear spin in a strong magnetic field. The fine structure in the frequency spectrum of the resonances can be used for studying the chemical environment of these atomic species.

*magnocellular layers Layers 1 and 2 of the primate lateral geniculate nucleus, containing large cells sensitive to motion and gross structure of the stimulus.

maturational window Critical period.

*medial Toward the midplane, relative to some landmark. Each nucleus can have a medial portion, such as the medial geniculate nucleus .

*membrane time constant The reciprocal of the rate at which a neuron's membrane passively charges or discharges. Defined as the product of the membrane's specific resistance and capacitance. Typically 2 msec.

metameric color match A side-by-side match of a patch of any given color to an adjacent patch composed of the three primary colors such that the boundary between the patches becomes minimally visible.

metapsychological problems Metaphysical problems in psychology beyond our grasp to understand them or to test them by scientific experiments.

missing fundamental Although pitch plays a basic role in speech, it is possible to filter it out and still have understandable speech. This is due to the nonlinearities of the auditory system.

monochromat A person who has only one cone system and perhaps cannot see any color.

*motion capture The illusion that a stationary foreground object containing many spatial frequencies moves in the same direction as a moving large-field background containing low spatial frequencies.

*motion parallax A monocular cue to depth that results from the fact that, when an observer moves, the images of closer objects pass more rapidly over the retina than the images of more distant objects.

*multiplexing Representation of more than one dimension of information in one sensory channel or population of units. In computers this is done by time slicing—each channel gets its turn.

multiple stable state A system that has more than one stable configuration for a single set of external parameters.

*myelination Wrapping of axons in layers of the lipid membrane of Schwann cells to provide electrical insulation. This means that the action potential has to be regenerated only at certain intervals along the axon (nodes of Ranvier), thus allowing faster transmission.

*nearest-neighbor method A method of representing similarity of examplars within a category. Exemplars with features in common are clustered together around a central prototype in similarity space. Distance from the prototype defines the degree of similarity of an exemplar (similarity metric). A neural network is naturally configured for this method of representation.

*Necker cube A two-dimensional line drawing of a three-dimensional cube that can be seen alternately two different 3-D configurations. The switch can be under conscious control, but both configurations cannot be seen simultaneously. Named after a Swiss crystallographer.

*neocortex A six-layered, convoluted sheet of cells forming the outer surface of the cerebral hemispheres. Composed primarily of spiny, excitatory pyramidal cells and smooth inhibitory cells. A recent development in evolution, associated with higher mammals. Thought to be the locus of cognition and complex sensorimotor processing.

neural net(works) Simulation of brain activity by neuron-like elements (neuromimes). Information processing takes place through excitatory and inhibitory interactions among a large number of such simple elements.

neurontropy (neural entropy) A term denoting the fact that fusion goes from order to disorder 10 times faster than vice versa.

*neurotransmitter A chemical signal, passed from one neuron to another at a synapse, that binds to receptors in the postsynaptic cell membrane, usually causing a conductance change.

*normalization Keeping the total activity in a system constant (e.g., by including feedforward inhibition), or keeping the sum of weights in a system constant. In a network undergoing learning, this prevents one unit or weight from responding to too many input vectors.

nth-order statistics A measure in integral geometry where the vertices of an n-gon are randomly thrown over an image and fall on certain colors. For instance, by throwing 2-gons (lines or dipoles) at random on an image one can harvest the dipole statistics.

*occipital lobe An area of the neocortex at back of brain involved in visual processing.

*ocular dominance columns Alternating vertical columns of cells in V1 within the center of which neurons respond only to stimulation in either the left or the right eye. The neurons at the borders respond to binocular stimulation.

olfactory bulb An outgrowth of the forebrain that receives all input from olfactory receptors and project directly to the olfactory cortex. It spatially segregates neuronal representations of different odors. The neocortex evolved at the expense of the olfactory bulb.

*open loop A neural circuit operating without error feedback. Allows fast response from simple circuitry, but at the cost of insensitivity to performance.

*operant conditioning Instrumental conditioning. Learning by association of an organism's own behavior with a subsequent reinforcing or punishing environmental event.

*optic nerve A fiber tract carrying axons of retinal ganglion cells to many places in the brain, including the lateral geniculate nucleus and the superior colliculus. The center of the optic nerve carries an artery into the eye to supply the retina.

*optimization Finding the best solution to a problem bounded by a number of constraints (such as the traveling-salesman problem). Solutions can be found by relaxation of a suitable network such as the Boltzmann machine to a global energy minimum.

*orientation columns Vertical columns of cells in V1 tuned to a stimulus bar of a particular orientation. Organized in patches of continuously varying orientation, punctuated by discontinuities and singularities.

orthonormal (base) functions A set of functions that may be used to represent a complex function as a set of more elementary functions which are mutually independent (i.e., orthogonal). Best-known are the cosine and sine functions in Fourier analysis.

palinopsia Imagery of textures after prolonged stimulation to them (e.g. being surrounded by shrubs, berries, or sand). Even people who have never had eidetic imagery can experience palinopsia.

*Panum's fusional area A region about 10–20 arc min behind and in front of the horopter where mildly disparate images can be fused by the visual system to yield perceptions of single objects. With slow pulling and a random-dot stereogram it can be extended up to 120 arc min.

parallel distributed processing (PDP) A theory assuming that information processing takes place through excitatory and inhibitory interactions among a large number of simple processing units. Hypotheses and concepts—particularly hidden units and backpropagation—are represented as the distributed activity of many units.

*parietal lobe An area of the neocortex concerned with language, somatic sensation, visuospatial processing, and representation of space in general.

*parvocellular layers Layers 3–6 of the primate lateral geniculate nucleus, containing small cells sensitive to the detailed spatial structure and wavelength of the stimulus.

*perceptron A feedforward network using binary threshold units. Has one layer of modifiable weights between the input and output layers. The perceptron learning rule for the weights can be used to improve performance.

*plasticity Changes in the nervous system that can occur as the result of experience or damage. Plasticity can occur as synaptic modification, growth of axons and dendrites. and changes in the densities and kinetics of ion channels.

*positron-emission tomography (PET) An imaging technique based on detection of radiation emitted by radioactive isotopes inhaled by the subject. The flow of (isotope-containing) blood increases at sites of increased electrical activity, so a dynamic picture of neural processing is possible. Resolution is limited to a few minutes and a few millimeters.

power spectrum A representation showing the amount of energy of a stimulus at each frequency. This representation can be produced by calculating the Fourier transform of the stimulus or taking the Fourier transform of the autocorrelation of the stimulus.

*primary auditory cortex (AI) Located in superior temporal gyrus. Receives input from medial geniculate nucleus. Contains tonotopic frequency maps and is organized in columns in an analogous way to primary visual cortex, area V1.

*primary motor cortex (M1) Area 4 of neocortex, precentral gyrus. Main output of the cortical motor system. Organized topographically into a distorted motor map of the whole body. Contains giant layer-5 pyramidal cells (Betz cells) that project via the pyramidal tract onto motor neurons in the spinal cord.

*primary visual cortex (V1) Striate cortex (also called area 17). Region of neocortex at pole of occipital lobe receiving input from lateral geniculate nucleus. Contains cells responsive to oriented bars of light or spots of different wavelengths.

priming (cueing) Short-term facilitation of performance by the prior presentation of particular stimuli (words, arrows, etc.). Can be subconscious, and spared in amnesia. Often it is assumed that priming shifts focal attention prior to the onset of the stimulus.

*principal-component analysis Mathematical method of analysis that finds the most important directions of variance in the data in a linear fashion. Applicable to neural networks with linear hidden units, finding the subset of vectors that is the best linear approximation to the set of input vectors. Data containing higher-order statistical properties can be characterized by nonlinear hidden units.

*principal curvatures Directions of maximum and minimum curvature along the surface of a curved object. These directions are always at right angles to each other. Together with the orientation of the axes, they provide a complete description of the local curvature.

*procedural memory Nondeclarative memory occurring as changes in the way existing cognitive or motor operations are carried out. Many brain areas could be involved. These forms of memory are spared in amnesia.

*process In anatomy, any linear extension of a neuron, such as a dendrite or an axon. Also called a *neurite*. In computer science, a program that runs on a computer.

*prosopagnosia A type of agnosia in which the subject cannot recognize previously familiar faces. Reported to extend to recognition of individual animals, such as a pet cat, and unique cars. Associated with damage to a specific area in extrastriate cortex in which cells responding specifically to faces have been reported.

*psychophysics A branch of psychology based on treating a perceptual system (e.g. the visual system) as a black box, giving the system a characterized input, and observing the output (often a verbal response). These data are then used to infer principles of operation of the system.

*Purkinje cell Output cell of cerebellar cortex. Large inhibitory neuron with extensive dendritic arbor confined to a single plane. May receive more than 100,000 synapses from parallel fibers running perpendicular to arbor. Named after a nineteenth-century physiologist.

qualia (sensations) quality of experience associated with stimulating a particular nervous-system "component" (i.e., a hypothetical functional "unit"). The problem—at present metapsychological—is to be able to specify how a given response of the nervous system gives rise to a particular kind of experience (e.g., pain, pleasure, motion, color), i..e, how the neural properties relate to epistemic properties.

random-dot stereogram (RDS) A pair of images made up of random patterns of black and white dots. The images are identical except that in one image some set of dots has been displaced to the right or the left by a few dot widths. When fused by the two eyes, the displaced dots appear to be at a different depth plane from the background. Only with computers can one ensure that no monocular imperfections yield some cues.

*rapid eye movement (REM) sleep A stage of sleep associated with profound loss of muscle tonus, desynchronized electroencephalogram, and broad sympathetic activation. Dreaming is thought to occur during REM sleep.

*recency effect A phenomenon whereby the last few items on a list are recalled better than words from the middle of the list. Attributed to the fact that the last items are stored in short-term memory.

receptive field A map of a cell's sensitivity profile. For cells reponding to some form of visual input, this map is typically created by stimulating some region of the retina with some visual stimulus (e.g. spots or bars of light) and recording whether the firing rate of a neuron is either increased or decreased. The former indicates excitation, the latter inhibition. Often surrounded by a sensory region, called the *nonclassical receptive field,* that can modulate the central response.

*refractory period A period after an action potential, or a burst of action potentials, during which the threshold for firing spikes is infinite or at least increased. Results from inactivation of depolarizing currents such as that carried by sodium and residual activation of hyperpolarizing currents such as that carried by potassium.

*relaxation A process undergone by neural networks to reach an optimal solution to a problem bounded by a number of constraints (constraint satisfaction). Constraints are embodied in the network as the pattern and strength of connections (weights) between units. Relaxation involves convergence to a steady level of global network activity through repeated local interactions.

*resolution The minimum distance between two stimuli in some sensory space that is needed to distinguish them as two separate stimuli. Not to be confused with accuracy.

*retina The sensory transducer of the visual system. Three layers of neurons at the back of the eye containing five basic cell types, including photoreceptors and retinal ganglion cells.

*retinal ganglion cell Projection cell of the retina. Receives indirect input from photoreceptors and projects out of the retina to many sites, including the lateral geniculate nucleus, the superior colliculus, nuclei in the accessory optic system, and hypothalamic structures.

retinal slip Movement of the visual image across the retina. Serves as the input driving the smooth-pursuit eye-movement system. Also occurs when the gain of certain eye movements, such as the VOR, is not correct. Provides an error signal to the VOR system to correct its gain. Also used in stabilized vision when the close-fitting contact lens that holds a mirror (or light source) inadvertently slips.

*rod A photoreceptor in the retina with a low absolute threshold to light. Its response adapts in normal daylight, where cones are most sensitive. Peak wavelength sensitivity around 510 nm, responsible for photopic (night) vision.

*rostral Toward the nose of the organism.

*reaction time Time elapsed between presentation of a stimulus and elicited response of a subject.

*saccade High-speed ballistic eye movement used to direct the fovea to a target of interest in the visual field. Occurs, on average, three times a second.

*scaling problem A general issue in complexity theory: How does the time taken to solve a problem increase with the size of the problem? In the context of networks, the issue is how long it takes to train a network as a function of the number of weights and amount of data.

segmentation problem Separation of information in an input (e.g., a visual image) into separate batches for separate processing. *Figure-ground segmentation* refers to the separation of one coherent object in an image from the background, a task that requires global analysis of the whole image. *Motion segmentation* refers to the separation of all components of an object that are moving together, though not necessarily with the same velocity. *Early vision* emphasizes segmentation by simple processes based on stereopsis, motion, and texture discrimination, and ignores the higher semantic processes.

*semantic memory The division of declarative memory concerned with knowledge of the world; i.e., organized information, such as facts, vocabulary, and concepts. This reference memory has no temporal structure.

*serotonin 5-hydroxytryptamine, an indoleamine neuromodulator found in raphe nuclei. A variety of post-synaptic receptors have been identified, but the effects of serotonin are still unclear.

*sharp waves Irregular high-amplitude field potentials at 0.02–3 Hz recorded in the hippocampus of rats that are eating, grooming, resting, or in slow-wave sleep. Proposed as a natural stimulus that might induce long-term potentiation.

short-term memory A system that retains information temporarily in a particular status while it is transformed into a more stable, long-term memory. Information in this form is immediately accessible to consciousness.

*simple cells Neurons found in cortical area V1 with linear response properties. The receptive field is made up of discrete excitatory and inhibitory subfields with a specific axis of orientation.

*simulated annealing An optimization technique for finding a global energy minimum. Can be used with a network such as a Boltzmann machine to find solutions to constraint-satisfaction problems. Based on allowing increases in energy of the network early on during relaxation to jump out of local energy minima into the global minimum. As the relaxation process progresses, the temperature is gradually lowered so that the system moves down to the bottom of the global minimum.

single-microelectrode neurophysiology In current neurophysiology, a single microelectrode is placed near a neuron in order to record electrical activity. The cat or monkey is anesthetized and immobilized, and some visual stimulus (e.g. an oriented bar) is moved across the field until the selected neuron is activated. [Recently mokeys with a sealed opening in their skulls (installed weeks before experimentation) have been trained to fixate at a marker. Since the brain is devoid of pain detectors, neurophysiologists can penetrate the brain with their microelectrodes hundreds of times (until the dura hardens) and measure neural activity in the *alert* monkey.] The specific local area with the proper orientation and aspect ratio that elicits the largest activity is

the *receptive field* of the selected neuron. Some neurons require some complex trigger features to become activated, and the spatial concept of the receptive field is inadequate to describe the behavior of these complex and hypercomplex feature analyzers.

*smooth pursuit Moving the eyes to track a moving object in order to keep the retinal image stabilized on the fovea.

*spin glass A substance characterized by unpaired electrons with spin, either up or down, in mixtures of attractive and repulsive interactions. The properties of spin glasses are similar to those of associative Hopfield nets.

split-brain paradigm A method of studying human patients who have had their corpus callosum severed, usually performed to control epileptic seizures. The corpus callosum contains the primary connections between the two hemishperes of the brain. Such methods usually involve restricting some sensory input to a particular hemisphere of the brain and evaluating the nature of the information available to the two hemispheres.

*stereopsis A term literally meaning "solid vision" but taken as referring just to binocular depth perception, which is 3-D perception arising from the retinal disparity of images in the two eyes.

*stereoscope A device that presents a different image to each eye. If the images are identical except that elements of one scene are shifted slightly to the left or right with respect to the other, then the resulting retinal disparity produces stereoscopic vision of the scene.

strabismus Cross-eyedness. When it is not corrected at an early age, one of the eyes becomes nonfunctional, resulting in stereo blindness.

structuralism A school of psychology that sought to experimentally investigate the structure of conscious experience. Structuralists held that concious experience could be decomposed into a set of elementary sensations which could be deduced through introspection.

*superior colliculus A midbrain structure receiving projections from the visual, auditory, and somatosensory systems in register with neurons that drive saccadic eye movements. Responsible for orienting the subject to salient sensory stimuli. Homologous to the optic tectum in birds.

*synapse Functional contact between two cells, consisting of a presynaptic terminal bouton separated by a narrow gap (the synaptic cleft) from an area of postsynaptic membrane containing receptors. Electrical synapses are physical connections between cells, usually allowing bidirectional flow of ions. At a chemical synapse, a release of neurotransmitter from the presynaptic terminal carries a signal to the receptors on the postsynaptic membrane. Autoreceptors on the presynaptic terminal may be affected as well, and if the transmitter escapes from the synaptic cleft it may influence other nearby glial cells and neurons.

*temperature A parameter used in simulated annealing to determine the probability of a unit's making a state change that decreases the energy of the system. The temperature is gradually decreased during the annealing process, causing the system to settle to the bottom of the global energy minimum.

*temporal lobe Area of the cortex concerned with auditory processing, visual learning, declarative memory, and emotions.

texture gradient A local change in textural properties, also called a *texton gradient*. Also, a pattern formed by a regularly textured surface extending away from the observer. Elements in the texture gradient that are far from the observer appear small relative to corresponding elements that are close.

*thalamus The "gateway" to the neocortex, through which all sensory information bound for the cerebral cortex passes. May perform attentional gating on the flow of information to the cortex.

*topographic map A representation used by many sensory modalities in the nervous system. The cortical surface (e.g. primary sensory cortex) contains an orderly spatial map of receptive fields (e.g., of the visual field or the body's surface). Probably serves to reduce wiring and

delays by placing areas that need to communicate close together.

trichromacy A theory of color vision stating that all the visible colors may be constructed from three basic or primary colors. Today this theory is understood as a reasonable representation of the three types of retinal receptors (cones) believed to underlie color vision.

*tuning curve A description of the selectivity of a unit (neuron) to a dimension of the stimulus (e.g. orientation). Many neurons respond best to one particular orientation, though they also respond significantly to other orientations with broad tuning curves.

Turing imitation game A procedure (also called the *Turing test*) whereby the behavior of a machine (algorithm) and a human are compared.

Turing machine An infinite-state abstract automaton, invented simultaneously by A. M. Turing and E. L. Post in 1936, consisting of a control box containing a finite program, a potentially infinite tape, and devices under the command of the box that can scan, print, erase, and move the tape.

Universal Turing Machine The most general class of Turing (Post) machines.

V1 The primary visual cortex in the monkey (analogous to Brodman's Area 17 in the cat).

V2 The extrastriate visual cortex in the monkey (analogous to Brodman's Area 18 in the cat).

V3 The extrastriate visual cortex in the monkey (analogous to Brodman's Area 19 in the cat).

V4 See *extrastriate visual cortex.*

vector An ordered set of numbers. Functions performing vector-to-vector mapping are used to model the evolution of the state of a network with time. In contrast, a scalar has just a single value.

ventral Toward the front, or belly, of the organism.

vergence Disjunctive movements of the eyes to foveate objects that are moving in depth. When the object moves closer, the eyes converge; when it moves away, they diverge.

very-large-scale integration (VLSI) The fabrication of a complex electronic circuit consisting of millions of components on a single piece of silicon.

*vesicle Membranous sacks, thought to contain neurotransmitter, which are located inside presynaptic terminals and which fuse with presynaptic membrane upon entry of calcium into the terminals. After fixation of the tissue for electron microscopy, excitatory synaptic terminals usually contain round vesicles, and inhibitory synapses have flattened vesicles.

*vestibulo-ocular reflex Short-latency movement of the eyes, in the direction opposite to head movement, which stabilizes the image on the retina.

Weber's Law $kI = \Delta I$, where k is a constant, I is the intensity of a stimulus, and ΔI is the smallest change in stimulus intensity that may be discriminated (i.e., the just-noticeable difference). This law states that the just-noticeable difference in the intensity of a stimuli is proportional to the intensity of the stimulus. Weber believed that that $\Delta I/I$ (known as -the Weber fraction) was a constant for a given sensory modality.

winner-take-all The unit in a group responding most strongly to an input has its activation increased, and that of the other units decreases. This process, the basis of vector quantization, can be combined with a learning rule in competitive learning networks.

working memory A term (proposed by Baddeley and Hitch) referring to a memory buffer in which Information is maintained while it is being processed. Now thought of as a collection of temporary capacities associated with different modalities. Usually it is acoustic and based on rapid rehersal (e.g. repeating a telephone number before dialing). Not to be confused with iconic memory and echoic memory, whicht are less than 500 msec in duration.

zero crossing A point along a dimension at which the value is zero, changing from positive to negative or vice versa.

REFERENCES

Note: The author's publications are listed and commented on in appendix B.

Abeles, M. 1982. *Local Cortical Circuits: An Electrophysiological Study*. Springer-Verlag.

Abeles, M. 1991. *Corticonics: Neural Circuits of the Cerebral Cortex*. Cambridge University Press.

Adelson, E., and Bergen, J. 1985. Spatio-temporal energy models for the perception of motion. *Journal of the Optical Society of America* 2: 284–299.

Amit, D. 1989. *Modeling Brain Function*. Cambridge University Press.

Anderson, B. 1992. Hysteresis, cooperativity, and depth averaging in dynamic random-dot stereograms. *Perception and Psychophysics* 51 (6): 511–528.

Anderson, B., and Nakayama, K. 1994. Towards a general theory of stereopsis: Binocular matching, occluding contours, and fusion. *Psychological Review* 101: 414–445.

Anderson, C., and Van Essen, D. 1987. Shifter circuits: A computational strategy for dynamic aspects of visual processing. *Proceedings of the National Academy of Sciences* 84: 6297–6301.

Anstis, S. 1978. Apparent movement. In *Handbook of Physiology,* vol. VIII: *Perception,* ed. R. Held, H. Leibowitz, and H. Teuber. Springer-Verlag.

Aschenbrenner, C. 1954. Problems in getting information into and out of air photographs. *Photogramm. Eng.* 20 (3): 398–401.

Babington-Smith, B. 1977. A wartime anticipation of random-dot stereograms. *Perception* 6: 233–234.

Barkow, B. 1973. Foundations of visual psychoanatomy. *Contemporary Psychology* 18 (11): 515–516.

Barlow, H. 1990. A theory about the functional role and synaptic mechanism of visual after-effects. In *Vision: Coding and Efficency,* ed. C. Blakemore. Cambridge University Press.

Barlow, H., Blakemore, C., and Pettigrew, D. 1967. The neural mechanism of binocular depth discrimination. *Journal of Physiology* 193: 327–342.

Barlow, H., and Mollon, J., eds. 1982. *The Senses*. Cambridge University Press.

Baumgartner, G. 1960. Indirekte Grössenbestimmung der rezeptiven Felder der Retina beim Menschen mittels der hermannschen Gittertäuschung. *Pfluegers Archiv* 272: 1–21.

Ben-Av, M., Sagi, D., and Braun, J. 1991. Visual attention and perceptual grouping. Technical report CS91–22, Weizmann Institute.

Bergen, J., and Adelson, E. 1988. Early vision and texture perception. *Nature* 333: 363–364.

Bernstein, J. 1984. *Three Degrees Above Zero*. Scribner.

Bishop, P. 1963. Neurophysiology of binocular single vision and stereopsis. In *Handbook of Sensory Physiology,* vol. 7, ed. R. Jung. Springer.

Bishop, P.. and Pettigrew, J. 1986. Neural mechanisms of binocular vision. *Vision Research* 26 (9): 1587–1600.

Blakemore, C. 1969. Binocular depth discrimination and the nasotemporal division. *Journal of Physiology* 205: 471–497.

Blakemore, C., and Campbell, F. 1969. Adaptation to spatial stimuli. *Journal of Physiology* 200: 11–13.

Blakemore, C., and Cooper, G. 1970. Development of the brain depends on the visual environment. *Nature* 228: 477–478.

Blum, H. 1967. A new model for brain function. *Perspectives in Biology and Medicine* 10 (3): 381–408.

Blum, H. 1973. Biological shape and visual science, part I. *Journal of Theoretical Biology* 38: 205–287.

Blum, H. J., and R. Nagel. 1978. Shape description using weighted symmetric axis features. *Pattern Recognition* 10: 167–180.

Boff, K., Kaufman, L., and Thomas, J. 1986. *Handbook of Perception and Performance,* vol.1: *Sensory Processes and Perception.* Wiley.

Boynton, R., ed. 1986. Reprinted version of *Vision Research* 26 (9): 1601–1629.

Braddick, O. 1974. A short range process in apparent motion. *Vision Research* 14: 519–527.

Braddick, O. 1980. Low-level and high-level processes in apparent motion. *Philosophical Transactions of the Royal Society of London* B 290: 137–151.

Braitenberg, V. 1984. *Vehicles: Experiments in Synthetic Psychology.* MIT Press.

Braun, J., and Sagi, D. 1990. Vision outside the focus of attention. *Perception and Psychophysics* 48: 45–58.

Bregman, A., and Campbell, J. 1971. Primary auditory stream segregation and perception of order in rapid sequence of tones. *Journal of Experimental Psychology* 89: 244–249.

Bregman, A., and Rudincky, A. 1975. Auditory segregation: Stream or streams? *Journal of Experimental Psychology: Human Perception and Performance* 1: 263–267.

Broadbent, D. 1958. *Perception and Communication.* Pergamon.

Bruce, V., and Green. P. 1985. *Visual Perception: Physiology, Psychology, and Ecology.* Erlbaum.

Buchsbaum, G., and Gottschalk, A. 1983. Trichromacy, opponent colours coding and optimum colour information transmission in the retina. *Proceedings of the Royal Society* B 220: 89–113.

Bülthoff, H., and Mallot, H. 1990. Integration of stereo, shading, and texture. In *AI and the Eye,* ed. A. Blake, and T. Troscianco. Wiley.

Burbeck, C. A., and S. M. Pizer. 1994. Object representation by cores. *Invest. Ophth. Vis. Sci.* 35: 1626.

Burr, D. 1980. Sensitivity to spatial phase. *Vision Research* 20: 391–396.

Burt, P., and G. Sperling. 1981. Time, distance, and feature trade-offs in visual apparent motion. *Psychological Review* 88: 171–195.

Caelli, T., Hoffman, W., and Lindman, H. 1978. Subjective Lorentz transformations and the perception of motion. *Journal of the Optical Society of America* 68: 402–417.

Campbell, F., and Robson, J. 1968. Application of Fourier analysis to the visibility of gratings. *Journal of Physiology* 197: 551–566.

Cavanagh, P., and Mather, G. 1989. Motion: The long and short of it. *Spatial Vision* 4: 103–129.

Chargaff, E. 1978. *Heraclitean Fire: Sketches from a Life before Nature.* Rockefeller University Press.

Churchland, P. S. 1986. *Neurophilosophy. Toward a Unified Science of the Mind-Brain.* MIT Press.

Churchland, P. S., and T. Sejnowski. 1992. *The Computational Brain.* MIT Press.

Cornsweet, T. 1970. *Visual Perception.* Academic Press.

Crick, F., and Koch, C. 1990. Towards a neurophysiological theories on consciousness. *Seminars in Neurosciences* 2: 263–275.

Crick, F., and Koch, C. 1990. Some reflections on visual awareness. *Cold Spring Harbor Symposia on Quantitative Biology* 55: 953–962.

Darian-Smith, C., and C. S. Gilbert. 1994. Axonal sprouting accompanies functional reorganization in adult cat striate cortex. *Nature* 368: 737–740.

Desimone, R., and Ungerleider, L. 1989. Neural mechanisms of visual processing in monkeys. In *Handbook of Neurophysiology,* vol. 2, ed. F. Boller and J. Grafman. Elsevier.

Dev, P. 1975. Perception of depth surfaces in random-dot stereograms: A neural model. *International Journal of Man-Machine Studies* 7: 511–528.

Dev, P. 1974. Segmentation processes in visual perception: A cooperative neural model. Technical report 74C-5, Computer and Information Science, University of Massachusetts, Amherst.

De Weert, C., and Sadza, K. 1983. New data concerning the contribution of colour differences to stereopsis. In *Color Vision,* ed. J. Mollon and T. Sharpe. Academic Press.

Devancy, R., Goldberg, L., and Hubbard, J. 1986. Dynamical approximation to the exponential map by polynomials. Technical report 10019–86, Mathematical Sciences Research Institute, Berkeley.

De Valois, R., Albrecht, D., and Thorell, L. 1978. Cortical cells: bar detectors or spatial filters? In *Frontiers of Visual Science,* ed. S. Cool and E. Smith. Springer.

Dodwell, P. 1983. The Lie transformation model of visual perception. *Perception and Psychophysics* 34: 1–16.

Edelman, G. 1989. *The Remembered Present: A Biological Theory of Consciousness.* Basic Books.

Edelman, G., Gall, W., and Cowan, W., eds. 1984. *Dynamic Aspects of Neurocortical Function.* Wiley.

Egeth, H., and Blecker, D. 1971. Differential effects of familiarity on judgements of sameness and difference. *Perception and Psychophysics* 9: 321–326.

Egeth, H., and Dagenbach, D. 1991. Parallel versus serial processing in visual search: Further evidence from subadditive effects of visual quality. *Journal of Experimental Psychology* 17 (2): 551–560.

Enns, J. 1986. Seeing textons in contex. *Perception and Psychophysics* 39: 143–147.

Eriksen, C., and Spencer, T. 1969. Rate of information processing in visual perception: some results and methodological considerations. *Journal of Experimental Psychology* 79: 1–16.

Erdös, P., and Rényi, A. 1959. On random graphs, I. *Publ. Math. Debrecen* 6: 290–297.

Erkelens, C. J. 1988. Fusional limits for large random-dot stereograms. *Vision Res.* 28: 345–353.

Erkelens, C., and Collewijn, H. 1986. Eye-movements in relation to loss and regaining of fusion of disjunctively moving random-dot stereograms. *Human Neurobiology* 4: 181–188.

Falk, D. S., Brill, D. R., and Stork, D. G. 1986. *Seeing the Light: Optics in Nature, Photography, Color, Vision, and Holography.* Harper and Row.

Farrel, B., and Pelli, D. 1993. Can we attend to large and small scale at the same time? *Vision Research* 33 (18): 2757–2772.

Fiorentini, A. 1989. Differences between fovea and parafovea in visual search processes. *Vision Research* 29: 1153–1164.

Flanagan, J. 1972. *Speech Analysis, Synthesis, and Perception.* Academic Press.

Fodor, J., and Pylyshyn, Z. 1988. Connectionism and cognitive architecture: A critical analysis. In *Connections and Symbols,* ed. S. Pinker and J. Mehler. MIT Press.

Fogel, I., and Sagi, D. 1989. Gabor filters as texture discriminators. *Biological Cybernetics* 61: 103–113.

Földiák, P. 1992. The 'Ideal Homunculus': statistical inference from neural population responses. In Proceedings of the Computation and Neural Systems Conference, San Francisco.

Fox, R., Aslin, R., Shea, S., and Dumais, S. 1980. Stereopsis in human infants. *Science* 207: 323–324.

Gabor, D. 1946. Theory of communication. *Journal of the Institute of Electrical Engineers (London)* 93: 429–457.

Gazzaniga, M. 1989. Organization of the human brain. *Science* 245: 947–952.

Georgopoulos, A., Kettner, R., and Schwartz, A. 1988. Primate motor cortex and free arm movements to visual targets in three-dimensional space. II. Coding of the direction of movement by a neuronal population. *Journal of Neuroscience* 8 (8): 2928–2937.

Gibson, J. 1950. *The Perception of the Visual World.* Houghton Mifflin.

Gilbert, C. D., and T. W. Wiesel. 1992. Receptive field dynamics in adult primary visual cortex. *Nature* 356: 150–152.

Glass, L. 1969. Moiré effect from random dots. *Nature* 223: 578–580.

Gorea, A., and Papathomas, T. 1993. Double-opponency as a generalized concept in texture segregation illustrated with color, luminance and orientation defined stimuli. *Journal of the Optical Society of America* 10A (7): 1450–1462

Gorea, A., Papathomas, T., and Kovacs, I. 1993a. Motion perception with spatiotemporally matched chromatic and achromatic information reveals a 'slow' and a 'fast' motion system. *Vision Research* 33 (17): 2515–2534.

Gregory, R., ed. 1987. *The Oxford Companion to the Mind.* Oxford University Press.

Gregory, R. 1990. *Eye and Brain: The Psychology of Seeing.* Princeton University Press.

Grimson, W. E. L. 1981. *From Images to Surfaces.* MIT Press.

Grinberg, D., and Williams, D. 1985. Stereopsis with chromatic signals from the blue sensitive mechanism. *Vision Research* 25: 531–537.

Grinvald, E. E., E. E. Lieke, R. D. Frostig, and R. Hildesheim. 1994. Neural correlates of figure-ground segregation in primary visual cortex: Cortical point-spread function by real-time optical imaging of macaque monkey primary visual cortex. *J. of Neuroscience* 14 (5): 2545–2568.

Grossberg, S., ed. 1988. *Neural Networks and Natural Intelligence.* MIT Press.

Grossberg, S., and Mingolla, E. 1985. Neural dynamics of perceptual grouping: Textures, boundaries, and emergent segmentations. *Perception and Psychophysics* 38: 141–171.

Gurnsey, R., and Browse, R. 1987. Micropattern properties and presentation conditions influencing visual texture discrimination. *Perception and Psychophysics* 41: 239–252.

Hadani, I., Ishai, G., and Gur, M. 1978. Visual stability and space perception in monocular vision: A mathematical model. Biomedical engineering technical report, Israel Institute of Technology.

Hadani, I., Ishai, G., and Gur, M. 1980. Visual stability and space perception in monocular vision: Mathematical model. *Journal of the Optical Society of America* 70: 60–65.

Hadani, I., Ishai, G., Kononov, A., and Fisch, H. L. 1994. Two solutions to 3-D reconstruction for an eye in pure rotations. *J. Opt. Soc. Am.* 11 (1): 1–11.

Harris, C., ed. 1980. *Visual Coding and Adaptability.* Erlbaum.

He, Z., and Nakayama, K. 1994. Perceiving texture: beyond filtering. *Vision Research* 34 (2): 151–162.

Hebb, D. 1949. *The Organization of Behavior.* Wiley.

Hecht, S., Shlaer, S., and Pirenne, M. 1942. Energy, quanta, and vision. *Journal of General Physiology* 25 (6): 819–840.

Heilman, K., Watson, R., Valenstein, E., and Goldberg, M. 1987. Attention: behavior and neural mechanisms. In *Handbook of Physiology,* section 1, volume V, ed. V. Mountcastle, F. Plum, and S. Geiger. American Physiological Society.

Heitger, F., Rosenthaler, L., von der Heydt, R., Peterhans, E., and Kübler, O. 1992. Simulation of neural contour mechanisms: From simple to end-stopped cells. *Vision Research* 32 (5): 963–981.

Held, R., and Hein, A. 1963. Movement-produced stimulation in the development of visually guided behavior. *Journal of Comparative and Physiological Psychology* 56: 872–876.

Helmholtz, H. von. 1896. *Handbuch der Physiologischen Optik. Dritter Abschnitt, Zweite Auflage.* Voss. English translation: *Helmholtz's Treatise on Physiological Optics,* tr. J. Southall (Optical Society of America, 1924; Dover Publications, 1962).

Hering, E. 1878. *Zur Lehre vom Lichtsinn* Gerold's Sohn.

Hildreth, E. 1984. *The Measurement of Visual Motion* MIT Press.

Hillis, D. 1985. *The Connection Machine.* MIT Press.

Hirsch, H., and Spinelli, D. 1970, Visual experience modifies distribution of horizontally and vertically oriented receptive fields in cats. *Science* 168: 869–871.

Hoffman,, D., and Richards, W. 1988. Representing smooth plane curves for recognition: Implications for figure-ground reversal. In *Natural Computation,* ed. W. Richards. MIT Press.

Hoffman, W. 1970. Higher visual perception as prolongations of the basic Lie transformation group. *Mathematical Biosciences* 6: 437–471.

Hogg, J. 1854. *The Microscope: Its History, Construction and Application.* London.

Hopfield, J. 1984. Neural networks and physical systems with emergent collective computational abilities. *Proceedings of the National Academy of Sciences* 79: 2554–2558.

Horn, B., and Brooks, M. 1985. The Variational Approach to Shape from Shading. Memo 813, MIT Artificial Intelligence Lab.

Hubel, D. 1988. *Eye, Brain, Vision.* Freeman.

Hubel, D., and Wiesel, T. 1960. Receptive fields of optic nerve fibres in the spider monkey. *Journal of Physiology* 154: 572–580.

Hubel, D., and Wiesel, T. 1962. Receptive fields, binocular interaction and functional architecture in the cat's visual cortex. *Journal of Physiology* 160: 106–154.

Hubel, D., and Wiesel, T. 1968. Receptive fields and functional architecture of the monkey striate cortex. *Journal of Physiology* 195: 215–243.

Hubel, D., and Wiesel, T. 1970. Stereoscopic vision in the macaque monkey: Cells sensitive to binocular depth in area 18 of the macaque monkey cortex: Stereoscopic vision in the macaque monkey. *Nature* 225: 41–42.

Hubel, D., and Wiesel, T. 1974. Uniformity of monkey striate cortex: A parallel relationship between field size, scatter, and magnification factor. *Journal of Comparative Neurology* 158: 295–306.

Humphreys, G., and Bruce, V. 1989. *Visual Cognition: Computational, Experimental, and Neuropsychological Perspectives.* Erlbaum.

Ichiro, F., Tanaka, K., Ito, M., and Cheng, K.. 19XX. Columns for visual features of objects in monkey inferotemporal cortex. *Nature* 360: 343–346.

James, W. 1890. *The Principles of Psychology* (republished in 1925 by Dover Publications).

Johansson, G. 1973. Visual perception of biological motion and and a model of analysis. *Perception and Psychophysics* 14: 201–211.

Judd, S. 1987. Learning in networks is hard. In Proceedings of the First IEEE International Conference on Neural Networks, vol. II.

Kabrisky, M. 1966. *A Proposed Model for Visual Information Processing in the Human Brain.* University of Illinois Press.

Kac, M. 1985. *Enigmas of Chance.* Harper & Row.

Kandel, E., and Schwartz, J. 1985. *Principles of Neural Science,* second edition. Elsevier North-Holland.

Kanizsa, G. 1976. Subjective contours. *Scientific American* 234 (4): 48–52.

Karni, A., and Sagi, D. 1990. Where Practice Makes Perfect in Texture Discrimination. Technical report CS90-02, Weizmann Institute of Science.

Kleffner, D., and Ramachandran, V. 1992. On the perception of shape from shading. *Perception and Psychophysics* 52 (1): 18–36.

Kelly, J., Jr. 1956. New interpretation of information rate. *Bell System Technical Journal* 35: 917–926.

Kelly, D. 1960. Jo stimulus patterns for visual research. *Journal of the Optical Society of America* 50: 1115–1116.

Kelly, D., ed. *Visual Science and Engineering: Models and Applications.* Marcel Dekker.

Koenderink, J., and van Doorn, A. 1992. Affine structure from motion. *Journal of the Optical Society of America* 82: 377–385.

Koffka, K. 1935. *Principles of Gestalt Psychology.* Harcourt, Brace.

Kolers, P., and Pomerantz, J. 1971. Figural change in apparent motion. *Journal of Experimental Psychology* 87: 99–108.

Krauskopf, J., and Srebro, R. 1965. Spectral sensitivity of color mechanisms: Derivation from fluctuation of color appearance near threshold. *Science* 150: 1477–1479.

Kröse, B. 1987. Local structure analysers as determinants of preattentive pattern discrimination. *Biological Cybernetics* 55: 289–298.

Kubovy, M. 1981. Concurrent pitch-segregation and the theory of indispensable attributes. In *Perceptual Organization,* ed. M. Kubovy and J. Pomerantz. Erlbaum.

Kuffler, S. 1953. Discharge patterns and functional organization of mammalian retina. *Journal of Neurophysiology* 16: 37–68.

Kuhn, T. 1962. *The Structure of Scientific Revolutions.* University of Chicago Press.

Langton, C. 1992. Artificial life. In *Artificial Life: Proceedings of an Interdisciplinary Workshop on the Synthesis and Simulation of Living Systems,* ed. C. Langton. Addison-Wesley.

LeDoux, J., and Hirst, W., eds. 1986. *Mind and Brain: Dialogues in Cognitive Neuroscience.* Cambridge University Press.

Lehky, S., and Sejnowski, T. 1990. Neural model of stereoacuity and depth interpretation based on a distributed representation of stereo disparity. *Journal of Neuroscience* 10: 2281–2299.

Leith, E., and Upatnieks, J. 1962. Reconstructed wavefronts and communication theory. *Journal of the Optical Society of America* 52:1123–1130.

Lettvin, J., Maturana, H., McCulloch, W., and Pitts, W. 1959. What the frog's eye tells the frog's brain. *Proceedings of the IRE* 47:1940–1951.

Leyton, M. 1992. *Symmetry, Causality, Mind.* MIT Press.

Livingstone, M., and Hubel, D. 1984. Anatomy and physiology of a color system in the primate visual cortex. *Journal of Neuroscience* 4: 309–356.

Luneburg, R. 1950. The metric of binocular visual space. *Journal of the Optical Society of America* 40: 627–642.

MacAdam, D. 1970. *Sources of Color Science.* MIT Press.

Mach, E. 1886. *The Analysis of Sensations and the Relation of the Physical to the Psychical.* Republished by Dover Publications in 1959 using the fifth German edition revised and supplemented by S. Waterlow.

Mahowald, M., and Delbrück, T. 1989. Cooperative stereo matching using static and dynamic image features. In *Analog ELSI Implementation of Neuro Systems,* ed. C. Mead and M. Ismail. Kluwer.

Malik, J., and Perona, P. 1990. Preattentive texture discrimination with early vision mechanisms. *Journal of the Optical Society of America* 7 (5): 923–932.

Marr, D. 1982. *Vision*. Freeman.

Marr, D., and Poggio, T. 1976. Cooperative computation of stereo disparity. *Science* 194: 283.

Marr, D., and Poggio, T. 1979. A theory of human stereopsis. *Proceedings of the Royal Society* B 204: 301.

Mayhew, J., and Frisby, J. 1979. Convergent disparity discriminations in narrow-band-filtered random-dot stereograms. *Vision Research* 19 (1): 63–71.

Melzak, Z. 1976. Mathematical Ideas, Modeling and Applications. Volume II of *Companion to Concrete Mathematics* . Wiley.

Miller, G. 1956. The magic number of seven, plus or minus two. *Psychological Review* 63 (2): 81–97.

Mitchell, D. 1980. The influence of early visual experience on visual perception. In *Visual Coding and Adaptability*, ed. C. Harris. Erlbaum.

Moore, E. 1961. Machine models of self-reproduction. *Proceedings of Symposia on Applied Mathematics* 14: 17–33.

Moran, T., and Desimone, R. 1985. Selective attention gates visual processing in the extrastriate cortex. *Science* 229: 782.

Mountcastle, V. 1979. An organizing principle for cerebral function: The unit module and the distributed system. In *The Neurosciences: Fourth Study Program*, ed. F. Schmidt and F. Worden. MIT Press.

Mowforth, P., Mayhew, J., and Frisby, J. 1981. Vergence eye movements made in response to spatial-frequency-filtered random-dot stereograms. *Perception* 10 (3): 299–304.

Müller, J. 1844. *Handbuch der Physiologie des Menschen*, fourth edition. J. Hölscher.

Nakayama, K. 1985. Biological image motion processing: A review. *Vision Research* 25: 625–660.

Nakayama, K. 1990. The iconic bottleneck and the tenuous link between early visual processing and perception.

In *Vision: Coding and Efficency*, ed. C. Blakemore. Cambridge University Press.

Nakayama, K., and Mackeben, M. 1989. Sustained and transient components of focal visual attention. *Vision Research* 29: 1631–1647.

Nakayama, K., and Silverman, G. 1986. Serial and parallel processing of visual feature conjunctions. *Nature* 320: 264–265.

Nelson, J. 1975. Globality and stereoscopic fusion in binocular vision. *Journal of Theoretical Biology* 49: 1–88.

Nothdurft, H. 1985. Sensitivity for structure gradient in texture discrimination tasks. *Vision Research* 25: 1957–1968.

Ogle, K. 1964. *Researches in Binocular Vision*. Hafner.

Ogle, K., and Wakefield, J. 1967. Stereoscopic depth and binocular rivalry. *Vision Research* 7: 89–95.

Olive, J., Greenwood, A., and Coleman, J. 1993. *Acoustics of American English Speech: A Dynamic Approach*. Springer-Verlag.

Paillard, J., ed. 1977. The Lie transformation group model for perceptual and cognitive psychology. *Cahiers de Psychologie* 2 (entire issue).

Papathomas, T., and Gorea, A. 1988. Simultaneous motion perception along multiple attributes: A new class of stimuli. *Behavioral Research Methods, Instruments and Computers* 20: 528–536.

Papathomas, T., and Gorea, A. 1989. A new paradigm for testing human and machine motion perception. *Proceedings, SPIE-International Society for Optical Engineering* 1077: 285–291.

Papert, S. 1961. Centrally produced geometrical illusions. *Nature* 191: 733.

Penrose, R. 1989. *The Emperor's New Mind* Oxford University Press.

Pentland, A. 1986. Shading into texture. *Artificial Intelligence* 29: 147–170.

Petrig, B. 1980. Nachweis von Stereopsis bei Kindern mittels stochasischer Punktstereogramme und der zuhörigen evozierte Potenziale. Ph.D. thesis, ETH, Zürich.

Pettigrew, J. 1974. The effect of visual experience on the development of stimulus specificity by kitten cortical neurones. *Journal of Physiology (London)* 237: 49–74.

Pettigrew, J. 1990. Is there a single, most efficient algorithm for stereopsis? In *Vision: Coding and Efficiency,* ed. C. Blakemore. Cambridge University Press.

Piantanida, T. 1986. Stereo hysteresis revisited. *Vision Research* 26: 431–437.

Poggio, G. 1984. Processing of stereoscopic information in primate visual cortex. In *Dynamic Aspects of Neocortical Function,* ed. G. Edelman, W. Gall, and W. Cowan. Wiley.

Poggio, G., Gonzalez, F., and Krause, F. 1988. Stereoscopic mechanisms in monkey visual cortex: Binocular correlation and disparity sensitivity. *Journal of Neuroscience* 8: 4531–4550.

Poggio, T., Torre, V., and Koch, C. 1989. Computational vision and regularization theory. *Nature* 317: 314–319.

Polanyi, M. 1969. *Knowing and Being.* University of Chicago Press.

Polat, U., and Sagi, D. 1993. Lateral interaction between spatial channels: suppression and facilitation revealed by lateral masking experiments. *Vision Research* 7: 993–999.

Pollack, I. 1952. The information in elementary auditory displays. *Journal of the Auditory Society of America* 24: 745–749.

Pollack, I. 1953. The information in elementary auditory displays. II. *Journal of the Auditory Society of America* 25: 765–769.

Posner, M. 1978. Orienting of attention. *Quarterly Journal of Experimental Psychology* 32: 3–25.

Pylyshyn, Z. 1984. *Computation and Cognition: Toward a Foundation of Cognitive Science.* MIT Press.

Ramachandran, V. 1988. Perception of shape from shading. *Nature* 331: 163–166.

Ramachandran, V. 1990. Visual perception in people and machines. In *AI and the Eye,* ed. A. Blake and T. Troscianco. Wiley.

Ramachandran, V., and Gregory, R. 1978. Does colour provide an input to human motion perception? *Nature* 275: 55–56.

Regan, D. 1989. *Human Brain Electrophysiology.* Elsevier.

Regan, D., and Beverley, K. 1985. Visual responses to verticity and the neural analysis of optic flow. *Journal of the Optical Society of America* 2: 280–283.

Reichardt, W. 1961. Autocorrelation, a principle of evaluation of sensory information by the central nervous system. In *Sensory Coding,* ed. W. Rosenbluth. Wiley.

Reichardt, W., and Egelhaaf, M. 1988. *Naturwissenschaften* 75: 313–315.

Rényi, A.. 1964. A Socratic dialogue on mathematics. *Physics Today* (December): 24–36.

Resnikoff, H. 1987a. *The Illusion of Reality.* Springer-Verlag.

Resnikoff, H. 1987b. Concurrent computation and models of biological information processing. In *Advances in Cognitive Science,* ed. M. Kochen and H. Hastings. Westview.

Richards, W., ed. 1988. *Natural Computation.* MIT Press.

Richards, W., and Kay, M. 1974. Local versus global stereopsis: Two mechanisms? *Vision Research* 14: 1345–1347.

Rock, I. 1984. *Perception.* Freeman.

Rock, I., and Palmer, S. 1990. The legacy of gestalt psychology. *Scientific American* 12: 84–90.

Ronchi, L., and Bottai, G. 1964. Simultaneous contrast effects at the center of figures showing different degrees of symmetry. *Atti della Fondazione G. Ronchi* 19 (1): 84–100.

Rosenblatt, M., and Slepian, D. 1962. Nth order Markov chains with any set of N variables independent. *J. Soc. Indus. Appl. Math.* 10: 537–549.

Rubenstein, B., and Sagi, D. 1990. Spatial variability as a limiting factor in texture- discrimination tasks: implications for performance asymmetries. *Journal of the Optical Society of America* 9: 1632–1643.

Rumelhart, D., McClelland, J., and the PDP Research Group. 1986. *Parallel Distributed Processing: Explorations in the Microstructure of Cognition* (two volumes). MIT Press

Sagi, D. 1988. The combination of spatial frequency and orientation is effortlessly perceived. *Perception and Psychophysics* 43 (6): 601–603.

Sagi, D. 1990. Detection of an orientation singularity in Gabor textures: Effect of signal density and satial-frequency. *Vision Research* 30 (9): 1377–1388.

Sakai, K., and Y. Miyashita. 1990. Form correlation detectors in the temporal cortex. An alternative to grandmother detectors. *Nature* 250: 152–155.

Saltzman, Z., Britten, K., and Newsome, W. 1990. Cortical microstimulation influences perceptual judgements of motion direction. *Nature* 346: 589.

Schade, O. 1948. Electro-optical characteristics of television systems. I. Characteristics of vision and visual systems. *RCA Review* 9: 5–37.

Schroeder, M. 1986. *Number Theory in Science and Communication*. Springer-Verlag.

Schumann, F. 1904. Einige Beobachtungen über die Zusammenfassung von Gesichtseindrucken zu Einheiten. *Psychol. Stud.* 1: 1–32.

Schwartz, E. 1980. Computational anatomy and functional architecture of striate cortex: A spatial mapping approach to perceptual coding. *Vision Research* 20: 645–669.

Sekuler, R., and Blake, R. 1985. *Perception.* Knopf.

Selfridge, O. 1958. Pandemonium: A paradigm for learning. In *Mechanization of Thought Processes.* HMSO.

Shepard, R., and Metzler, J. 1971. Mental rotation of three-dimensional objects. *Science* 171: 701–703.

Shiffrin, R., and Gardner, G. 1972. Visual processing capacity and attentional control. *Journal of Experimental Psychology* 93: 72–82 .

Shiffrin, R., Gardner, G., and D. Allmeyer. 1973. On the degree of attention and capacity limitations in visual processing. *Perception and Psychophysics* 14: 231–236 .

Shiffrin, R. 1975. The locus and role of attention in memory systems. In *Attention and Performance,* ed. Rabbitt and Dornic.

Snowden, R., and Braddick, O. 1990. Differences in the processing of short-range apparent motion at small and large displacements. *Vision Research* 30: 1211–1222.

Sokoloff, L. 1984. *Metabolic Probes of Central Nervous System Activity in Experimental Animals.* Sinauer.

Sperling, G. 1970. Binocular vision: A physical and neural theory. *J. Am. Psychol.* 83: 461–534.

Sperling, G. 1978. The Goal of Theory in Experimental Psychology. Technical memo 78–1221–12, Bell Telephone Laboratories.

Sperling, G., Budiansky, J., Spivak, J., and Johnson, M. 1971. Extremely rapid visual search: The maximum rate of scanning letters for the presence of a numeral. *Science* 174: 307–311.

Sperry, R. 1982. Some effects disconnecting the central hemispheres. *Science* 217: 1223–1226.

Sternberg, S. 1966. High speed scanning in human memory. *Science* 153: 652–654.

Sun, J., and Perona, P. 1993. Preattentive perception of elementary three-dimensional shapes. *Investigative Ophthalmology and Visual Science* 34 (4): 1865.

Teller, D. 1980. Locus questions in visual science. In *Visual Coding and Adaptability,* ed. C. Harris. Erlbaum.

Theraulax, G., and Deneubourg, J.-L. 1992. Swarm intelligence in social insects and the emergence of cultural swarm patterns. Working paper 92-09-046, Santa Fe Institute.

Thompson, P. 1980. Margaret Thatcher: A new illusion. *Perception* 9: 483–484.

Tootell, R., Silverman, M., Switkes, E., and De Valois, R. 1982. Deoxyglucose analysis of retinotopic organization in primate striate cortex. *Science* 220: 737–739.

Townsend, J. 1972. Some results on the identifiability of of parallel and serial processes. *British Journal of Statistical and Mathematical Psychology* 25: 168–199.

Townsend, J. 1976. Serial and within-stage independent parallel model equivalence on the minimum completion time. *Journal of Mathematical Psychology* 14: 219–238.

Townsend, J. 1990. Serial vs. parallel processing: sometimes they look like tweedledum and tweedledee but they can (and should) be distinguished. *Psychol. Sci.* 1: 46–54.

Treisman, M. 1964. Selective attention in man. *British Medical Bulletin* 20: 12–16.

Treisman, A. 1985. Preattentive processing in vision. *Computer Vision Graphics and Image Processing* 31:156–157.

Treisman, A., and Gelade, G. 1980. A feature-integration theory of attention. *Cognitive Psychology* 12: 97–136.

Treisman, A., and Gormican, S. 1988. Feature analysis in early vision: Evidence from search asymmetries. *Psychological Reviews* 95: 15–48.

Treisman, A., and Paterson, R. 1984. Emergent features, attention and object perception. *Journal of Experimental Psychology: Human Perception and Performance* 10: 12–31.

Trotter, Y., Celebrini, S., Stricanne, B., Thorpe, S., and Imbert, M. 1992. Modulation of neural stereoscopic processing in primate area V1 by the viewing distance. *Science* 257: 1279–1281.

Ts'o, D., Frostig, R., Lieke, E., and Grinvald, A. 1990. Functional Organization of Primate Visual Cortex Revealed by High Resolution Optical Imaging. *Science* 249: 417–420.

Tyler, C. W. 1991. Cyclopean vision. In *Vision and Visual Disfunction,* ed. D. Regan. CRC Press.

Ulam, S. M. 1976. *Adventures of a Mathematician.* Scribner.

Ullman, S. 1977. The Interpretation of Visual Motion. Ph.D. thesis, Department of Electrical Engineering and Computer Science, MIT.

Ullman, S. 1979. *The Interpretation of Visual Motion.* MIT Press.

Ullman, S. 1984. Visual routines. *Cognition* 18: 97–159.

Uttal, W. 1990. On some two-way barriers between models and mechanisms. *Perception and Psychophysics* 48: 188–203.

Van de Grind, W., Van Doorn, A., and Koenderink, J. 1983. Detection of coherent movement in peripherally viewed random-dot patterns. *Journal of the Optical Society of America* 73: 1674–1683.

van den Enden, A., and Spekreijse, H. 1989. Binocular depth reversals despite familiarity cues. *Science* 244: 959–961.

van Santen, J., and Sperling, G. 1985. Elaborated Reichardt-detectors. *Journal of the Optical Society of America* A2: 451–473.

Victor, J. 1994. Images, statistics, and textures: A comment on triple correlation uniqueness for texture statistics and the Julesz conjecture. *Journal of the Optical Society of America* 11 (5): 1680–1684.

Volkman, F. 1962. Vision during voluntary saccadic eye movements. *Journal of the Optical Society of America* 52: 571–578.

von der Heydt, R., Peterhans, E., and Baumgartner, G. 1988. Illusory contours and cortical neuron responses. *Science* 224: 1260–1262.

von Schelling, H. 1956. Concepts of distance in affine geometry and its applications in theory of vision. *Journal of the Optical Society of America* 46: 309–315.

Voorhees, H., and Poggio, T. 1988. Computing texture boundaries from images. *Nature* 333: 364–367.

Wallach, H., and O'Connell, D. 1953. The kinetic depth effect. *Journal of Experimental Psychology* 45: 205–217.

Watson, A., and Ahumada, A. 1985. Model of human visual-motion sensing. *Journal of the Optical Society of America* A2: 322–342.

Watt, R. 1988. *Visual processing: Computational, Psychophysical, and Cognitive Research*. Erlbaum.

Weichselgartner, E., and Sperling, G. 1987. Dynamics of automatic and controlled visual attention. *Science* 238: 778–779.

Weisstein, N., and Harris, C. 1974. Visual detection of line segments: An object-superiority effect. *Science* 186: 752–755.

Werkhoven, P., Snippe, H.P., and Koenderink, J. 1990. Metrics for the strength of low-level motion perception. *Journal of Visual Communication and Image Representation* 1: 176–188.

Westheimer, G. 1979. Cooperative neural processes involved in stereoscopic acuity. *Experimental Brain Research* 36: 585–597.

Wigner, E. 1960. The unreasonbable effectiveness of mathematics in the natural sciences. *Communications on Pure and Applied Mathematics* 13: 1–14.

Williams, D., and Julesz, B. 1992. Perceptual asymmetry in texture perception. *Proceedings of the National Academy of Sciences* 89: 6531–6534.

Williams, D., Phillips, G., and Sekuler, R. 1986. Hysteresis in the perception of motion direction: Evidence for neural cooperativity. *Nature* 324: 253–255.

Wilson, F., Scalaidhe, S., and Goldman-Rakic, P. 1993. Dissociation of objects and spatial processing domains in primate prefrontal cortex. *Science* 260: 1955–1958.

Woodward, P. 1960. *Probability and Information Theory, with Applications to Radar*. Pergamon.

Wohlgemuth, A. 1911. On the aftereffect of seen movement. *British Journal of Psychology Monographs* 1: 1–117.

Wolfe, J. 1992. Effortless texture segmentation and parallel visual search are not the same thing. *Vision Research* 32 (4): 757–763.

Wolfe, J., and Cave, K. 1990. Deploying visual attention:The guided search model. In *AI and the Eye*, ed. A. Blake and T. Troscianco. Wiley.

Zadeh, L. A., and Ragazzini, J. R. 1950. An extension of Wiener's theory of prediction. *J. Appl. Physics* 21: 645–655.

Zeki, S. 1980. The representatioon of color in the cerebral cortex. *Nature* 284: 412–418.

Zohary, E. 1992. Population coding of visual stimuli by cortical neurons tuned to more than one dimension. *Biological Cybernetics* 66:265–272.

INDEX